YOGA FOR A NEW AGE

Bob Smith has been a student of yoga since 1969 and has been teaching it since 1973. He is the founder of the Hatha Yoga Center, a private studio for yoga instruction, in Seattle, Washington.

Bob's graduate work at the University of Washington was in philosophy and kinesiology. His Bachelor of Arts degree was in sociology.

Linda Boudreau has studied yoga since 1970 and has instructed since 1973. Linda has also been involved in the healing arts for many years. She is a Licensed Massage Therapist and a Certified Postural Integrationist.

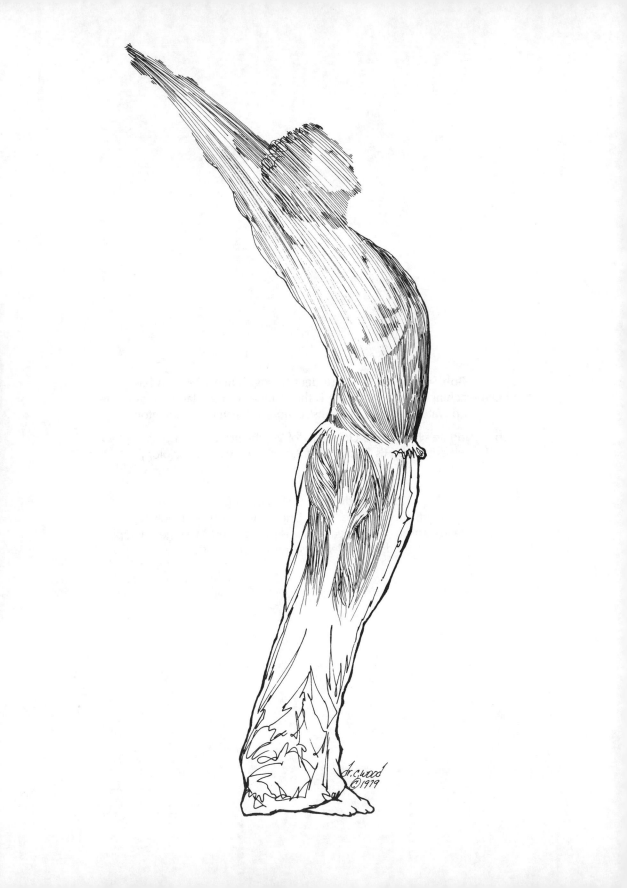

A MODERN APPROACH TO HATHA YOGA

yoga
for a new age

BOB SMITH
LINDA BOUDREAU

photographs by Helen P. Smith
medical illustrations by Charles D. Wood, Ph.D.

SMITH PRODUCTIONS, Seattle, Washington

Library of Congress Cataloging in Publication Data 86-090391

SMITH, BOB (date). 8/25/48   Smith, Linda Boudreau   7/06/48
   Yoga for a new age.

   A Smith Productions Book
   Bibliography: p.
   Includes index.
      1. Yoga, Hatha.   I. Smith, Helen (date)
II. Wood, Charles D. (date).   III. Title.
RA781.7.S64   613.7'046   81-11911
                           AACR2

ISBN 0-9616545-0-3

This Smith Productions Book can be made available to businesses
and organizations at a special discount when ordered in
quantities. For more information, contact

Smith Productions, 4550 11th Ave. N.E.
Seattle, WA 98105

"The first edition of Yoga for a New Age
was created by the book publisher,
Prentice - Hall, Inc, in February of 1981."

Interior design and page layout by Christine Gehring Wolf
Editorial/production supervision by Eric Newman(1st edition),
Helen P. Smith (Revised edition)
Cover design by Ira Shapiro

10 9 8 7 6 5

contents

I

NEW-AGE YOGA

2

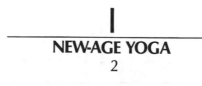

ONE

new-age yoga

5

IV

WORKBOOK FOR THE BEGINNING, INTERMEDIATE, AND ADVANCED STUDENT OF YOGA
86

FIVE
standing postures
89

SIX
inverted postures
133

SEVEN
twists
163

EIGHT
backbends
183

NINE
forward stretches
205

V

MEDITATION
228

TEN

ego, mind,
and meditation
231

appendix
243

index

When yoga first arrived in America earlier this century,
considerable importance was placed upon studying under an Asian master,
learning his language, adopting the eating and clothing habits
of his culture, receiving from him a new and foreign name,
and, if possible, making a pilgrimage to his land. All of these peculiarities
bespeak the hidden assumption that the real yoga
exists over there in Asia and that what we have here is a pale reflection,
having lost much through cultural translation. At the same time
that the imitation trend continues among many Western practitioners
of yoga, an innovative trend is just now beginning
to emerge, a trend toward adaption of Asian yoga beliefs and practices
to the Western cultural milieu—a trend,
if you will, toward formation of an authentically
"American yoga" in which Asian and Western elements merge.

RAEBURN S. HEIMBECK, PH.D.

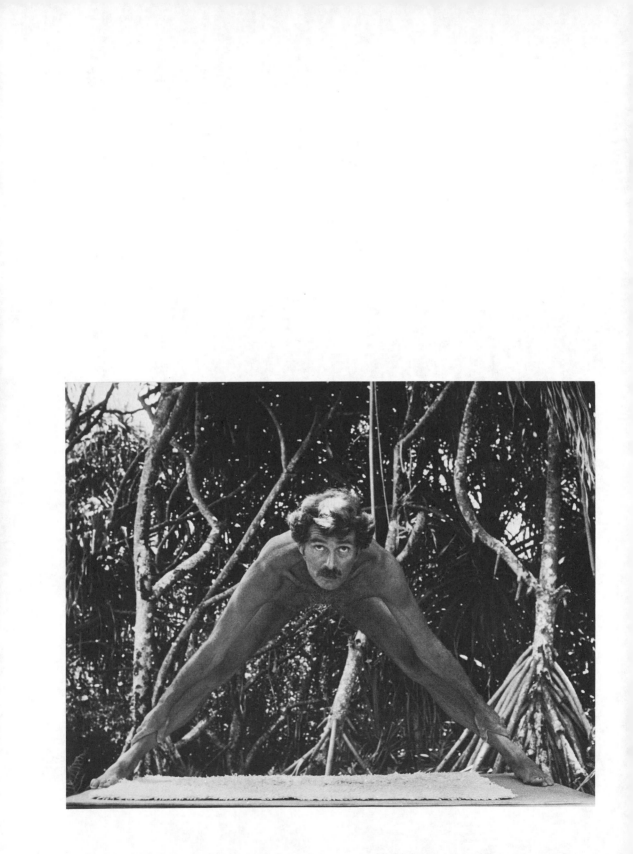

foreword

Whether or not an Aquarian Age is dawning for the world at large, yoga today is experiencing a rebirth. It is happening not in Asia, as one might expect, but in the United States largely as part of the global culture some say is now forming here. Yoga has only recently become ensconced in the West, within our own century, in fact. By venturing westward, yoga has found itself immersed in a powerful new matrix of transformation. But then, yoga is no stranger to change. Even a quick glance at its complex history reveals it to have always been a growing, organic thing—branching out, adapting to new environments, surrendering to pruning and reshaping, never static and at no point finalized in form.

The fecundity of yoga through the ages could be anticipated from the richness of the term itself. The Sanskrit word *yoga,* as is well known, means "union," although "reunion" is perhaps closer to actual usage. "Reunion" implies a reconnection of factors earlier joined but subsequently separated. This Asian word, therefore, in meaning resembles the European word *religion,* which according to its Latin roots signifies "that which binds back together again." The comparison is apt, for *yoga* in Asia has been used to name just about every sort of religious practice known to man.

The richness of the term, then, is matched by the astonishing diversity of practices and beliefs with which yoga has been associated. Through twenty-five centuries of religious experiments and innovations, yoga in India (connected there with the Hindu, Buddhist, and Jaina traditions) came to include mind-altering meditation, chanting of sacred sounds (mantras), ascetic austerities, devotional study of revealed scripture, disinterested performance of daily work, ritualistic worship, channeling of mystical energy up the spine, ecstatic sexuality, actions patterned on geometrical diagrams (mandalas), bizarre bodily purifications, dietary observances, exotic bodily postures, breathing exercises, and more, to list them in sequence of appearance from about 500 B.C. to A.D. 1000. Chinese or Taoist yoga, over the same time period and resulting from similar explorations of human spirituality, has encompassed, in addition to meditation, outrageous alchemical experiments, alterations of diet, conservation and recirculation of breath and semen, and training in martial arts such as Kung Fu and T'ai Chi Ch'uan. From this itemization it is apparent that yoga practice through the ages has been manifold rather than monolithic.

Now the full Asian heritage of yoga is available to Americans right in our own backyard. In but a few brief decades and in what must go down as the swiftest transcontinental importation in the history of human spirituality, all of the above-mentioned yogic practices and beliefs are being purveyed on a mass scale across the land, embraced by enthusiastic multitudes, and rapidly assimilated into the ever-evolving American culture. Bob and Linda Smith's book, *Yoga for a New Age,* fits into the broader picture of yoga in America—as a stepping stone into a yoga authentically American.

The photographs in their book convincingly document that the authors have become adept at the most difficult Hatha Yoga postures through years of arduous, disciplined work. Yet they have managed to accomplish this while maintaining their cultural identity and integrity. They have become yoga adepts while remaining refreshingly American. They have brought yoga into the very heart of their American experience; they have not shed their culture for another in order to become yogis. They have not changed their names or their manner of dress. They call the yoga postures by their English rather than by their Sanskrit names. They have not been to India to study on soil sacred to yoga; they have learned their yoga right in Seattle, from European and American teachers mostly, though they have worked occasionally but briefly under the guidance of visiting Indian masters. And Bob continues in his private life—bless him—to vent his enthusiasm for Western sports—baseball, golf, and basketball, in particular; in fact, at one time his ambition was to become a professional athlete.

A further evidence of the accommodation of yoga to Western culture in Bob and Linda's book is to be found in its wonderfully simple, clear, intelligible explanations, both of how to do the postures and breathing exercises of Hatha Yoga and also of what happens physiologically while they are being done. Human biology is brought to bear upon the understanding of yoga. In order to offer their reader this kind of Western-oriented understanding, the Smiths have taken the trouble to learn human anatomy, physiology, and kinesiology, and to learn them well. They have conferred at length with medical people about the bodily processes invoked by yoga work. Most importantly, they have together conducted a searching, sensitive, experiential examination of what happens within their own bodies as they perform the postures and breathing exercises of yoga; here they have broken new ground and gone well beyond anything similar in English print.

One more point about Bob and Linda Smith's book as a giant stride toward an original American yoga; it has to do with the philosophical context within which they root their Hatha Yoga. Borrowing from the inspirational thought of Pir Vilayat Inayat Khan, leader of the Sufi Order of the West (a syncretic movement incorporating all the wisdom traditions), Bob Smith proceeds to visualize the role of Hatha Yoga in relation to the philosophical principals of Cosmic Evolution and of Totality. When he envisions yoga as the primary instrument for the future evolution of the human "bodymindspirit" (they are inseparable according to our author) until the Divine Consciousness itself is perfectly brought to embodiment on Earth, he joins minds with Sri Aurobindo Ghose, the greatest Indian philosopher and (some say) the most accomplished yogi of modern times. Aurobindo conceived an Integral Yoga, which bonds together all the traditional yoga systems of India plus the physical and intellectual disciplines of Western origin—in my opinion the greatest contribution to the ongoing yoga tradition since the inception of Hatha Yoga itself about a thousand years ago. Aurobindo's metaphysics have been compared to those of Pierre Teilhard de Chardin, Alfred North Whitehead, and Henri Bergson on the basis of the Cosmic Evolution theme common to all four; what gives Aurobindo's metaphysics its distinctiveness among this company is his attempted synthesis of the monastic philosophy of the Upanishads with Western scientific thought as exemplified by evolutionism. Through Pir Vilayat, Bob Smith's yoga philosophy links up with the thought of Aurobindo, in particular his idea that humankind is evolving toward Supermind (the Divine Life on earth).

Pir Vilayat serves to mediate yet another stunning metaphysical principle in the formulation of Bob Smith's yoga philosophy—the Principle of Totality, associated with certain Indian Buddhist texts and Chinese Buddhist schools. According to the Totality doctrine, since everything is present in everything else to form one grand unity, the Eternal can be experienced Now, and the Spirit is forever imminent in physical existence. Bob Smith relates to the Totality Principle by advancing the belief that yoga leads neither to the transcendence of earthly existence nor to earthly existence without transcendence, but to a transformation of consciousness at the spiritual level that must be brought back down and worked out under the terms of our present, earthly existence.

My point in suggesting these deeper philosophical connections is that they bring out the full flavor and richness of Bob Smith's yoga philosophy. The value of that philosophy to Westerners is its compatibility with Western science. It is a yoga philosophy that is at once both spiritual and "scientific" in the sense of having high valence with modern philosophy of science; it is, in other words, a yoga philosophy that resonates harmoniously with Western thought preferences and tolerances.

What I read in *Yoga for a New Age,* to sum it up, speaks to me of a new age for yoga, of the emergence of a uniquely American yoga now forming and assuming its place at the forefront of the long development of yoga through the ages. Such a yoga will not be the ultimate yoga but simply its present version in an ongoing process promising surprises yet to come. But it speaks to me, too, about the prospect of a new age for humankind, based upon a truly global culture in which this new yoga will make an even larger contribution to the human spirit.

RAEBURN S. HEIMBECK, Ph.D.
Professor of Religious Studies
Central Washington University

preface

Yoga is a means of preventive medicine. It is more than three thousand years old, and it is still with us today only because it does, in fact, provide a road to better health and greater peace of mind. As more and more scientific research on the physical effects of yoga is conducted, it looks better and better. Indeed, it may prove to be the most complete form of exercise that mankind has yet devised. People of all ages are taking it up to relieve or prevent backaches, headaches, tiredness, insomnia, high blood pressure, heart disease, nervousness, digestive disorders, ulcers, kidney problems, constipation, obesity, varicose veins, mental depression, menstrual disorders, sterility, impotency, anemia, arthritis, bursitis, asthma, bronchitis, lack of mental clarity, emotional imbalances, hormonal imbalances, glandular problems, allergies, epilepsy, spinal disc problems, knee problems, fallen arches, hypoglycemia, hyperglycemia—the list goes on and on.

Incredible as its physical benefits may be, yoga is infinitely more than a complete exercise program—it is a way of life that frees the mind and the spirit. Yogis have taught for thousands of years that the materialistic life is not the true road to inner peace. There is a deep despair that persists in each of us until we actually feel a reality that goes beyond the limited body–mind–personality complex. Yoga has the power to lead us to this timeless reality.

In the first chapter of *Yoga for a New Age,* the role of hatha yoga postures is discussed, the classical eightfold path of yoga is outlined, and a new-age yoga philosophy is expounded. Highlighting this chapter is a quote by Pir Vilayat Inayat Khan regarding the ultimate experience in life. The philosophical discussion begun in Chapter 1 is completed in Chapter 2 as ancient yoga metaphysics is compared with modern yoga metaphysics. The second chapter, entitled "Yoga, Communication, and Relationships," concerns itself with the question: How can the practice of yoga actually improve our daily relationships?

In Chapters 3 through 10, the focus is on specific teachniques that bring health to the body and clarity to the mind. Detailed discussions on how to breathe, stand, walk, and sit correctly are given in Chapter 3, "Body Alignment and Breath." A rich supply of photographs and medical illustrations pictorially show the muscular work that is a prerequisite to deep breathing and proper body alignment. A few simple postures are recommended in Chapter 3; these can do wonders for anyone whose work requires several hours of sitting each day.

Chapter 4, "Yoga for Beginners," was written by Linda Boudreau, who has a particular gift for teaching the beginning yoga student. At the end of Chapter 4, six sample routines are presented, providing a concrete program for beginning students. There are countless levels of beginning yoga postures, and we definitely do not wish to limit new students to those postures presented in Chapter 4.

All of the postures in Chapters 5 through 9 have been classified as beginning, intermediate or advanced, and all students are encouraged to look through the entire book for postures that could help them. Chapters 5 through 9 divide the Hatha Yoga postures into five groups: standing, inverted, twists, backbends, and forward stretches. The correct way to work in the postures, their benefits, and the way to use a wall, bar, strap, or partner are shown and described in these five chapters. Sixteen sample routines for beginners with some experience and for intermediate and advanced students are listed in the appendix, but these are intended only to serve as springboards for your own creative routines. This book can serve as a reference for years without exhausting the countless routine possibilities.

The final chapter, "Ego, Mind, and Meditation," contains important instructions on maintaining a meditative frame of mind while out and about in the world and concludes with a personal meditation experience.

In *Yoga for a New Age*, we have attempted to relay the highest yogic teachings of our age, outlining a step-by-step road not only to improved health but also to inner harmony. We have drawn quite strongly upon the philosophic teachings of Pir Vilayat Inayat Khan in this book. No religious dogma is contained herein; it is equally appropriate to Christian, Jew, Hindu, Buddhist, Muslim or Sufi.

Yoga can be practiced by people of all ages, from little children to the very elderly. It is my hope that you will find inspiration and guidance here, whatever your age and whatever your previous yoga experience. Above all, we wish you to understand that this ancient yet modern discipline is more than a form of total exercise for the body, and it is more than a subject for the mind to theorize upon—it is an experience that is capable of changing your life.

DEDICATION

Western-born yoga teachers owe an immeasurable debt to present-day gurus from India who have shared with us what was for centuries a secret discipline. Many of us who teach yoga are specifically indebted to B.K.S. Iyengar, whose disciples have spread his teaching methods throughout the world. His book *Light on Yoga* has set meticulous standards for precision and accuracy as well as added creatively to the storehouse of Hatha Yoga postures. Although I have not met Mr. Iyengar, much that I know about the yoga postures was learned studying under his disciples and poring over his book.

A large amount of the new-age philosophy presented in this book has come from the teachings of the Sufi leader Pir Vilayat Inayat Khan. Without question, Pir Vilayat is presently the person who has become my main guide. The message that he relays is that we have all emerged from the same source; that, in essence, all religions and all beings are one.

Add to this list the name of Ram Das, whose words have over the past sixteen years helped me through many a difficult situation. The honesty of his being has been a deep inspiration to me.

Although I readily acknowledge the influence these three leaders had upon my book, I wish to express particular gratitude to the teacher who above and beyond all others affected what is written herein. Marie Svoboda started me on the path of yoga and nurtured my development as a student and teacher of yoga for seven years.

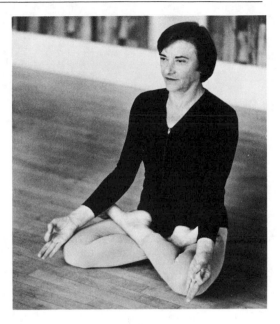

Formerly a ballerina, then a ballet instuctor, Marie met Indra Devi, who taught her the Hatha Yoga postures. Marie was so impressed by the benefits of yoga that she decided to devote her life to it. She went to the East to study under many yoga teachers before returning to the United States to teach the ancient science.

It was Marie who taught me not only the postures of yoga, but the attitude and philosophy of yoga, as well. She will always occupy a special place in my heart, and it is to her that I dedicate this book.

about the pictures

We were very fortunate to enlist the creative artistry of Dr. Charles Wood, whose unique medical illustrations illuminate the effect that yoga postures exert upon the body.

The photographs were taken by Helen Smith, a professional photographer who also happens to be my mother. She combed the parks of Seattle, found settings that were pleasing, and took several thousand yoga pictures over a period of two years. In the summer of 1978 I conducted a retreat with fourteen students at Hana on the beautiful island of Maui, Hawaii, and this, too, she duly recorded on film.

We are appreciative of our good friends at Price Photo Service in Seattle, who developed all the film for this book and printed many of the photos.

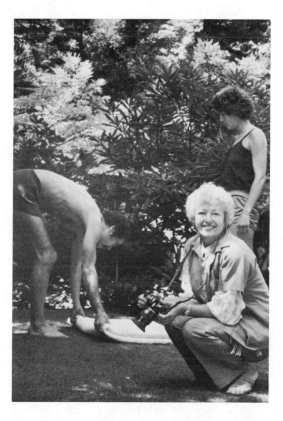

Photo by Trisha Brennen

YOGA FOR A NEW AGE

I

NEW-AGE YOGA

The main focus of this book is upon the postures of Hatha Yoga, which are pictured and described in fine detail in Chapters 4 through 9. The ultimate goals and underlying philosophy must be considered before practice of the postures makes sense, however. Part I, comprising Chapters 1 and 2, describes the basic stages of yoga practice and lays the metaphysical foundation for the other four parts of the book. Part I is mainly concerned with how yoga fits into the modern world.

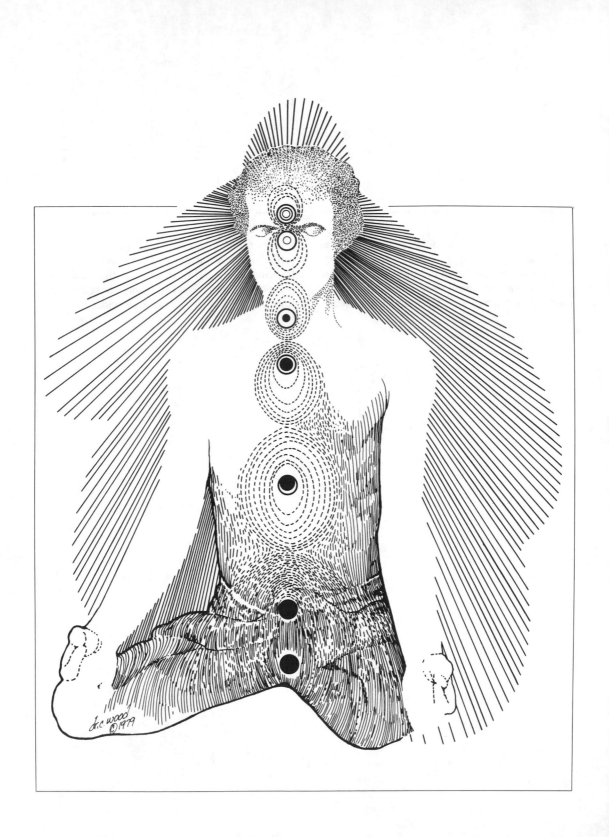

ONE
new-age yoga

INTRODUCTION

Since the sunrise of our sojourn on earth we humans have sensed that we are spiritual as well as physical beings. We have questioned why spirits that are eternal are housed in bodies that are temporal. We have wondered what is the purpose of life. Over the past three thousand years there has evolved a way to deal with these questions, and this way is called *yoga*. The premise of yogic philosophy is that the physical and spiritual aspects of our being cannot be separated. In the following pages I will present a practical technique that can help you to attain a healthier body, a more peaceful mind, and a deeper understanding of the nature of life. This technique is a new-age approach to yoga.

Yoga is a means of self-discovery. It gives us a way to discover how the blood, oxygen, and nerve energy move throughout the body. It enables us to understand the manner in which our breath and posture affect our mental processes. Yoga should be approached more as an experience than as a philosophy. Yoga practice provides a tangible process that allows us temporarily to withdraw from the chaos of the world and find a quiet space within. It is the zone of peace that surrounds the yogi that I am interested in helping you discover for yourself.

Most people begin yoga practice primarily to improve the health of their physical body. Improved health comes about through increased circulation of blood, oxygen, and nerve energy, which results from the opening of tight joints and from the stretch and relaxation of tight muscles. Through the posture work of Hatha Yoga our muscular, respiratory, circulatory, digestive, eliminative, reproductive, endocrine, and nervous systems all become more efficient.

The second most important reason people become involved in yoga practice is to calm the mind. If a great deal of muscular tension is present, it may be accompanied by undue amounts of mental and emotional tension. Mental anxiety and negative emotions must somehow find a channel of release if we are to feel peaceful. Through the postures and breathing techniques of yoga, mental and emotional tension can be discharged. Thus, peace of mind then becomes more attainable.

The third reason for yoga involvement is

to increase spiritual awareness. According to the yoga masters, consciousness is not bound by space or by time. Through meditation we can go beyond the limited perspective and reach direct awareness of universal laws, archetypal imagery, and cosmic truths. The way to attain spiritual realization is through the expansion of consciousness that the yoga path embraces. Yoga is not a religion, however. Yoga must be thought of as a method of physical, mental, emotional, and spiritual attunement to the cosmic order of life.

Yoga provides a way to understand how the body functions from the inside out. The transformation of the body–mind–spirit continuum is a long and difficult task, and yoga does not propose a fast, easy solution. Release of muscular and mental tension begins with one's very first yoga posture, but the all-out transformation of consciousness is a lifetime pursuit. Yoga is, however, a road to freedom that is available to one and all.

The "bible" of yoga, Yoga Sutras, was written somewhere around 200 B.C. by a man named Patanjali. The main problems Patanjali dealt with in the Yoga Sutras are the same problems that we deal with today. Strong desires for material satisfaction pervade our society, and the impossibility of fulfilling these insatiable desires creates anxiety and tension. It has been my observation as a yoga teacher that many of the problems that lead people to medical doctors or psychiatrists can be solved or prevented through daily practice of yoga.

Yoga practice affects us at the deepest level possible and most certainly will reflect out into our daily life. When we are beset with many duties and responsibilities, they can overwhelm us. Before we realize it, our basic outlook on life, relationships, and work can be undermined by outer circumstances. We need to stop periodically and look within ourselves to understand the causes behind the effects, then look further to find the causes behind the causes, and then look deeper to uncover the roots of the situation we are in-

volved in. Yoga practice can help us to understand our relationship with ourselves, with others, and with the world. Ultimately, yoga can help us to expand our consciousness and to unveil the purpose for our life here on this earth.

YOGA—YESTERDAY AND TODAY

Yoga is an ancient practice that has historically centered in India. For three thousand years yoga was a technique of spiritual training passed down from generation to generation through master–disciple relationships. During this period yogic knowledge was held sacred, and its well-guarded transmittal kept it from the masses. In the past eighty years the manner of yogic transmittance has changed, until today we find it is the pupil who shops around and decides who his teacher will be, rather than the master who personally selects a handful of students.

This being an age of mass communication, the teachings are now openly presented through books, tapes, and many yoga centers throughout the world. As knowledge of yoga spreads throughout the globe, new devices are added to the teaching techniques. Though the main asanas (postures) of Hatha Yoga remain the same, there is an evolving approach to the training of the body so that the student can move further into the poses. Changes within the small wave (Hatha Yoga) reflect changes within the larger wave (yoga as a whole).

Mainly through the inspiration of B.K.S. Iyengar, author of Light on Yoga, new tools have been added to help the practitioner of Hatha Yoga. Though his book does not mention most of these teaching devices, he has instructed many student teachers in the use of such aids to posture work as walls, bars, straps, blocks of wood, chairs, and tables. I would like to add to new-age yoga my own emphasis, this being partner work to facilitate one's asana involvement.

I do encourage a self-expressive approach to Hatha Yoga practice. I believe that the postures should be performed as a dance, not as calisthenics. Precision must be demanded in the yoga asanas, but freedom of individual expression can be found in the midst of the discipline. If yoga practice is to move us toward the flow of cosmic harmony, it must be presented in a way that awakens the creative, spontaneous impulse of the soul. The body that is vibrating harmoniously draws to it more positive, creative energy, whereas a body that is vibrating unharmoniously draws to it more negative, destructive energy. Yoga gives us a way to attune the physical organism to a positive flow of energy. It gives us a way to dispel the clouds that hide our true nature, leading us to peace within.

HATHA YOGA

Hatha Yoga translates as "sun–moon union." Hatha Yoga presents a series of postures that can help to balance the right and left sides of the body and the right and left hemispheres of the brain. Through the demanding work of trying to balance the body, the mind will begin to find balance as well. Once the mind moves toward harmony, one's spiritual essence can begin to unveil itself. The message of yoga is that body, mind, and spirit cannot be separated and that the threefold aspect of our being must unfold and evolve as a unit.

Before discussing the philosophy of the yoga path, I want to briefly focus on the aspect of yoga that will be the main concern of this book—the postures of Hatha Yoga. There are hundreds of yoga postures, which aim not only at balancing the two sides of the body but also at making the body limber, strong, and straight. Muscles that are well toned and

joints that are flexible are prerequisites for maintaining good body alignment throughout the day. A well-rounded set of yoga asanas carries each joint through a full range of movement and stretches and contracts all the body's major muscle groups.

According to the yoga masters, straightening the spinal column is prerequisite work to acquiring a clear and quiet mind. The most obvious reason the yogis are so concerned with straightness of the spinal column is that sitting or standing with a crooked spine for a prolonged period leads to backaches. The majority of backaches occur in the lumbar vertebrae, because much of the weight of the torso sinks into the lower part of the back if we fail to lift through the spine properly. The person whose body is trained to sit, stand, and walk with the spinal column well aligned throughout the day will be much better able to concentrate for long periods than the person who slouches when sitting, standing, or walking. However, the person whose spine has been crooked for years must first change the manner in which the muscular system works, and this realignment may involve a great deal of initial postural work.

The yogi aligns the body in order that proper breathing can occur. A caved-in, sunken chest constricts one's lung capacity very markedly. A collapsed rib cage does not allow the main breathing muscles, the diaphragm and intercostal muscles, to work properly. If the exhale is incomplete day in and day out, a toxic buildup of carbon dioxide occurs. If the inhale is incomplete, there is a shortage of oxygen throughout the cells of the body, including the brain cells. One of the main keys to healthy living is proper intake of oxygen and proper expulsion of carbon dioxide.

Since it is blood that distributes oxygen to the cells of the body and blood that takes carbon dioxide away from the cells, it is absolutely essential that the circulatory system of the body be made as efficient as possible.

Proper circulation of the blood depends upon periodic movement of the muscles. Thus, stretching the muscles becomes a matter of simple practicality and common sense. A body that is not used stiffens up, creating circulatory constriction and oxygen deprivation.

YOGA ASANAS (POSTURES)

There are six main groups of yoga asanas: standing postures, inverted poses, twists, backbends, forward stretches, and meditational poses.

1. The standing postures bring strength to the legs and exercise the key muscles of the entire body to counteract the effect of gravity. The standing postures have a very grounding and centering effect upon the mind.

2. The two key inverted postures are headstand and shoulderstand.

    a. Standing on one's head brings extra blood into the brain, pituitary, and pineal gland. The change of blood flow provides an elevated feeling, improves one's thinking power, helps to bring the whole endocrine system into balance, and helps the legs, heart, and internal organs.

    b. Shoulderstand, like headstand, reverses the way in which gravity works on the body and is also very helpful for the legs, heart, and internal organs of digestion, elimination, and reproduction. Shoulderstand draws blood into the throat, where the thyroid and parathyroid glands are located, improving the body's metabolism.

3. Twisting postures greatly aid the digestive organs, loosen and strengthen the back muscles, help to relieve backaches,
and spread the ribs away from each other so that strong intercostal breathing can take place.

4. Backbends open the chest, loosen the shoulder joints, and help one to take a deeper, fuller breath. Backbends are very invigorating postures.

5. Forward stretching action lengthens the calf, hamstring, and back muscles. Better blood circulation throughout the entire body results from forward stretches.

6. Meditational poses help one to calm the body and calm the mind. A basic principle of meditation is that the mind will move toward clarity as the body stills in a well-aligned position.

The standing postures and backbends are, for the most part, very active postures in which the body must work very hard. The mind must move toward forcefulness and assertiveness while performing these postures. On the other end of the scale are the meditational poses, which move the mind toward quietness and receptivity. Forward stretches, on the whole, require one to develop a submissive, yielding mental attitude. Inverted postures and twists require a blend of assertiveness and of letting go into the pose.

My advice to all interested in Hatha Yoga is to practive a few of each of the six main groups of yoga asanas as part of one's daily workout. The physical, mental, and emotional balance we seek comes about through a well-rounded set of yoga asanas that takes one through active and forceful work as well as submissive and passive work.

Performing a well-rounded set of yoga postures improves the functioning of every muscle, nerve, and gland throughout the body. As the sexual glands, the adrenal glands, the pancreas, the thymus, the thyroid and parathyroid glands, the pineal, and pituitary gland all begin to work more efficiently and harmoniously, greater emotional stability results.

The body–mind dichotomy looses its extreme polarity as we learn how the body works from the inside out. In practicing the yoga postures, we come to understand how oxygen enters the lungs, how carbon dioxide is expelled, how blood pulsates through the circulatory system, how the joints can be loosened, how nerve impulses are transmitted throughout the body, how the breath and thought patterns are directly related, and how the posture the body assumes can greatly influence the type of thoughts that move through the mind. The work of Hatha Yoga is an exploration of one's own body and mind.

PARTNER WORK

Numerous partner adjustments will be shown in this book. I have found partner work to be a very powerful way to speed the process of Hatha Yoga development. The partner adjustments shown are, for the most part, safe means to help one stretch, twist, or arch more fully. It has been my experience that partners facilitate the release of tension in the muscles and the joints much faster than can be done on one's own. The work is safe if awareness and close communication take place during the process of the adjustment.

The attitude with which you approach partner work is extremely important. The person having the adjustment done must depend upon the adjuster to work carefully, precisely, and slowly. Trust must be built into the work. The adjustment will be especially helpful if a feeling of unified purpose is found in the newly formed relationship.

The person adjusting must, at first, be very gentle and find the correct placement of his or her body in relation to the partner's. Firmness can proceed out of gentleness in many of the adjustments. If the two work together as one body, then the adjustment will

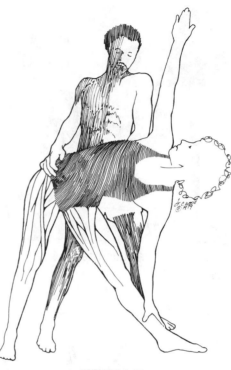

FIGURE 1.1A

not only be helpful physically for the person receiving the adjustment, but both persons will benefit emotionally as well. Both individuals must focus attention upon the breath, as the breath is the key to moving more deeply into the work. If each individual can develop a rhythmic flow of breath, the work will proceed with much less resistance on all levels.

The partner work shown in Chapters 4 through 9 is directed not only to teachers of yoga but to each and every student as well. It is a tremendous learning experience to work with others in the performance of the postures. Adjusting another can help you understand your own as well as another's body and mind at a much deeper level. The real reward of partner work, however, is the unity found between two who work closely together as one.

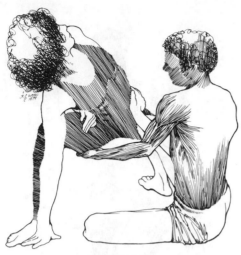

FIGURE 1.1B

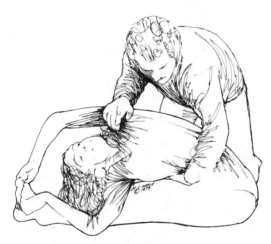

FIGURE 1.1C

MACROCOSM WITHIN THE MICROCOSM

Ultimately, yoga practice is the process of discovering who we are, and how and why we continue to exist. Through yoga practice our consciousness can be raised to a new vantage point from which to view life. Yoga theory conveys to us that we must look within our own physical bodies and our own minds to find truth. The process of uplifting our consciousness begins by uplifting the energy level of the body. Our natural heritage is one of cosmic consciousness, but this can be realized only as we remove the dust of the body and illusions of the mind, say the yoga masters.

Discipline is the key to yoga. To discipline our minds, we must give the thought process a concrete focus. We can accomplish this by watching the internal rhythms of the body. As internal harmony is reached, we begin to understand that the external world is guided by laws similar to those of the internal world. The paradox is that the totality of the universe is contained within each of the individual units of the universe. The yogi believes that it is through the individual body that one realizes divine consciousness. The yogi works in a very concrete way on physical and mental attunement. It is said that the body and the mind must become pure vessels for the divine to clearly manifest within the individual.

THE EIGHTFOLD PATH OF YOGA

As we noted earlier, around 200 B.C. a man named Patanjali wrote what has come to be the "bible" of yoga. The *Yoga Sutras* (*sutras* means "aphorisms") of Patanjali describe the eightfold path of yoga as: (1) yama, (2) niyama, (3) asana, (4) pranayama, (5) pratyahara, (6) dharana, (7) dhyana, and (8) samadhi.

Steps one and two, *yama* and *niyama,* consist of moral restraints and ethical observances and are somewhat similar to the Ten Commandments of the *Bible.*

The third step of yoga is *asana,* which translates as posture control. The main focus of *Yoga for a New Age* is upon this third step of yoga. Hatha Yoga is a discipline that is primarily concerned with the third step of the yoga path.

The fourth step, *pranayama,* translates as breath control.

Pratyahara, the fifth step of yoga, concerns itself with the withdrawal of the senses from the outside world and a refocusing of attention within the body.

Dharana, the sixth step, translates as concentration. Dharana is concerned with the development of a one-pointed mind through special concentration techniques in which the mind is brought to focus on the internal world.

The seventh step of yoga, *dhyana,* translates as contemplation. In the dhyana stage the meditator merges with the object or image of concentration and contemplates its many-splendored attributes.

Yogic meditation culminates in the eighth and last step of yoga, *samadhi,* which means union with the supreme.

Meditation provides a way to escape the prison of the limited self. In the process of meditating, one begins to realize that the individual ego and personality function at only one level of reality and that there are far more encompassing levels of reality. Through the process of meditation, the meditator can begin to contact the life force that moves throughout the entire universe. In the samadhi state an inexhaustible supply of cosmic energy can be tapped into.

Samadhi is the ultimate goal of classical yoga. In samadhi one identifies with the unchanging aspect of reality. Master yogis have told us that everlasting peace and harmony can be found only by losing oneself in the advanced state of samadhi. It is through dedicated practice of concentration, contemplation, and meditation that one can move toward samadhi.

The path of yoga is the path of mastery. Patanjali begins the *Yoga Sutras* by stating that the oscillating tendency of the mind must be brought under control. The mind is said to be like a wild horse that needs to be reined

and harnessed. Through the development of yogic concentration, one can develop tremendous will power. The will must control the mind, and the mind must control the body.

NEW-AGE YOGA

The objective of new-age yoga differs from that of classical yoga. The goal of new-age yoga is to experience the reality beyond creation right in the midst of creation. To state the difference simply, classical yoga aims toward detachment from the physical universe, whereas new-age yoga aims toward bringing the divine consciousness down to earth. The classical yoga approach presents a wonderful technique to help lead one to a level of consciousness beyond the everyday problems of the world, but it does not tell us how to make a smooth reentry into the physical universe. New-age yoga provides a technique for descending from samadhi, for reentering the world renewed in body, mind, and spirit.

It is the new-age way to focus on the experience of life on earth rather than to deny the reality of physical existence. This is not to say that to experience samadhi is not essential. If we hope to ever be free, we must realize that behind the aspect of reality that is changing there exists an aspect of reality that is unchanging. The despair of humankind comes about because we get caught on a level where our perspective is limited, and we think this narrow view is all there is to life. We need to experience samadhi if we are to gain access to the highest vantage point possible, but through our experience on the earth we can consciously evolve the spiritual aspect of our being. We should return from the samadhi experience with an enhanced appreciation of the beauty of the physical existence.

Through contact with other beings we can fulfill the desire to know who we are. We must realize that a net gain for the evolution of humanity occurs through the communication of human souls on earth. However, we limit the level of communication with other beings when we confine ourselves to ego consciousness. If we are to adopt the divine point of view, we must attune to the collective mind of humankind.

Once we have experienced the unity behind the outward appearance of the physical universe, we can begin to participate in the manifestation as illuminated souls. New-age meditation provides a way to exist simultaneously above and within the physical universe. We come to realize that our individual evolvement is dependent upon the spiritual evolvement of the whole of humanity. We must bring the unity and the ecstasy of the higher spheres down into the world of action.

Through meditation we can get in touch with feelings of peace, harmony, and ecstasy. In samadhi it is possible to view the perfection of the universe and to realize that even the frustration, anxiety, and despair of humans are part of this perfection. In the meditative state we can call upon the collective mind of the universe to help us understand our earthly problems and the problems of those around us. Once we gain new insight, we can come back to free others rather than bind them to us. After we see the light of unity, we are no longer so trapped by the limitations of our body–mind–personality complex and can help one another unconditionally.

Pir Vilayat Inayat Khan describes the meditation of the new age as a four-stage process.[1] The first stage is to withdraw from everyday thoughts, concentrate within, and move into an impersonal state of mind in which a higher will takes over the individual will. This stage corresponds to the fifth, sixth, and seventh steps of the classical yoga path: withdrawal of the senses,

concentration, and contemplation.

The second stage of new-age meditation is the expansion up and out of one's consciousness into a transcendental realm. This stage could be likened to the samadhi state of classical yoga. Here we experience the one and only consciousness, which lies behind all of life.

The third stage is to bring cosmic truth right down onto the earth. Here we experience the cosmic consciousness descending into human form and accepting the limitations of this human form.

The fourth stage involves the spreading of cosmic intelligence and pure love into the physical world in whatever way it can be received. This stage will be the main subject of Chapter 2, "Yoga, Communication, and Relationships."

Pir Vilayat speaks of three kinds of samadhi: (1) samadhi as defined by the classical yogis, (2) samadhi with open eyes, and (3) omega samadhi. In the direct quote that follows, he begins by describing the classical notion of samadhi:

When you're involved in events, you can't see the causes, you just see the occurrences. It's like when you're walking in the streets, you can't see the lie of the land, but if you climb to the top of the mountain and you overlook the town or the city, of course you can see the distribution of streets and the general configuration. In the same way, in samadhi you see the interrelationship between events, what one could call the programming behind the events. But of course the events are blurred.

It's like with a camera. Either you can see a vast panorama, but then you can't see the detail, or you can focus the lens in such a way that you see the detail, but then you don't see the vast panorama. So you have the choice between the two.

In samadhi you're in what I call the sleep in the night of time, so you're able to reach very, very high up. I would say, even beyond the planning. But you lose sight of the detail. We said that already.

[1]Pir Vilayat Inayat Khan, "New Age Meditation" (cassette tapes M7801 and 7802). Copyright © 1975, Sufi Order, New Lebanon, New York.

Now samadhi with open eyes would be a state in which you're still attuned to this very high state and you see the details again. One could call it stereoscopic consciousness. It is like seeing two dimensions at the same time that are superimposed on one another.

... So perhaps we could [in samadhi with open eyes] say that one never just sees events, but one is always seeing what is beyond it. Like, for example, when you look at a person, you are always conscious of the eternal qualities that are ready to come through in that person. You don't just consider the personality, but you are always conscious of all the possibilities, and so on. You are always looking at that which transpires behind that which appears.

Now omega samadhi is more difficult to explain. I think we could put it this way. Let's say the archetypes of all things are like the seeds, and all things seem to be like the plant. So you could say your nature, your personality, is like the plant. It expresses, it unfolds, let us say, a certain part of all the richness of that which is contained in the seed, which is your eternal being.

So you could say that if you were in a state of samadhi, you would be able to experience your eternal being; and if you were in your ordinary consciousness, you would be able to experience your personality. But the fact is there's more in the personality than was present in the seed, because your personality has come into contact with other personalities and has enriched itself with those other personalities. And if that is so, then life on earth adds something to the way things were right up there. Something is gained by the interfusion of the parts of the totality. Something is gained that wasn't there in the beginning. Otherwise, there would not be a purpose in life at all.

... You don't expect that God's consciousness is just in samadhi, beyond creation. The Divine Consciousness permeates through creation. So why do you try to discover the meaning of things [only] by getting into a state beyond creation, when this experience of creation is so important? So omega samadhi is experiencing the Divine Conscousness right down in physical matter.[2]

Please realize that yoga is but one way, and certainly not the only way, to reach the state of consciousness that Pir Vilayat calls *omega samadhi*. Realize also that it will most likely take the most dedicated of spiritual seekers the better part of a lifetime to attain this high state of consciousness. The unwrapping of innumerable layers shrouding the soul is a very involved task. However, what ambition could be more worthy than aspiring to become a fit vehicle to meet the challenges of the physical world in a spiritual light?

[2]Pir Vilayat Inayat Khan, "New Age Meditation" (cassette tape, recorded August 30, 1978). Copyright © 1978, Sufi Order, New Lebanon, New York.

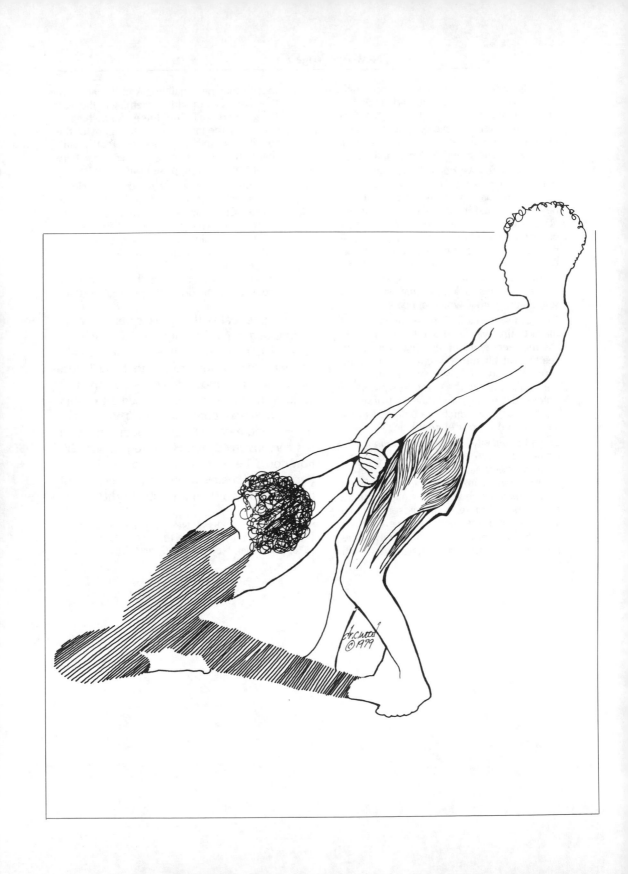

TWO
yoga, communication, and relationships

ANCIENT YOGA METAPHYSICS

According to ancient yoga theory we are *sat-chit-ananda* (existence, knowledge, and bliss). It is said that our birthright is one of eternal existence, infinite knowledge, and supreme bliss.

The classical teachings go on to say that the reason we have not recognized *sat-chit-ananda* is that we have become too enamored of the physical world, which has only a transitory existence. We have elevated our temporary, lower nature to the point where we actually believe that we exist only as separate egos, apart from all other egos. We have been caught in an illusion and have come to believe that the illusion is reality.

The ancient yogic notion is that each person is born of pure intentions and that all we have to do to achieve enlightenment is return to our original pure state. The soul longs to return to the immaculate state. There can be no lasting peace in the world of forms until we recognize our original state of eternal existence, infinite wisdom, and supreme bliss. The essence of classical yoga philosophy is that the purpose of life on earth is to gain conscious understanding of what we already unconsciously know.

SALVATION BY SECLUSION?

The new-age yoga message accepts the classical teachings, but it goes one step further to state that we have been placed upon earth to aid in the evolvement of creation. Modern technology and mass communication have made it very clear that we are all interconnected in a world community, and it appears that personal salvation is not to be achieved through seclusion. The new-age message is that we must claim our divine heritage while relating to this world rather than turning our back to it, that a net gain for the collective consciousness of humankind can be achieved through this process of interaction.

What I want to transmit to you is the assurance that our life *is* guided by an omniscient presence and that by attuning to it we can go beyond the veil of despair into peace and unity. However, to carry forward the new mode of life that is unfolding in our time, a new depth of consciousness must emerge. It is our choice whether to become a part of the vast synchronized intelligence that moves toward light or to sink in despair in our own personal suffering.

The path of yoga provides a means of physical, mental, emotional, and spiritual attunement to the higher order. The yoga way of life awakens within us a recognition of the divine qualities of our own being as well as the divine qualities within others. Through yoga practice and meditation we can go beyond the veil and tap into an inner world where all beings resonate as one.

In *Yoga and Psychotherapy: The Evolution of Consciousness* the authors discuss the concept of a united consciousness:

> At the highest states of consciousness, as described in yoga, experience is not only similar, it is shared. In other words, we might think of the hierarchy of consciousness as similar to a pyramid. At the base there's a wide area where diversity exists. . . . At the peak of the pyramid all paths must come together and the consciousness and perspective that is gained there is identical. This is not a "loss of consciousness" nor a slipping back into an undifferentiated state. From this point any part of the surrounding area can be viewed clearly.[1]

Before inner fulfillment occurs, we must strike the chord that vibrates in harmony with all other souls. Whenever we relate to another being at the soul level, the whole of life is uplifted and transformed. We must realize, however, that only the higher nature of our being can unite with others at the soul level. We must look within the depths of our own being to find harmony and order, then bring peace into the outer world. The first testing ground for maintaining this harmony is in our homes and places of work. We are tested most by those closest to us—our family, friends, and working companions.

COMMUNICATION

Behind our need for communication lies the deeply rooted longing of the soul to share love with other souls. In a very close relationship the loss of our separateness is crucial, as it is through this relinquishment that two people form a new whole greater than the sum of the parts.

Relating to others at the soul level satisfies an inner longing, but it is also the most difficult and risky of all undertakings. In a close relationship we have a need to maintain a certain degree of autonomy, as we must remain true to our highest ideal; this is combined with the need to unite and lose ourselves in the formation of a new unit. It is the attempt to find balance between the opposing poles of autonomy and mergence that makes friendship challenging. Though the relationship of husband and wife is perhaps the most rewarding and most difficult relationship of all, people in all relationships must deal with the same central issue: how to unite, change, and maintain stability all at the same time.

Words from the genius of Kahlil Gibran shed light on the subject of the love relationship. In *The Prophet,* Gibran directly addresses the issue of marriage, yet his remarks apply to all love relationships:

> Then Almitra spoke again and said, And what of Marriage, master?
> And he answered, saying:
> You were born together, and together you shall be forevermore.
> You shall be together when the white wings of death scatter your days.
> Ay, you shall be together even in the silent memory of God.
> But let there be spaces in your togetherness, And let the winds of the heavens dance between you.

---

[1]Swami Rama; Rudolph Ballentine, M.D.; and Swami Ajaya (Allen Weinstock, Ph.D.), *Yoga and Psychotherapy: The Evolution of Consciousness* (Glenview, Illinois: Himalayan International Institute of Yoga Science & Philosophy of USA, 1976), p.126.

Love one another, but make not a bond of
love:
Let it rather be a moving sea between the
shores of your souls.
Fill each other's cup but drink not from one
cup.
Give one another of your bread but eat not
from the same loaf.
Sing and dance together and be joyous, but
let each one of you be alone,
Even as the strings of a lute are alone though
they quiver with the same music.
Give your hearts, but not into each other's
keeping.
For only the hand of Life can contain your
hearts.
And stand together yet not too near together:
For the pillars of the temple stand apart,
And the oak tree and the cypress grow not
in each other's shadow.[2]

DETACHMENT

Although we need to engage in social inter-
change some of the time, on occasion each
individual needs to withdraw from others to
contemplate upon the meaning of life.
Though we do benefit from the mutual exchange of thoughts, at times we need to be
still enough to hear our own inner voice.
Through contemplation and meditation we
can gain new perspectives, see new horizons,
and fill our bodies and minds with light and
hope. From this experience we can find a way
to bring greater harmony to our relationships.
Once we have learned to consistently attune
to this infinite flow of energy and illuminated
state of mind, nothing that others do can
change our love for their eternal being.

It may appear paradoxical, but through
detachment we can become more involved in
the richness of a relationship. Both parties in
a relationship are destined to suffer until each

[2]Reprinted from *The Prophet,* by Kahil Gibran, by per-
mission of Alfred A. Knopf, Inc. Copyright 1923 by Kahil
Gibran and renewed 1951 by Administrators C.T.A. of
Kahil Gibran Estate, and Mary G. Gibran.

gains a sense of self-reliance. In unhealthy
relationships the overly needy person drains
the energy of those upon whom he or she is
dependent, causing the stronger person to
pull away in self-defense, manipulate the
other person in a domineering way, or resent-
fully cater to the weakness of the other. All
three reactions can result in distress, not only
to the weaker person but to the stronger person as well. The most effective way to heal a
relationship that is based on clutching, cling-
ing dependence is to replace it with love that
is divinely inspired. Divine love allows one to
love another being without absolutely requir-
ing a like return of love.

Many of our problems arise because we
expect too much of others and do not rely
enough upon our own inner strength. It is a
mistake to try to mold the behavior of another
to fit our needs. If we try to make those close
to us conform to our expectations, we are
destined to be upset constantly. In return, our
companions will rebel against the patterns we
try to impose upon them, and this will only
lead to further dissension and conflict.

Yoga practice moves us toward a high
state of consciousness in which we experience the freedom of our own being, which
allows us to free others. After a transcending
experience we can come back to family and
friends not to take from them or to try to
change them, but to share with them the richness and beauty of our realizations. For if we
are fulfilled in our own being, our self-suffi-
ciency paradoxically allows us to become
more deeply involved with others.

Faith and trust are sacred bonding
agents that unite two beings, but it is difficult
to maintain faith and trust in our loved ones
when they act in a discordant way. When
someone close to us performs an act that
seemingly threatens the harmony of the relationship, meditation can be our salvation.
From the cosmic perspective we can see that
we (and all others) are actually free souls.
From a detached viewpoint we can see the

relativity of the problems before us. Once we get a broad perspective of the situation the best solution to the problem should come to us. It is intelligent guidance that we all seek and meditation can help to attune us to this divine guidance. Once we glimpse the solution to our most pressing problem, still, we must work things out in a very concrete way on the physical plane. This means a certain amount of suffering will be involved, but the key point is that meditation can help us to act with greater clarity and greater assurance.

The message of new-age yoga is not to detach away from all our problems and let these problems work themselves out. We must meet the great challenges of life in a very conscious, direct way. From an egocentric viewpoint we will never be able to see the whole picture; therefore, periodically we must let go of our limited view in order to gain a broader view. Our duty is then to come back and meet the challenges before us in the most honest and sincere way we can.

GUILT

Until all our debts are cleared on all levels of existence, with all beings, we will be bound. If we have been unjust to any person, in any way, we must ask and receive forgiveness from that person before our mind can be set at peace. Our conscience will imprison us until we have set things right.

The difficulty arises when a friend will not release us in spite of our efforts. If we have done everything in our power to repay all debts to this person and, still, that person refuses to acknowledge our sincere effort at reconcilation, we may have to accept that now it is our friend who is performing the unfair act. Each person must deal with their own unjust acts. We can only take full responsibility for our own.

After we have done everything possible to rectify the situation, we must let go of our guilt, blame, and self-persecution. If we are to free our conscience, we have to be able to forgive ourselves. The quality of compassion can then become the focus of our being. Out of compassion, we can see beyond our and our friends' expressed attitudes and manifested actions. We then rise above the prison that once bound us, and we are free to love ourselves and others.

SUFFERING

Life's most puzzling question is: Why is there so much suffering on earth? The answer can come only from the cosmic perspective. From this high viewpoint we can see through the temporary illusion of suffering. We suffer because we think we exist only as separate, individual egos, apart from all other beings. We suffer because we try to overpower others rather than unite with them. We suffer because we try to trap a flow of energy that cannot be stopped. Stated simply, we suffer because we hold onto our lower nature and stifle our higher nature.

Only as we attain a panoramic viewpoint do we come to realize that it was part of the perfection of life that we should become bound by the limitations of our lower nature for a long while before we could accept the message of the all-pervading intelligence. We regressed time and time again before we were ready to embrace the truth of ultimate unity. This being our own experience, we come to realize that all other manifested souls will have to go through a similar maturation process. Unqualified acceptance of our loved ones becomes our greatest asset in relating to them.

To the dismay of the ego-centered self, all life on earth must eventually succumb to death. We cannot change the fact that physical-plane reality will continue to involve an immense amount of pain and sorrow because of death and disease and transiency. Transcendence of physical reality is the only way to triumph over suffering. Unfortunately, a desire to transcend is usually not felt until we have suffered deeply.

There is a kind of "grace" involved in suffering, according to Ram Dass. The grace of suffering that he speaks about concerns the fact that an intense experience of pain forces the sufferer to look inward for a way out. Ram Dass says:

> Next you begin to realize that although they are all equal in teaching quality, some of your experiences seem to shake you more than others, that the model which you are stuck in, sometimes so subtly you don't even know it, is shaken by pain and suffering and all the negative qualities. At that point you recognize the bizarre phenomenon that suffering is grace.[3]

There are numerous levels of reality, and Ram Dass speaks of the free being as one who maintains equilibrium at each level of consciousness:

> . . . So we have the paradox that on channels one and two and three there is an incredible melodrama going on, and you are an actor within it. There is a great deal of suffering, and when you're locked into channel one and you're hungry, and there's no food, that's real suffering, it's not fake suffering. But from channels four and five you can look at one, two and three and all the individual differences and all the melodrama and say, "Look at the perfection of the dance. Look at the perfection of the flow of the Divine Law—including the will of man which can go against the Will of God. Look at the perfection of it all."
>
> But it's not freedom for the being attached to channels four or five who, when you are hurting, says, "It's not real, don't worry, you're the Buddha, it's all an illusion." That's no more liberated than the person who's caught in one, two and three and says, "There's only pain and suffering everywhere and it's hell, life is terrible and ugly." The free being lives within all those realities simultaneously. He understands paradoxically

that when there is suffering, you must do everything you can to alleviate it. While at the same time, the suffering is perfection itself and your doing everything you can to alleviate it too is part of the perfection. Because ultimately you understand when you are free to move without attachment from level to level of reality, that the only reason you stay in form is to alleviate suffering or bring others to the light, to consciousness, to liberation, to God. What a paradox! Is it perfect? Sure. Is it Hell? Sure. Both at the same moment.[4]

How, in fact, can we comfort friends who are suffering great amounts of physical, mental, or emotional pain? As Ram Dass implies, it would be a mistake for the aware being to come up to those in great pain with a big smile and tell them their problem is only an illusion. As he says, those engulfed in intense suffering are caught in a space in which the pain they are experiencing is the most real thing in the world. At such a time it would be futile to tell them that all is one, that there is nothing but love, and that life is an exquisite projection of God.

The only way you will be able to reach friends who are anguishing is to enter the plane on which they dwell, so you can speak to them in their terms. Before they will look to you for help, they must sense that you actually understand their problem. You must feel their pain, but not let it become your personal pain. The critical issue is that you must, in some way or another, transmit hope, light, joy, peace, and healing vibrations at the same time you are feeling the suffering of your friend.

THEMES FOR MEDITATION

The principle of meditation is that we must lose ourselves in order to find ourselves. We must lose the armor we have built around us —the envy, fear, mistrust, impatience, self-pity, guilt, deceit, frustration, anger, hatred.

---

[3]Ram Dass and Stephen Levine, *Grist for the Mill* (Santa Cruz, Cal.: Unity Press, 1976), p. 42.

[4]Ibid., pp. 56–57.

These are defense mechanisms, personal emotions and habits of thought that we have acquired along the way, but they are not our real selves. These are qualities of our lower nature self; they strain our relationships and cause us grief and sorrow. The beauty of yoga is that it gives us a straightforward, time-tested technique that allows us to rise above and to discard our lower nature (the possessive aspect of our being) while nourishing our higher nature (the universal aspect of our being).

To fulfill our highest calling we must spread our wings and fly above the earth-plane. Yet, in rising above the physical reality, we must maintain proper perspective regarding our involvement with family, friends, and work. It it our duty to awaken within those close to us a realization of the almost limitless possibilities of their being. We are here to communicate with other souls in the deepest way possible.

Contemplation and meditation upon the divine aspects of our friends can be of great benefit. If soul-level communication is to take place between ourselves and others, we must recognize the universal characteristics within our friends—qualities that go beyond the limited ego-centered personality traits that those persons may be manifesting. Everyone has untapped reservoirs of creativity, understanding, compassion, patience, perseverance, purity, love, joy, beauty, peace, humility, honesty, inner strength, and many other attributes. Each person manifests at least one or two of these qualities quite obviously. Look at the most shining characteristic of your friend; then begin to look more deeply and recognize the latent qualities.

Not only can you meditate upon the divine nature of your friend, you can also scrutinize your own personality from a detached viewpoint and realize that there is much more truth, patience, understanding, purity, honesty, love, compassion, joy, and peace that you could reveal in your daily life. Go through these traits very slowly and care-fully and let them become a conscious part of your being.

While in a meditative state you can send out waves of love and peace to your friends. It may be easier to relate to others meaningfully while in a meditative state than when talking to them in person. Ego conflicts build barriers, and during meditation we begin to see the shortcomings of ego games. As we put these and other hindrances aside, we are enabled to communicate with friends and loved ones from a more universal aspect of our being.

If, however, we have the feeling that we are separate from our friends, even if we are sending them waves of love, we are not yet one with them. Trying to view the world through the eyes of those about us is a highly recommended technique that can take us beyond ourselves. Begin by trying to view your relationship through the eyes of the other person, and proceed until you are eventually able to experience the world as it is perceived by your friend.

The intrinsic value of this kind of meditation is that, if we can see through the eyes of one other person, we can then begin to see through the eyes of many people. In meditation we are not limited by our body or by our personality. Although communication in the everyday world is subject to time-bound limitations, communication while in a meditative state of mind takes place on another level of reality; it springs from a different order of existence. From the inner level of our mind we can make a deep connection with vast numbers of people. By attuning to the inner light of our own being, we are attuning to the very light of the universe. The ultimate truth is that all beings are one.

In the following quotation, Pir Vilayat Inayat Khan speaks of this reality where all beings resonate as one. In the midst of Pir Vilayat's words are two direct quotes from his father, Pir-O-Murshid Hazrat Inayat Khan. Pir Vilayat is relaying the message that his father espoused, and he is bringing the light of the new to it.

> When you realize you are all beings, that means you love all beings, of course. Or when you love all beings, you realize you are all beings. These are two thoughts that are completely attuned to one another. "No one will sacrifice for another except when he is oneself. If this feeling develops, it extends further—not only to the friends and to the neighbor, but to the stranger and to the beast, to the bird, and to the insect. One is at one with all beings, and it gives one as much insight into another as the other person has into himself."

> You see, this is really the point that the Masters reach in the end, and, that is, one is all beings and one sees oneself in all beings. It's not like you love a being, but at least that being seems other than yourself. It goes to the point where you are all beings. You are the mother you are the brother and you are the father and so on. And so, Murshid says, at the end, after renouncing, you have reached a point in which you don't care for this or you don't care for that. You become like the saint who reaches the point when you offer him a wonderful thing, and that's okay; and he doesn't have anything to eat, and that's okay too. That's real renunciation. It doesn't matter—whatever happens, you're happy.

> You reach the point when you're just part of all beings. And you come back from that state of detachment into life, and you enjoy the game of the children of the world. You just enjoy it. And you feel happy because they're happy, and you're sad if they're sad, and so on. But you do not try to get anything for yourself out of it. If you're seeking for liberation, you're seeking for something for yourself.

> That's why Murshid says the secret to all of this is, "What is made for man, man may hold, but man must not be held by it." So you don't have to leave the world, but you do not let yourself be held by it.[5]

The enlightened being, the one with cosmic vision, sees that beyond all suffering exists the peace and bliss of unity. What I would like to add from my personal experience is that once we find a way out of the bondage of our personal suffering, we will quite naturally be moved to help those around us to find freedom. We will simply and unequivocally be driven from deep inside to work toward the alleviation of suffering as soon as we see the way through our own turmoil. What I have learned from Pir Vilayat is that we can help beings about us realize that they are free souls by sharing divine love with them.

It seems to be the case that only by losing ourselves through trust in others do we begin to break through the prison of our separateness. Not only do we evolve our spiritual nature through soul communion, but the whole of humanity evolves as well through this crucial process of people helping each other to discover the unity behind manifested life. This concept has never been more aptly expressed than by the Christian apostle Paul in I Corinthians 13:

> 1 If I speak in the tongues of men and of angels, but have not love, I am a noisy gong or a clanging cymbal. 2 And if I have prophetic powers, and understand all mysteries and all knowledge, and if I have all faith, so as to remove mountains, but have not love, I am nothing. 3 If I give away all that I have, and if I deliver my body to be burned, but have not love, I gain nothing.

> 4 Love is patient and kind; love is not jealous or boastful; 5 it is not arrogant or rude. Love does not insist on its own way; it is not irritable or resentful; 6 it does not rejoice at wrong, but rejoices in the right.

> 7 Love bears all things, believes all things, hopes all things, endures all things.

> 8 Love never ends; as for prophecy, it will pass away; as for tongues, they will cease; as for knowledge, it will pass away.

> 9 For our knowledge is imperfect and our prophecy is imperfect; 10 but when the perfect comes, the imperfect will pass away.

> ... 13 So faith, hope, love abide, these three; but the greatest of these is love.[6]

[5]Pir Vilayat Inayat Khan, "New Age Meditation" (cassette tape H7502, Side 1). Copyright © 1975, Sufi Order, New Lebanon, N.Y.

[6]From the *Revised Standard Version of the Bible,* copyrighted 1946, 1952, © 1971, 1973.

II
POSTURE
AND BREATH AWARENESS
IN THE EVERYDAY WORLD

The way we stand, walk, sit, and breathe throughout the day must be looked at very carefully. Poor posture habits and poor breathing patterns can result in serious physical, mental, or emotional problems. On the other hand, good body alignment and deep, slow, rhythmic breathing can lead you toward improved health and clearer thinking patterns.

Chapter 3, "Body Alignment and Breath," analyzes how to stand, walk, sit, and breathe properly. Keeping a constant check on our posture and breathing habits can help us move toward a state of physical and mental health. What will strike you most about the yoga path is the practicality of it. With this chapter begins the discussion of the concrete physiological work of yoga.

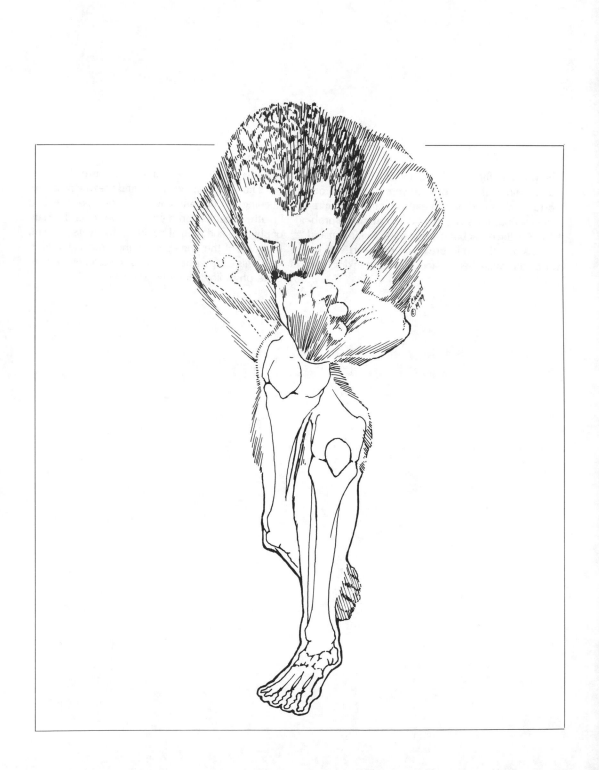

THREE
body alignment and breath

BODY ALIGNMENT

Standing Properly

It is unfortunate that most people in our society are not motivated to work on their postural habits until they have developed serious back, knee, or foot problems. To avoid such problems we must lift certain thigh and trunk muscles. To help relieve the downward stress upon the spinal vertebrae, we need to lift the abdominal and upper back muscles. It is important to create as much elongation and lift as possible through the legs and spine. The most efficient and healthy way to stand is with the legs and spine in a completely vertical position. How should the muscles work in order to bring the body to a vertically uplifted standing position?

Feet As any builder knows, one must begin the structure of a building at the bottom by laying a solid foundation, then work up. Let us now lay the foundation for the vertical standing posture. According to yoga principles, to stand in a perfectly erect way, you should bring the heels slightly apart and the base of the big toes together. From here press the balls of the big toes down, lift the toes, and spread them apart before placing them back onto the floor. Remaining centered on the heels, shift some of the weight to the outer edges of each foot, lifting the longitudinal and metatarsal arches of both feet.

Each foot should have three main points of floor contact when you are standing:

1. *The ball of the big toe.*
2. *The ball of the toes between the fourth and fifth toes.*
3. *The center of the heel.*

The weight should be distributed evenly on these three points.

The arches of the feet cannot lift effectively until the thigh muscles, abdominal muscles, and upper-back muscles lift as well. To put it simply, the feet have little chance to lift properly until the rest of the body begins to lift. This brings us to the next focus of attention, the legs.

Legs To overcome fallen arches, bunions, varicose veins, weak knees, and a weak back, we must build greater thigh strength. The *quadriceps* muscle group comprises the key

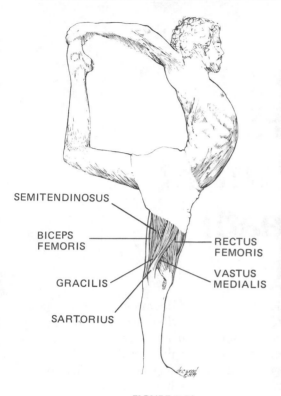

SEMITENDINOSUS

BICEPS
FEMORIS

GRACILIS

SARTORIUS

RECTUS
FEMORIS

VASTUS
MEDIALIS

FIGURE 3.1A

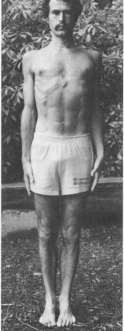

FIGURE 3.1B   **FIGURE 3.1C**

working muscles of the thighs. This group is composed of four muscles that act together as a unit: the vastus medialis, vastus intermedius, vastus lateralis, and rectus femoris. Quadriceps action directly controls the lifting action of the knees and indirectly controls the lifting of the foot, ankle, and abdominal muscles.

Turning the knees inward and locking them backward should definitely be avoided, as it leads to the following unwanted results:

1. *Bad pressure is exerted on the inner ligaments of the knee joints.*
2. *Too much weight is carried by the heels. This in turn causes the arches to collapse.*
3. *It becomes difficult to lift the quadricep muscles.*
4. *The back becomes swayed.*

5. *The abdominal muscles become lax.*
6. *The chest may begin to sink and collapse.*

To work the quadriceps properly, first make certain that the knees are in correct alignment by bending them slightly and directing them over the center of the third toe, as shown here in Figure 3.1B. Then slowly straighten the legs by lifting the quadriceps muscles, continuing to keep the knees directed over the center of the foot. Make sure the weight is evenly distributed on both feet (Figure 3.1C). The lower-leg muscles should lift straight upward to provide ankle stability and arch support. The lower-leg muscles should not have to do too much work if the quadriceps muscles work properly, however.

The kneecaps should be lifted, but not locked back, and should face straight for-

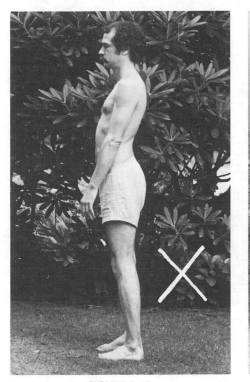

FIGURE 3.2A   FIGURE 3.2B

ward. The knee joints are hinge joints and are not constructed in a way that allows them to rotate to either side safely. If you have been placing too much stress on the ligaments of the knee while standing, the solution is to strengthen the quadriceps muscles so that the knees can be lifted and pointed in the right direction. Often a person who has lazy quadriceps muscles has lazy outer-thigh, abdominal, and buttock muscles as well. To keep the knees in their proper place, the outer-thigh, buttocks, and abdominal muscles must work in conjunction with the quadriceps.

Pelvic Tilt If the hip socket is allowed to internally rotate, causing the knees to turn in toward each other, swayback and sagging abdominal muscles most likely will result (Figure 3.2A).

If the hip socket is opened through con-traction of the outer-buttocks muscles, and if the outer-thigh muscles are held in, there is a much greater chance that the pelvic girdle can be tucked under (Figure 3.2B). By working the outer-thigh and outer-buttocks muscles, one can bring the pelvis and lumbar vertebrae into better alignment. (See Figure 3.2C to understand the position of the sacral, lumbar, thoracic, and cervical vertebrae and their relation to one another.)

Proper alignment of the spinal cord depends on the angle at which the sacrum connects into the lowest lumbar vertebra. As illustrated by Figure 3.2C, the more vertical the position of the sacrum the better one's chance of lessening the arch of the lumbar curve. The more vertically the sacrum is situated the better one's chance of positioning the thoracic and cervical vertebrae in good alignment. Taking the discussion one step fur-

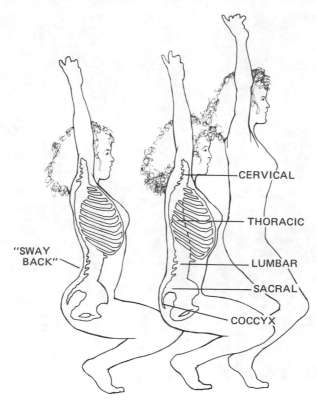

FIGURE 3.2C

ther, the more gradually the spinal cord curves in the lumbar, thoracic, and cervical regions, and the more the body lifts vertically upward, the less chance one has of suffering from backaches.

Sideways Curvature of the Spine Another serious problem that results from lazy outer-thigh and buttocks muscles is misalignment of the hips. It is a very common problem for one hip to be higher than the other. This often occurs because people stand around consistently on one leg or the other in the positions shown in Figures 3.3A and 3.3B. As one hip is thrown outward, most of the body weight is usually shifted onto the leg of that side and the knee locked back. This causes the lower spine to be pulled out of alignment. Foot, knee, and back problems can result. Avoid throwing one hip out when standing!

The hips should be leveled and should face squarely forward.

When the outer-thigh and buttocks muscles are drawn in during standing, the hips have a better chance of leveling and facing squarely forward. It is possible to bring most of the standing weight onto one foot and keep the hips level, but this is not too likely to happen unless you work at it in a very conscious way. The safest way to stand is evenly on both feet with the feet, hips, and shoulders all facing the same direction (Figure 3.3C).

Often those who have "saddlebags" on their outer thighs and a flabby bottom will have a swayback to go along with their excess fatty tissue. There is no better way to tone these problem areas than to contract the outer-thigh and outer-buttocks muscles when standing. Eliminating swayback, uneven

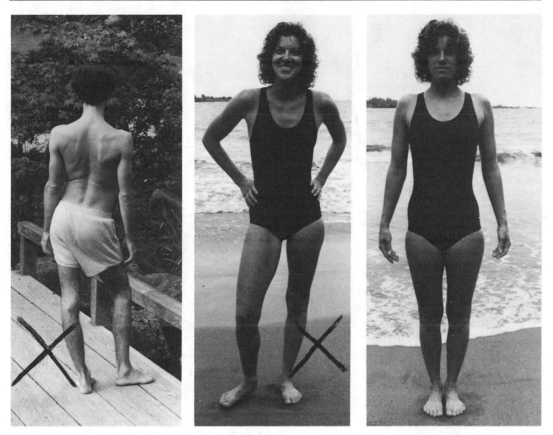

FIGURE 3.3A   **FIGURE 3.3B**   **FIGURE 3.3C**

hips, and sideways curvature of the lower spine and trimming down the outer thigh and bottom muscles all go together. Once the contractive work of the buttocks and outer thigh muscles has helped to bring the lower half of the body into good alignment, gradual relaxation of these muscle groups can occur.

As the hip socket opens to allow room for the pelvic girdle to tuck under, you should remain balanced on the triangular base of each foot and keep the feet parallel to each other. There is a tendency to roll to the outer edges of the heels as the hip sockets open through the contractive work of the outer thigh and outer buttocks muscles; avoid this by keeping the base of the big toes down and lifting up through the ankles. Both the inner and outer ankle must stabilize as the work in

the hip socket takes place; otherwise, the ankles will be overturned.

Rectus Abdominis The *rectus abdominis* muscle works in conjunction with the backside *erector spinae* muscles, and together they exert a significant influence on the pelvic tilt. As the rectus abdominis muscle

FIGURE 3.4A

ERECTOR SPINAE

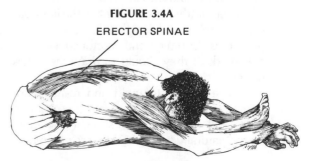

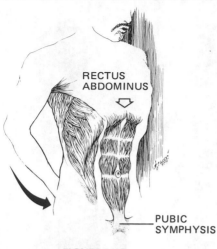

FIGURE 3.4B

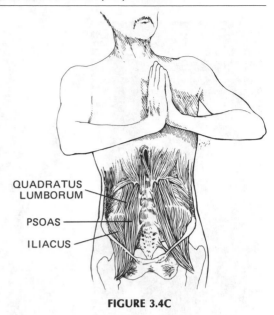

FIGURE 3.4C

contracts and pulls the pelvis under, the backside erector spinae muscles stretch, helping to elongate the lower spine (Figure 3.4A).

Figure 3.4B shows how to correct a swayed back. As the rectus abdominis muscle is drawn in and up, the lower-back muscles and the lumbar vertebrae quite naturally will lengthen. The pelvis is drawn under by means of a pulley system: the rectus abdominis muscles pulls up one way, and the erector spinae muscles go down the other way.

The *iliopsoas* and *quadratus lumbarum* muscles are shown in Figure 3.4C. The iliopsoas is composed of the iliacus and psoas muscles, which work together to flex the thigh when contracting. The *psoas* muscles attach to the sides of the lumbar vertebrae and cross through the pelvic girdle where they meet with the iliacus muscle. The *iliacus* attaches to the iliac crest at the top of the pelvic bone. The iliopsoas muscles insert at the top, inside of the femur (thigh bone). Only if the iliopsoas muscles relax and lengthen sufficiently can the rectus abdominis and erector spinae muscles work as they should to draw the pelvis under.

The goal is to mold and reshape our bodies to the point where the muscles and joints will maintain their straight alignment quite "naturally." It is the process of molding and reshaping that takes all the work. Remember that the most efficient way to stand is in a perfectly vertical position. Some of the contractive work of the thigh, buttocks, and abdominal muscles discussed earlier in this section can be released after one attains a well-aligned standing position. In the end far less muscular effort is needed to stand straight than to stand crooked.

Upper Back and Chest When we stand, the lower half of the body must receive help from the upper half in order to relieve some of the gravitational pressure upon the feet, legs, and lower back. We will see that the lift of the chest (Figure 3.5A) is a most important link in the chain of correct body alignment. As the chest is lifted, there is more freedom to move the lower spine into proper alignment, and less weight is placed upon the lumbar vertebrae, knees, ankles, and feet.

The active muscular work needed to lift the chest is done mainly through the contraction of the upper and middle-back muscles. As these muscles are drawn in toward the spine, the muscles across the chest will passively stretch and expand. An action I will

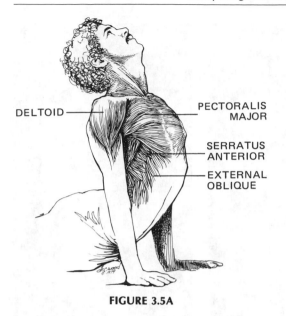

DELTOID —
PECTORALIS MAJOR

SERRATUS ANTERIOR

EXTERNAL OBLIQUE

FIGURE 3.5A

Arms   How should we carry our arms while standing around in conversation throughout the normal course of the day? For day-in-and-day-out standing arm positions, I highly recommend those shown in Figures 3.6A, B, and C. The principle is that one forearm goes behind the back, and the hand holds the forearm, the upper arm, or the inner elbow of the arm that hangs to the side of the body. This is comfortable, helps to bring the shoulders back and down, and keeps the chest lifted.

Holding one arm behind the back as in Figure 3.6A, gives you something to do with your nervous energy. The conscious act of drawing the shoulder blades in toward the spine must occur to expand the chest cavity fully, even in this position. The arm that goes behind the back also helps give those with swayback a reminder of how to straighten the lumbar curve, as the lower-back muscles can be pushed backward against the forearm.

As shown here in Figure 3.6B, when you are holding the inner elbow, you can use and move the free hand while in conversation. In order to keep the lower ribs in and to prevent an overarched lumbar region, it is best to breath backward against the forearm.

stress over and over again is that of rotating the shoulders back and down by drawing the shoulder blades in toward each other, as this brings the upper chest out and allows it to be lifted. To do this the middle trapezius, the rhomboideus muscles, and the latissimus dorsi muscles must all contract in conjunction with one another.

FIGURE 3.5B

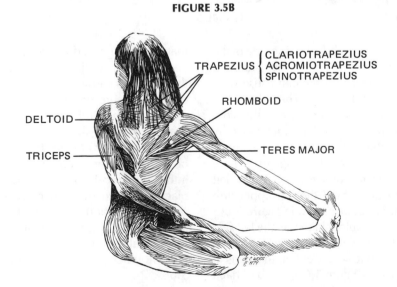

TRAPEZIUS { CLARIOTRAPEZIUS
ACROMIOTRAPEZIUS
SPINOTRAPEZIUS

RHOMBOID

DELTOID —

TERES MAJOR

TRICEPS —

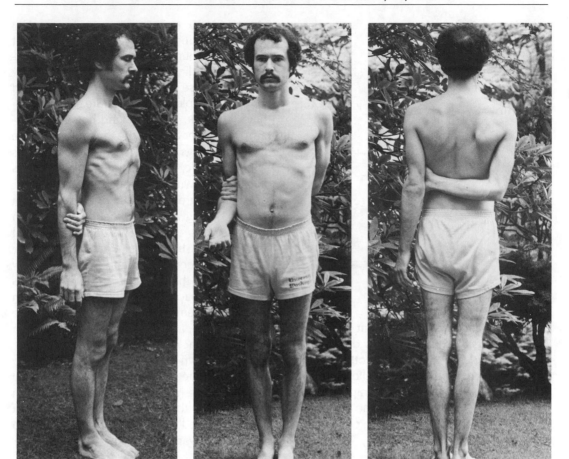

FIGURE 3.6A   FIGURE 3.6B   FIGURE 3.6C

Just about everybody has one side of the upper back tighter than the other side. An unbalanced muscular system can cause sideways curvature of the spine. The tightness in the muscles can be broken up and the sideways curve of the upper spine straightened by building the habit of holding the biceps muscle (upper arm muscle) of the tightest side. If you have a tight left upper back or tight left shoulder-joint area, hold the left upper arm with the right hand, as shown in Figure 3.6C. Notice how the shoulder blade on the left side has flattened in toward the body, activating the muscles of that area. Folding the arms in front, as shown in Figure 3.6D, is a bad habit

that leads to a caved-in chest, an overstressed neck, and spinal-disc compression. Sinking of the chest, as shown in the photo, also places excess pressure on the knees and feet.

For utmost relaxation in the standing position, the arms should be allowed to hang down gracefully next to the body. There will be little space between the arms and the torso if the shoulders have been drawn into proper placement and the arm muscles have been relaxed. The shoulders should be rolled back and down in a graceful manner rather than rigidly pulled back and down. Correct arm and shoulder positioning is shown in Figure 3.6E.

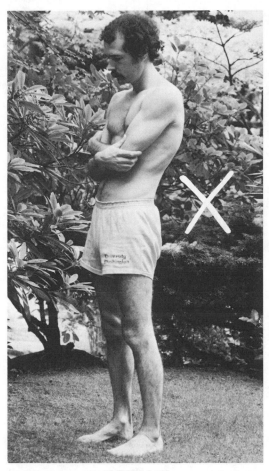

FIGURE 3.6D

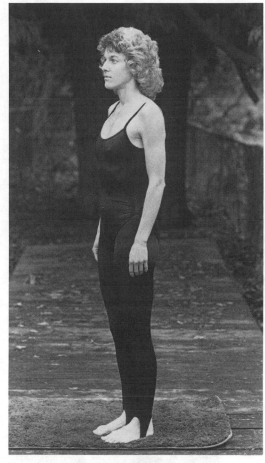

FIGURE 3.6E

Head and Neck A major and common mistake is improper carriage of the neck and head. Throughout most daily activities the hands, arms, and shoulders must go forward to perform specific tasks. Consider writing, typing, reading, carpentry, most sports activities, car riding, housecleaning, and yardwork, and you will realize that the hands, arms, and shoulders are required to move forward in these tasks. After hours, days, months, and years of this forward movement, there is a tendency for the shoulders to slump forward on a permanent basis.

The head tends to follow the forward movement of the shoulders, the negative re-

sult being too much sway in the neck (too much cervical curve). Poor head and neck carriage brings with it shoulder and neck tension, as well as headaches. However, one must realize that the neck cannot go into proper alignment until the shoulders are first drawn back and down. Once the shoulders have been fixed down, the back of the head can be lifted vertically upward to straighten the neck vertebrae.

The carriage of the head and neck demonstrated in Figure 3.7A is very poor. Notice how the shoulders have slumped forward and how the chin has gone far in front of the chest. This causes an extreme arch to occur along

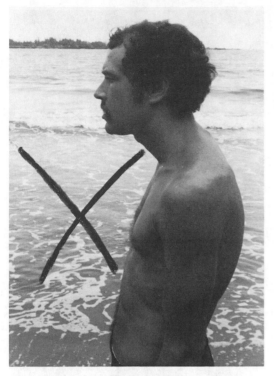

FIGURE 3.7A

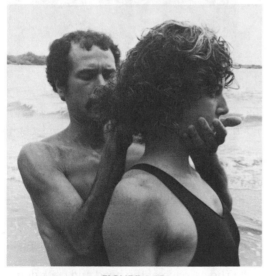

FIGURE 3.7B

the backside of the neck. Protrusion of the upper back and swaying of the lower back usually go hand in hand with excess curvature

of the neck, as can be seen in this figure.

In Figure 3.7B, I stretch the back of Linda's neck with one hand, as I gently bring her chin in with the other hand. To straighten the neck curve, concentrate on lifting the back of the skull straight up. To do this you must think down and in with the chin. This does not mean you should jam the chin back against the throat; it simply means you should gently bring it back. The main thought should be the upliftment of the back of the head. With good neck alignment the ear lobes will be positioned directly above the center of the shoulder joint. As a general rule the greater the vertical distance between the shoulders and the ears the better off we are.

The greatest curve in the neck generally occurs where the top two vertebrae of the neck and the back of the skull meet. Many people hold a large amount of tension at the top of the neck because of excess curvature here. It is a good idea to periodically massage that area of the neck to break up accumulated muscular tension. Usually one side of the neck will be tighter than the other side, and this can be found when massaging the neck. Another way to test your head carriage is to take notice if the head commonly pulls toward one side. Unless the head sits straight on top of the neck, an imbalance of energy will be created. Think about proper head carriage at intervals throughout the day, and try to find a way to maintain good neck alignment. We all have a lot of old postural habits that are very bad ones. We can break these crooked patterns of body carriage only by keeping a constant check on the body.

Standing Summary In looking at someone from the side, as in Figure 3.8, we can see good body alignment if the center of the hip joint is above the center of the foot and the legs are in vertical position. Good alignment means that the center of the shoulder joint is above the center of the hip joint and that the curves of the spine have been minimized. It

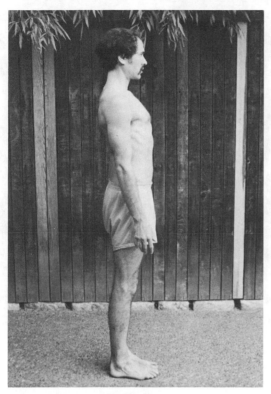

FIGURE 3.8

help you to strengthen the body's energy field and improve the clarity of your thinking.

Walking

To walk gracefully means to be light on the feet. Coming down hard on the heels is not only a jar to the nervous system but also stressful on the lower back, knees, and feet. You should keep the chest lifted and the spine as straight as possible while walking. You can overcome the downward force of gravity by lifting the leg, abdominal, chest, and back muscles.

Lifting and leaning out with the chest should precede each step. As the chest lifts and leans forward, one foot eventually must be brought forward to avoid falling. The forward movement of each leg should begin with a tucking action of the pelvis. The further the leg swings through, the more the pelvis tucks under. Thus, a subtle and gentle flexion of the lower spine occurs each time one leg is brought forward. Let the arms hang down to the sides, or let them swing very lightly. The main concern when walking should be on the upward lift of the spinal cord.

A person who walks around as in Figure 3.9A not only looks depressed, but actually becomes depressed. A caved-in chest and rounded upper back make for shallow breathing. Excess curvature in the upper and lower spine leads to backaches. Thrusting forward of the neck, as shown in the figure, eventually would cause a neckache.

Initiate each step by leaning the chest forward and lifting through the back of the head (Figure 3.9B). As you lean forward and lift the chest, lift strongly through the entirety to the standing leg. To take a step, tuck the pelvis, swing the back leg through, push off of the ball of the toes of the standing leg, and bring the weight onto the front foot (Figure 3.9C). Then lean the chest forward again and repeat the same process by swinging the other leg through.

means that the center of the ear lobe is above the center of the shoulder joint and that the chin forms a 90-degree angle to the throat. The arms can hang down next to the body and the hardness of the body softened by focusing upon deep, slow, rhythmic breathing.

Imagine that a string from above is attached to the back of the head, and try to picture this string as lifting the head and spine straight upward. As the vertical lift of the spine occurs, you can release some of the contractive work of the muscular system that was initially needed to bring the body into good alignment. Directing our attention to the straightness of the spinal column at regular intervals throughout the day helps to keep the whole body in better alignment and also helps to keep the mind more focused. Attuning to the flow of energy along the spine can

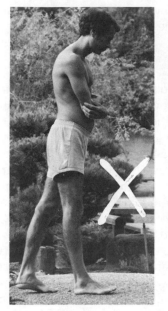 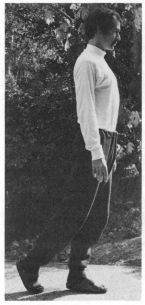 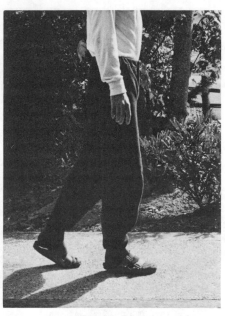

FIGURE 3.9A   **FIGURE 3.9B**   **FIGURE 3.9C**

FIGURE 3.9D   **FIGURE 3.9E**   **FIGURE 3.9F**   **FIGURE 3.9G**

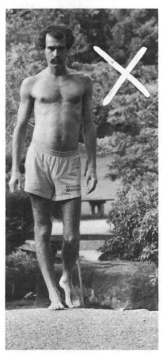 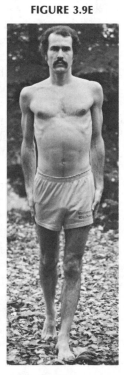 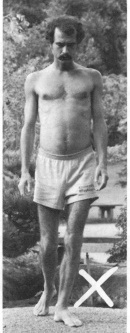 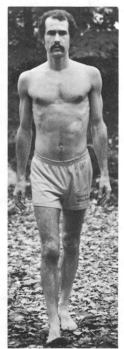

A common fault is swaying sideways with each step. As you can see in Figure 3.9D, side swaying causes the knees to turn inward and pulls the whole body out of alignment. Walking in this way can be harmful to the feet, knees, hips, pelvis, spine and neck. When walking, you should consciously contract the outer-thigh muscles of the planted leg as the other leg swings through. This will eliminate sideways swaying of the hips. The hips should face squarely forward, fairly level with each other, as shown in Figure 3.9E. The shoulders should stay as level as possible with each other above the hips.

Do not allow the feet to turn out when walking, as in Figure 3.9F; they should stay parallel to each other with each step. Turning the feet out can result in serious lower-back, knee, ankle, and foot problems.

As the body weight shifts forward onto the standing leg, the thigh muscles of that leg should be lifted. The abdominal, chest, and upper-back muscles should be lifted throughout all phases of the walk, as in Figure 3.9G. It may help if you imagine that a string is pulling the back of your head and your spine upward as your feet glide effortlessly along the ground.

Sitting

Most people give very little thought to the proper way to sit, even though they sit during most of their waking hours. With all the desk jobs and all the reading, television gazing, and car riding that people engage in, it is important that people learn how to sit with a straight spine. The prevalence of backaches in our society points to an obvious need for change in postural habits.

The key to sitting with a straight spine is to lift the chest and sit forward on the sitting bones. Letting the chest drop, the shoulders stoop forward, and the back round while sinking back onto the gluteus muscles for long periods is harmful to the neck and torso.

Backaches generally result when rounding of the back and sinking of the chest become habitual. The force of gravity weighs down heavily on the spinal discs and back muscles; this necessitates a strong lift upward to alleviate the compression that is caused. To sit properly one must lift the rib cage away from the pelvic girdle, lift the chest, drop the shoulders back and down, and then lift and align the spine on top of the two ischium bones (the sitting bones). The main muscular contraction when sitting should be to draw the muscles between the shoulder blades in toward the spine, as only then can the chest, upper back, and spine lift properly.

The problem is that after sitting at a desk for hours on end the natural tendency is for the back to round, the shoulders to stoop forward, and the chest to cave in, so that the lower back carries the weight of the upper back, chest, and head. Many jobs seemingly require one to hunch over the desk to do the work. Admittedly, it is a difficult task to keep the chest lifted and the shoulders back and down while doing desk work, but certainly in most situations it is not impossible. To help remind us of the muscular action that is needed to keep the chest lifted, the shoulders back, and the spine well aligned, we can do any of numerous yoga postures at work. Specifically, many twists, backbends, and forward stretches can be done while one is sitting in a chair. Doing a few simplified yoga postures periodically throughout the day brings awareness and life into the back muscles and helps break up tension that builds as we sit in the same position hour after hour.

As one performs chair backbends, twists, and forward stretches, the *pectoralis muscles* (chest muscles) and the *intercostal muscles* (the muscles between the ribs) are stretched, and the diaphragm area is freed to work without so much resistance. This allows deeper, fuller breathing. As an increased supply of oxygen is taken in through deeper inhalation, all the body systems begin to work more efficiently, including the brain cells and the nervous system. As more carbon dioxide is expelled through more complete exhalation, the body is relieved of toxic residues, and mental alertness is increased.

The legs and arms, too, seldom are stretched during a normal workday. We need to exercise the leg, ankle, and foot muscles as well as the arm, wrist, and finger muscles in order to keep a good flow of blood, oxygen, and nerve impulses moving throughout these areas of the body.

Another problem resulting from doing office work is that we generally write, file, type, or talk on the phone in a way that forces one side of the body to perform an action that the other side of the body is not performing. This unbalanced movement can cause the vertebrae to slip out of alignment if it is done without a counterbalancing movement. Once the vertebrae are misaligned, backaches result. If the spinal discs become so compressed that the nerves are pinched, extreme pain and immobility can result.

It is possible to put the vertebrae back in alignment by twisting to each side while sitting in a chair. This adjustment is safe *if the spine is lifted upward and kept vertical as you twist.*

Chair Twists

Of all the postures that can easily be done around an office, chair twists can relieve backaches the fastest. When done with an uplifted spine, chair twists are the safest of all yoga postures and can be done by the most inflexible of people. I recommend that chair twists be done by one and all periodically throughout the day. Incorporating a twist or two every hour is very helpful for both the body and the mind.

We look next at three simple chair twists. Each of these can be held safely from five to 20 seconds. To set the twist up, inhale, lift the chest, and elongate the spine; then exhale and twist the rib cage. Breathe deeply and slowly while in the twist pose. I reiterate:

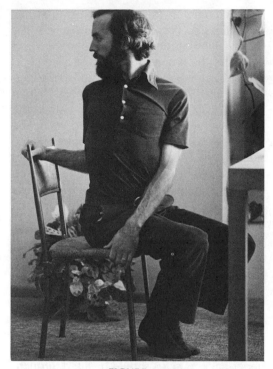

FIGURE 3.10A

do not try to twist until you first lift the chest and elongate the spine; then twist to your heart's content. For further explanation of the twisting postures, see the opening discussion in Chapter 7.

Figures 3.10A, B, and C demonstrate some of the many arm and hand positions that can be used while twisting in a chair. Whatever type of chair you have, twists can be done in it.

Note that as each man twists his rib cage, he does not twist his hips. With knees facing forward, he lifts his chest as he twists to either side. Also note how his hands are conveniently placed on the chair to grip, push against, or pull against. He maintains elongation through the backside of the neck as he turns his head over his back shoulder. Even though the rib cage turns 90 degrees or more, the spinal column should be as vertical as possible from the base of the spine to the top of the head.

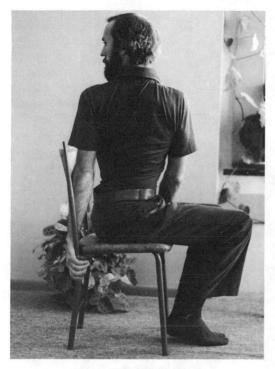

FIGURE 3.10B

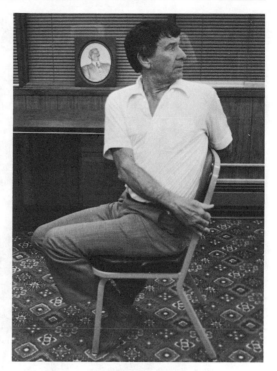

FIGURE 3.10C

Once in one of the twisting postures shown in Figures 3.10A, B, or C, pull the shoulder you have twisted toward down and back by contracting the shoulder-blade muscles of that side in toward the spine. Continue to lift through the lower part of the rib cage and expand and turn the chest. The abdominal muscles should pull across to aid the twist and to help keep the lower spine straight. After working one side for five to 20 seconds, breathing deeply the whole while, inhale, slowly come out of the pose, exhale, and repeat to the other side.

Office Yoga

Following are some postures that can be done at work. Study the pictures and try the postures one by one. Then decide which ones you want to incorporate into your daily office routine. It is a good idea to work in two or three minutes of office yoga for every hour of desk work. You will find that you will not get

as tired as you used to at the end of the day if you do these postures.

Your own flexibility and the privacy of your working conditions will determine which of these movements you can or cannot do at your office. *Do not hold any of these postures more than 20 seconds unless you have practiced yoga faithfully for six months or more. (other than foot and ankle exercises)*

Foot and Ankle Exercises It is a good idea to occasionally take one's shoes off during the day and exercise the ankle and foot muscles. The feet should be exercised and the ankles loosened daily. These simple movements can be done periodically throughout the day, as they do not impede desk work. The foot and ankle exercises will help keep the whole lower half of the body more awake. (Note in Figures 3.11A and B how John is sitting on a thickly folded blanket to help him maintain a straight back as he reads.)

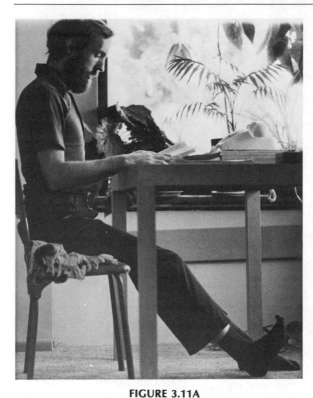

FIGURE 3.11A   **FIGURE 3.11B**

In Figure 3.11A, John is flexing and rotating his right ankle from side to side while stretching through the calf muscles. After doing this for a minute or so, he will move to the other foot and repeat the same loosening movements. This exercise can be done on numerous occasions throughout the day, as it does not disturb the work going on above the desk.

In Figure 3.11B, John is lifting both heels while gently pushing the balls of the feet down on the floor. This increases the blood circulation through the ankles and feet and helps to awaken the muscles of these areas. To do this exercise, lift the heels for a few seconds, then drop them gently down. This can be done over and over again.

Backbends To counteract the stooping tendency of the shoulders, the collapsing ten-dency of the chest, and the buildup of tension in the neck, shoulders, and back muscles, chair backbends are very helpful. Countless kinds of backbends can be done from a chair. For now let us look at three.

It is best to move into the backbends shown here on an inhale. Once in the pose, hold for a few seconds, take a couple of deep breaths, and then exhale to come out of the backbending position.

For the backbend in Figure 3.12A, sit on the front part of the chair, bring the heels of the hands to the back edge of the seat, inhale, push the straightened arms down, and lift the chest. Breathing deeply, pull the shoulders back and down, arch the upper back, look up, gently arch the neck, and let the bent legs relax. Work in the pose for a few seconds, come out slowly, rest, and then repeat.

For the backbend in Figure 3.12B, sit on

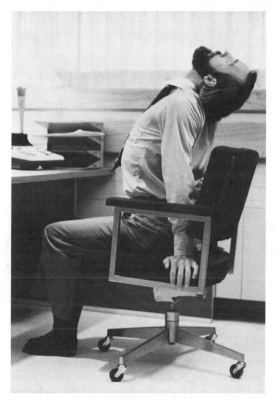

FIGURE 3.12A

the back part of the seat of the chair, inhale, and lift the upper back up and over the top of the backrest. Interweave the fingers, stretch the arms down, and rotate the inner wrist toward the chair (clockwise) until the heels of the hands are facing the floor with the fingers facing out. Continue stretching the arms and hands down and away from the chair. Breathe deeply, expand the chest, arch the upper back more, let the head fall back, and let the bent knees relax. Work for five to 20 seconds in the pose, come out of it slowly, rest, and then repeat.

In Figure 3.12C, Don demonstrates a simple back arch that loosens the shoulder joints, stretches the arm, chest, and abdominal muscles, and breaks up tension in the back muscles. To do the pose sit to the back of the chair, lift the upper back up over the backrest of the chair, inhale, interweave the fingers, and arch back over the chair. Notice how Don stretches upward through the heels of his hands, relaxes his neck backward, and lifts his chest. Yawning while in this arched position relaxes the jaw, eyes, and facial muscles and

FIGURE 3.12B

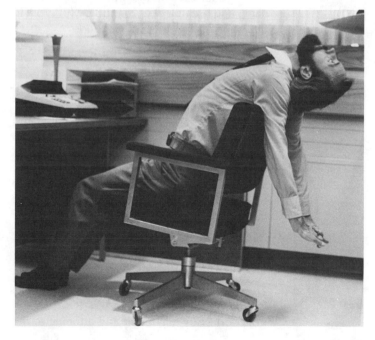

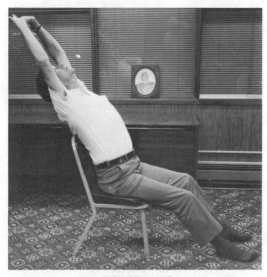

FIGURE 3.12C

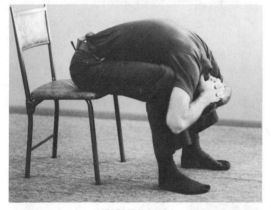

FIGURE 3.13A
FIGURE 3.13B

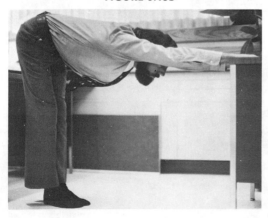

helps to oxygenate the brain. Work in the pose for five to ten seconds, rest, and repeat.

Forward Stretches Forward stretches increase the oxygen, blood, and nerve supply to the legs, arms, and back muscles. These postures stretch the spinal cord and help relieve tension in the back muscles. Exhale to move into a forward stretch, and breathe deeply while in the pose.

For the stretch in Figure 3.13A, sit on the front part of the chair with the knees bent and the feet shoulder-width apart. Exhale, fold the torso forward, and bring the chest between the knees. Interweave the fingers behind the neck, pull the elbows out, and stretch the neck and back muscles. Breathe deeply, hold for a few seconds, release, and come up slowly.

For the stretch in Figure 3.13B, bring the hands to the desk and slowly walk the feet back until the arms, spine, and legs can all stretch fully. Bring the hips above the feet, tilt the pelvis upward, elongate through the whole backside of the body, drop the rib cage, and breathe deeply and slowly. Work in the pose for ten to thirty seconds.

Quadriceps Strengthener Shown in Figure 3.14 is a simple way to strengthen the quadriceps muscles. While sitting on a chair, take one foot off the floor and straighten and stretch through the backside of the leg. Pull the kneecap up by contracting the quadriceps muscles and hold the contraction for a few seconds. Repeat to the other side, then do both sides again. This quadriceps strengthener can be done periodically throughout the day.

Conversational Posture

The way we sit, stand, and breathe affects greatly our attitude toward life. By maintaining good body alignment and attuning to the

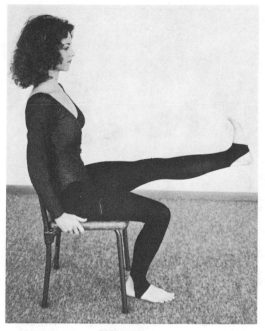

FIGURE 3.14

FIGURE 3.15A

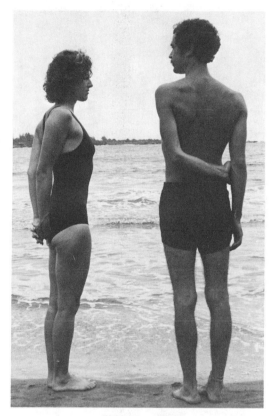

FIGURE 3.15B

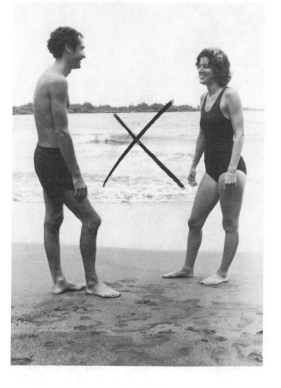

breath, we can remain centered and focused throughout the day. To awaken a deeper, clearer level of communication with others we should be conscious of our own body alignment and breath.

Figures 3.15A through 3.18C show examples of bad and good conversational posture. The A's are examples of poor conversational posture, whereas the B's and the C are examples of good conversational posture.

Poor posture habits will not be alleviated until conscious attention is brought to the body on a day-in and day-out basis. A small part of you, a witness, must keep a constant check on the condition of your posture throughout your waking hours if good posture habits are ever to be developed.

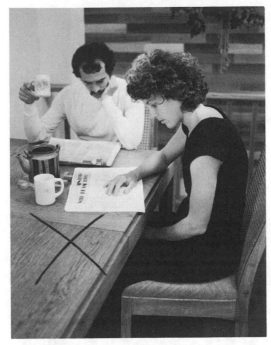

FIGURE 3.16A

FIGURE 3.16B

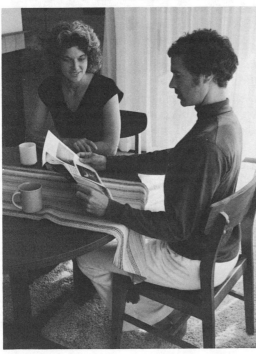

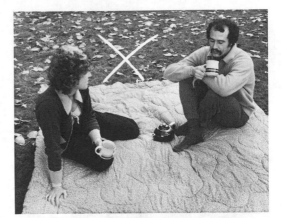

FIGURE 3.17A

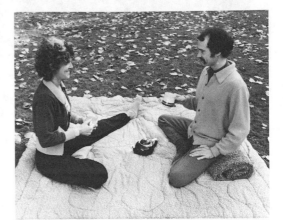

FIGURE 3.17B

FIGURE 3.18A

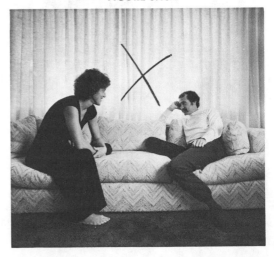

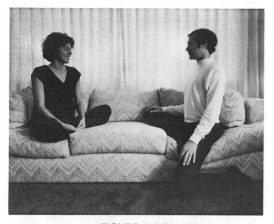

FIGURE 3.18B

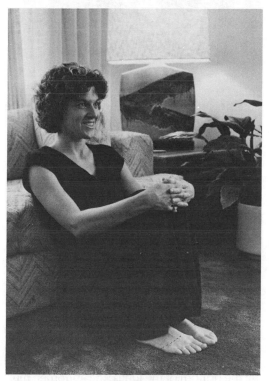

FIGURE 3.18C

PROPER BREATHING

It is important that you begin to carry over into your daily activities the opened-up feeling attained during Hatha Yoga practice.

Besides maintaining the length and straightness of the spinal column that the body has experienced in yoga practice, you need to be aware of proper breathing throughout the day.

Breath

Incredibly large amounts of tension can be released through deep, slow, rhythmic breathing. As soon as you have the presence of mind to notice your breath in a tense situation, you have taken the first step in releasing mental nervousness and physical tautness. I highly recommend the following as an effective antidote for an anxious mind:

1. *Breathe in slowly and deeply, counting to three slowly.*

2. *Pause momentarily.*

3. *Counting to three, slowly empty the air from the lungs.*

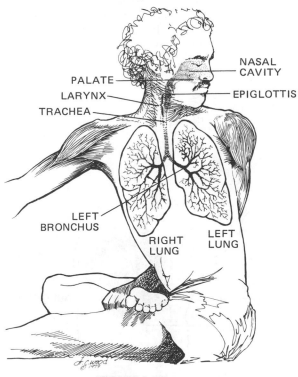

FIGURE 3.19A

Do this breath quite a number of times and watch the tension subside. Breathe in and out of the nostrils rather than the mouth.

Try to conceive of the lungs (Figure 3.19A) as two balloons that are located inside the chest cavity. Picture them expanding with the inhale and contracting with the exhale. The air moves in through the nose, down through the throat, and into the lungs on the inhale—and vice versa on the exhale. Inside the lungs themselves the main expansion and contraction occur in grapelike clusters of microscopic air sacs called *alveoli.* "It has been estimated that there are 300 million alveoli in the lungs and that the total area available for gas exchange is about 40 times the body surface."[1]

Inhalation The inhale begins as the diaphragm contracts and is drawn downward. The *diaphragm* is the domelike muscle that separates the chest cavity from the abdominal cavity (Figure 3.19B). Its contraction creates more space in the lungs, reducing air pressure there to the point where it is lower than atmo-

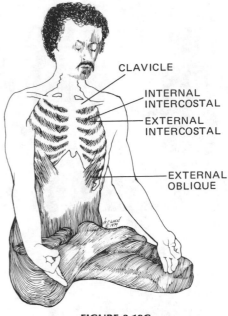

CLAVICLE

INTERNAL INTERCOSTAL

EXTERNAL INTERCOSTAL

EXTERNAL OBLIQUE

FIGURE 3.19C

spheric pressure. Thus, air from the outside rushes in to fill the vacuum.

Taking in a complete yoga breath means filling the lungs frontward, sideward, and backward from the bottom to the top. The dimension of breathing often neglected is sideways intercostal breathing. The *intercostal muscles* are the muscles between the ribs (Figure 3.19C). The complete yoga in-breath depends very strongly on the expansion of the rib cage through the action of intercostal muscles.

Three-Part Yoga Inhale Since the lungs are somewhat pear-shaped, the lower portion can expand more than the middle portion, and the middle portion more than the top. To fill the bottom of the lungs, the abdomen must round out. The expansion of the abdomen occurs as the diaphragm moves down, push-

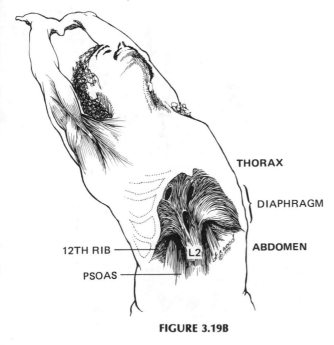

THORAX

DIAPHRAGM

ABDOMEN

12TH RIB

L2

PSOAS

FIGURE 3.19B

[1]Mary Griffiths, *Introduction to Human Physiology* (New York: Macmillan Publishing Co., Inc., 1974), p. 205.

ing the internal organs down and out. Figure 3.20A shows the abdominal muscles rounding out during the first third of the inhale.

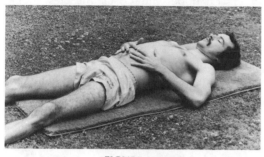

FIGURE 3.20A

Next, the air should move into the middle portion of the lungs, causing the lower and middle rib cage area to expand (Figure 3.20B). Unfortunately, the way to expand the lower rib-cage area has not been taught to most people. It is important to realize that only during the first third of the inhale should the abdomen round out. During the last two-thirds of the inhale, the abdomen should quite naturally flatten as this allows the middle and upper sections of the lungs to expand completely and fully.

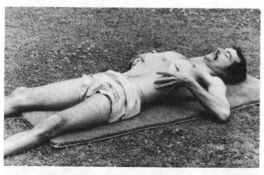

FIGURE 3.20B

The completed in-breath ends with the expansion of the upper chest (Figure 3.20C). The higher the air goes into the lungs, the more you should work on drawing the shoulders down away from the ears, as this allows the upper lungs to fill completely.

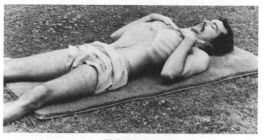

FIGURE 3.20C

Exhalation The exhale also begins with movement of the diaphragm, this time by an upward action. As the diaphragm passively moves back toward its rest position, the air at the bottom of the lungs will be pushed up and out. The air in the middle and upper lungs will be exhaled as the diaphragm continues to move upward.

With each normal breath the average person moves around 500 milliliters of air in and out of his lungs. Since the average person has a 5000-milliliter lung capacity, it should be obvious that the breath can be changed quite drastically. The key to bringing about this change is learning to exhale totally. A complete exhalation requires quite a lot of work by the abdominal muscles and the intercostal muscles. The contraction of these muscles must be done consciously if one is to overcome years of shallow breathing.

During the complete yoga out-breath, the air should empty from the bottom to the top of the lungs. This would appear to mean that the abdominal muscles should contract first, then the lower intercostal muscles should contract, and finally the upper intercostal muscles should come into play. However, the muscular action of exhalation is a bit more complicated than simply moving from the bottom to the top of the lungs. In the following description of the exhale, the correct muscular action will be discussed.

Complete Yoga Exhale Consciously, the initial action of the exhale should be to flatten the abdominal muscles, as this helps to

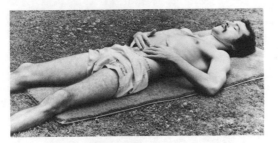

FIGURE 3.21A

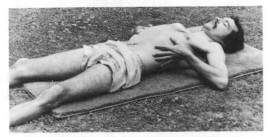

FIGURE 3.21B

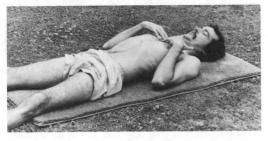

FIGURE 3.21C

push the air out of the lower part of the lungs and intiate the upward action of the diaphragm (Figure 3.21A). The abdominal muscles should continue to flatten throughout the entirety of the exhale if you seek to empty the lungs totally.

The second phase of the exhale should be to concentrate on the contraction of the lower and middle intercostal muscles (Figure 3.21B). *During the complete exhale, the main focus should be on the squeezing action of the lower rib-cage area inward by the intercostal muscles.* I find it helpful to imagine that the diaphragm is becoming more and more inverted inside the rib cage the longer I exhale. The diaphragm will move upward during the entire out-breath, but it will do so

optimally only if the lower intercostal muscles work in conjunction with the abdominal muscles.

The upper intercostal muscles should not have to do much work to complete the out-breath (Figure 3.21C). The air in the upper part of the lungs can, for the most part, be pushed out through the upward action of the diaphragm, squeezing action of the intercostal muscles in the lower ribs, and by the continual flattening of the abdominal muscles. This is not to say that upper intercostal action should be neglected entirely. It is best to get into the habit of exhaling as much carbon-dioxide-laden air as is comfortably possible, and contraction of the upper intercostal muscles can aid this process.

Intercostal Breathing Since the sideways expansion and contraction of the rib cage is often neglected, I urge you to give special attention to this aspect of breathing. While you lie on your back with the feet together and the knees dropped open, the abdominal muscles will naturally flatten so that you can focus exclusively on the sideways expansion of the rib cage. Placing the hands on the sides of the rib cage will help to bring awareness to the area. Note the expansion that has occurred on the inhale in Figures 3.22A and B and the contraction that has occurred on the exhale in Figure 3.22C.

FIGURE 3.22A

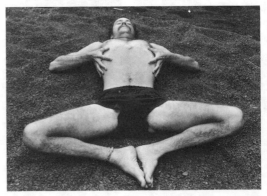

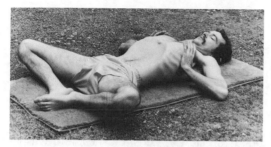

FIGURE 3.22B

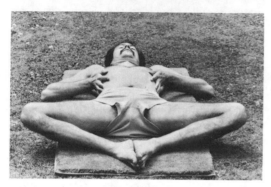

FIGURE 3.22C

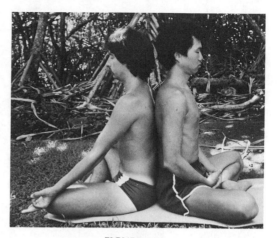

FIGURE 3.23

Breathing Up the Spine The air should fill the lungs frontward, sideward, and backward. Most people can accomplish the front-filling aspect of the breath without too much difficulty. Having specifically discussed how the sideways expansion of the breath can be practiced, let us now focus on the backward aspect.

A good way to practice breathing backward is to sit back-to-back with a partner, as in Figure 3.23. The idea is to sit very straight and breathe against your partner's back.

First, one person attunes to the other's inhalation as it moves up the back. After feeling the manner in which the breath moves along his or her partner's back for a few inhalations, the observer helps the breather by placing his hand(s) on the particular area of the breather's back where the breath is weak and gives verbal feedback as well. The breather then concentrates on moving the in-

hale up the back with emphasis on the weak area that has been pointed out.

The observer will not be able to feel the exhale as clearly as the inhale, but it should be observed in the same manner. Verbal feedback and hand placement again help the breather understand how to exhale more thoroughly. Switch roles after a few minutes.

Tight Jaws, Tense Throat Tight jaws and tense throat muscles restrict the breath. One way of relaxing the jaw and throat muscles is to keep the base of the tongue back in the throat. As this occurs the, top and lower teeth will separate, releasing jaw and throat tension.

Unless you are talking, the thick part of the tongue should be kept back in the throat throughout the day. By keeping the tongue back, you will better be able to control the degree to which the throat passage opens. Keeping the base of the tongue back is a trick that allows you to control the amount of air moving through the throat so that the inhale and exhale each will have a steady inflow and outflow of air from the beginning to the end. You should be able to hear the steady, continuous sound of the air moving through the back of the throat while you are breathing.

Summary of Yoga Breathing

Let us now summarize the main points of yogic breathing. The main focus of the complete yoga breath should be upon the exhale. Think of the exhale as a continual rising of the diaphragm. The higher the diaphragm rises, the more air is pushed out. Conceive of the complete yogic exhale as being mainly controlled by the muscles closest to the diaphragm—the abdominal muscles to begin the exhale, the lower intercostal muscles in the second phase of the exhale, and both the abdominal and intercostal muscles to complete the exhale.

The inhale, like the exhale, should be slow, deep, rhythmic, and thorough. The inhalation should fill the lungs from the bottom to the top, and the diaphragm should continue to move down throughout the entirety of the inhale. The abdominal muscles should round out only for the first third of the inhalation and should gradually flatten back for the last two-thirds. To fill the lungs fully, the shoulders should be drawn back and down through the work of the upper-back muscles. The lungs should expand three-dimensionally as the air is drawn in.

Retention of the in-breath is not recommended for day-in and day-out breathing. The in-breath can be retained on special occasions to help give psychological and physiological relief from anxiety or during special pranayama breathing. The breath should not be held in for long periods of time unless you have been trained by a pranayana teacher. If you are extremely tense, you may wish to hold an occasional in-breath for up to three seconds and then slowly release the air in a very conscious way.

Rhythmic Breathing

According to the yoga masters, practice of proper breathing is the most important physiological aspect of life. Since most of us have unconsciously fallen into bad breathing habits, we need to consciously focus on the process of breathing periodically throughout the day.

We should try to make the breath as rhythmic as ocean waves. With the base of the tongue back in the throat, the breath will actually begin to sound like ocean waves. Consider how a wave begins far out at sea, builds up slowly, curls, crashes, and washes its way up the shoreline; and then how the water is pulled back to sea. Each wave is a complete process from beginning to end.

Just as each wave must crest and crash and sweep its way up the beach, so the exhale must take place. We must release the stale air; otherwise, there will be a dangerous buildup of toxins within the body. Consider the power that a breaking ocean wave carries and the manner in which the water sweeps its way up the shoreline. Liken this to the carbon-dioxide-laden air that must be expelled from the lungs and be carried out of the nose and into the atmosphere.

The diaphragmatic action of the inhalation can be likened to the undercurrent that pulls the wave water back out to sea. The air that slowly fills the lungs can be compared to the buildup of a new wave, one that begins far out at sea and slowly moves in toward the shoreline. On the inhale we are building our supply of oxygen as we slowly increase the size of our lungs, somewhat like a wave that builds in size.

To help calm our mind during a particularly stressful situation, it may be helpful to retain the breath for a short while after the inhalation. The retention aspect of the breath can be compared to a wave that is on the verge of breaking into white water. The breath can be held for only a few seconds comfortably before the air must be expelled. Similarly, each wave builds up to the point where it simply must crest and crash to fulfill its purpose, but the moment just before it comes down can be a transcending moment.

Whenever we get out of harmony, we

must go back to the breath. Through deep, slow, rhythmic breathing, we can move toward a more peaceful state of mind. Attuning to the breath is the most reliable means of getting back into harmony with our innermost self. Whatever activity we are engaged in, we should feel the breath rhythmically moving in and out of the lungs, just like the constant ebb and flow of the ocean waves.

You should allow the balloon-like lungs to expand and contract fully within the rib cage. Once you have carefully trained the breathing muscles how to work in the complete yoga breath, deep, slow, thorough, rhythmic breathing becomes a very natural process. Notice in Figure 3.24 the incredible amount of space the lungs have to expand and contract within the rib cage. Pay attention to the breath at periodic times throughout the day and you will feel clearer and calmer.

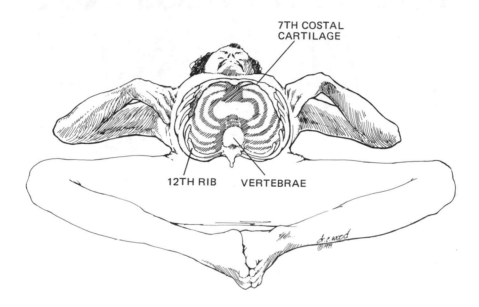

7TH COSTAL CARTILAGE

12TH RIB   VERTEBRAE

FIGURE 3.24

III

YOGA FOR BEGINNERS

Part III comprises a single chapter, which has been specifically designed for the beginner of yoga and yet will be very helpful to even the intermediate or advanced student. The postures given in Chapter 4 lay a solid foundation for the practice of Hatha Yoga. The basic postures introduced here will move the beginner toward a deeper understanding of the other yoga asanas discussed throughout the book. The main focus here is to show and describe asanas that bring flexibility to the spinal column and loosen the shoulder and hip-joint areas. Until the spine, back, shoulder, and hip areas of the body loosen, you will be limited not only in the yoga postures but also in daily life.

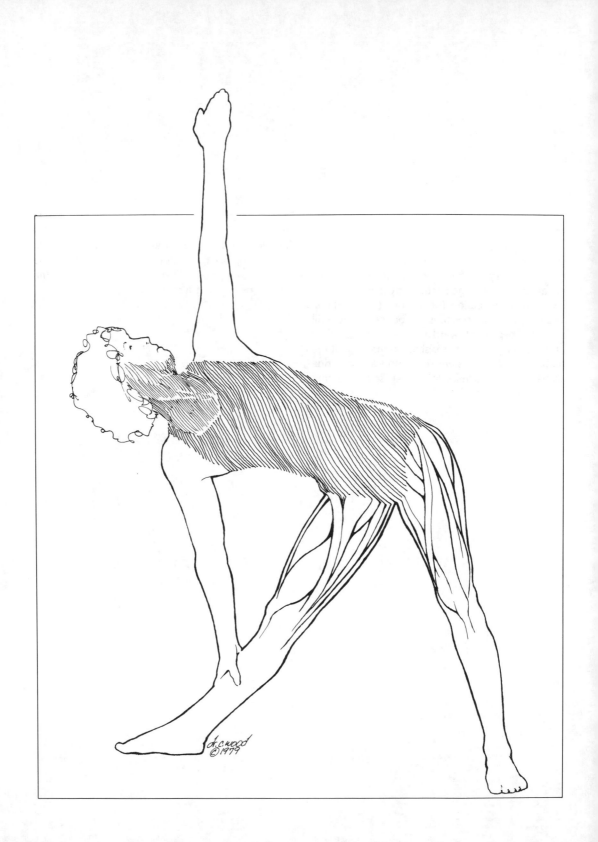

FOUR
yoga for beginners
co-written by Linda Boudreau

INTRODUCTION

How does one begin the practice of yoga? One begins by learning a few of the yoga postures well. It is important to start each practice session with postures that slowly loosen the muscles and joints, progress to postures that build strength and endurance, and end with those that calm the mind. Six sample routines are given near the end of this chapter. These routines have been designed with specific effects in mind. We recommend that you work through all the postures of this chapter by attempting to perform the routines one by one in a very thorough and conscious way.

There is no doubt that yoga practice is a difficult undertaking for the beginning student. Bringing about a change in body structure, breathing patterns, and thought patterns requires a persevering attitude and an open mind. The initial stages of yoga practice can be discouraging unless you look at the fact that it took years for the body, breath, and mind to reach their present condition and realize that it may take years to undo what has been done. It may help you develop the quality of patience if you recognize that yoga practice is not a competitive endeavor.

One thing that helps kindle enthusiasm is the positive transformation that begins with the very first yoga posture you perform. This positive transformation will continue as long as you remain dedicated to the practice of yoga.

Practice the yoga postures for fifteen minutes to one hour a day to begin with. A more vigorous set of asanas should be chosen for morning yoga practice than for the evening when a more calming, relaxing set should be chosen. Of course, as pointed out in Chapter 3, you should not limit the practice of yoga postures to a short period during the day and then forget about it the rest of the day. Stretching, backward arching, twisting, and loosening actions should be done periodically throughout the day.

Good body alignment is basic to good health, and the way to achieve it is through elongation of the spine. The prayer pose, dog stretch, triangle, warrior, lateral stretch, forward stretches, dancers' pose, twisting postures, and corpse pose shown in this chapter help to improve body alignment.

The cat–cow stretch, floor twists, sitting twists, shoulder looseners, standing rotations, sun salutation, bridge, bow, crow, shoulder-stand preparations, and slow-motion firming postures shown in this chapter help to bring flexibility to the body. These postures should be performed in a flowing, dancelike fashion. Moving into and out of these postures builds strength, stamina, endurance, flexibility, concentration, and rhythmic awareness. The rhythmic flow of the body naturally moves toward a recognition of the spirit within.

While working through the postures of this chapter, feel the stretching, feel the stimulation, feel the release of energy within, and feel the relaxation of the body. While you are doing the postures, the breath must become a part of the flow of each movement. You will notice that the inhale can give you energy to work in the postures, and that the exhale can be used to release tension so that the body can go more deeply into the pose.

Proper breathing is of great importance —indeed, it is the very key to life. We can live without food for a time, but we cannot live without breath. As it is the key to our physical existence, so too it is the key to our mental existence. By learning to breathe slowly, rhythmically, and deeply, we can experience a positive mental outlook and emotional stability.

Hatha Yoga revitalizes, reenergizes, and restores youthfulness. In the end the practice of yoga creates a harmonious flow between body, mind, and spirit. Let us now look into the individual postures that can help bring about the balance we all desire. Notice that all the main groups of postures are included in this chapter, including forward stretches, backbends, twists, standing postures, inverted preparations, and meditational postures.

HATHA YOGA POSTURES

Cat–Cow Flexibility of the spine is one of the keys to a long, healthy life. A stiff spinal

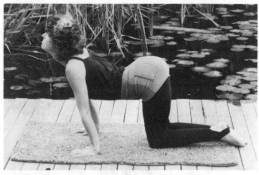

FIGURE 4.1A

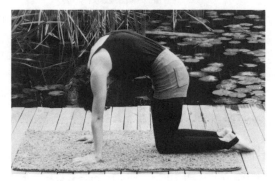

FIGURE 4.1B

column, caused by lack of movement and tightened muscles, not only will cause backaches but will hamper you in your daily activities. In time the shock absorbers of the spine become less efficient as the spine stiffens. For bringing flexibility to the spine and stimulating the spinal fluid, the continuous wavelike spinal movement of cat–cow has no equal.

Cat–cow releases excess tension in the digestive tract, so that the food breakdown can occur more efficiently. It stimulates the digestive system to release necessary hormones for further food digestion, aids the eliminative system, and greatly increases the efficiency of the nervous system.

Starting on all fours with the hands underneath the shoulders and the knees underneath the hips, inhale, drop the stomach, and let the back sway. Look up, expand the chest, and draw the shoulders down and back (Figure 4.1A). Now exhale, tuck under with the

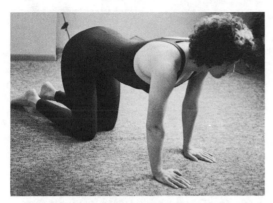

FIGURE 4.2A

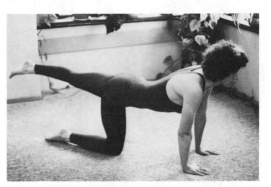

FIGURE 4.2C

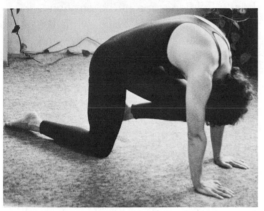

FIGURE 4.2B

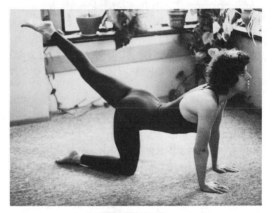

FIGURE 4.2D

pelvis, lift the abdominal muscles, arch the upper back, and bring the chin to the chest (Figure 4.1B). Go back and forth between these two poses three to ten times, rest, and repeat again.

Cat Stretch Cat stretch is done in a dance-like manner, flowing from one motion to another in rhythmic harmony with the breath. It brings flexibility to the spine, firms the buttocks and hamstring muscles, stretches the front side of the body, improves circulation, and stimulates the nerves along the spinal column.

Place the hands directly under the shoulders and the knees directly under the hips (Figure 4.2A). Pull the shoulders away from the ears. Inhale.

Exhale, draw the left knee to the forehead, contract the abdominal muscles, and arch the upper back (Figure 4.2B).

Inhale, stretch the left leg back, and feel an extension through the entire body (Figure 4.2C).

Keep the hips level as you lift the left leg and look up, still working for length through the body (Figure 4.2D).

Exhale, return to Figure 4.2A, repeat to the other side, and then repeat the whole series twice more.

Pose of the Child This very restful pose helps to relieve aches in the lower back by stretching the muscles along the spine. It allows the internal organs to relax and calms the nervous system.

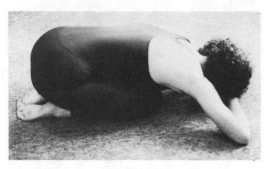

FIGURE 4.3

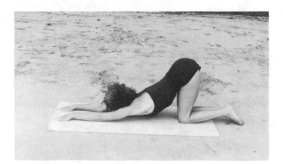

FIGURE 4.4

Begin by sitting on the heels in an upright position. Lean forward, lengthen the abdomen over the thighs, bring one hand on top of the other, and rest the forehead on the top hand (Figure 4.3). Breathe deeply and relax every muscle of the body. Hold for 20 seconds to one minute.

Bent-Knee Shoulder-Loosener This pose loosens the shoulder-joint, upper-back, and chest areas as it stretches the arm, shoulder, and back muscles. The position of the abdominal area while in this pose relaxes the internal organs so as to relieve digestive and eliminative problems and menstrual cramps.

From the pose of the child (Figure 4.3), stretch the arms straight out, bring the bottom off the heels, and slide the hands forward along the floor. Stop when the hips are directly over the knees. Extend through the spine, shoulders, and arms as you drop the chest toward the floor (Figure 4.4). An alternative is to fold the hands into the elbows, keeping the forearms above the head, and stretch through the elbows as you drop the chest toward the floor. This posture can be done at any time throughout your yoga practice.

Floor Twists Floor twists help to relieve lower-back aches, bring flexibility to the spine, stretch the abdominal muscles, and stimulate proper action of the digestive and eliminative systems. Perform the series shown here in a slowmotion, dancelike manner, briefly holding some of the positions.

Lying on the back with the arms stretched straight out to the sides and palms down, inhale, bend the knees, and bring them to the chest, lengthening the back of the neck. Exhale, bring the knees to the floor on the right side, and look toward the left hand with the feet off the floor (Figure 4.5A). Pull back and down with the left side of the rib cage and shoulder. Inhale, bring the knees to the chest, exhale, and repeat to the other side. Repeat both sides once again.

With both knees to the chest, straighten the right leg, and stretch through the heel. Place the left foot on the right knee or thigh (Figure 4.5B). Inhale.

Exhale, place the right hand to the outside of the left knee, and bring the knee toward the floor on the right side. As you bring the knee toward the floor, pull back and down toward the floor with the left side of the rib cage and left shoulder. Lengthen through both waistlines, and look to the left hand (Figure 4.5C). Work in the pose for ten to 20 seconds, breathing slowly and deeply. Repeat to the other side.

Raise the right leg to a 90-degree angle, stretch through the heels of the feet, draw the shoulders down, lengthen the back of the neck, and stretch the arms out to the sides (Figure 4.5D). Inhale.

Exhale, slowly bring the right foot to the floor on the left side of the body, lengthen

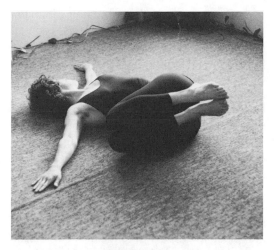

FIGURE 4.5A

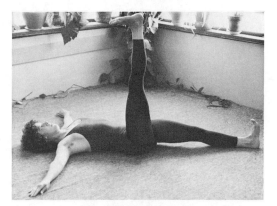

FIGURE 4.5D

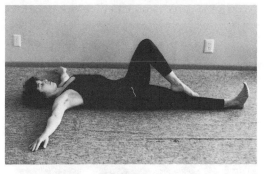

FIGURE 4.5B

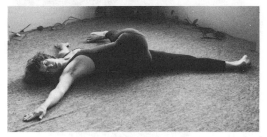

FIGURE 4.5E

FIGURE 4.5F

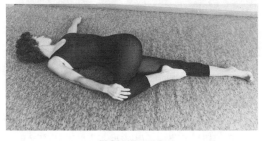

FIGURE 4.5C

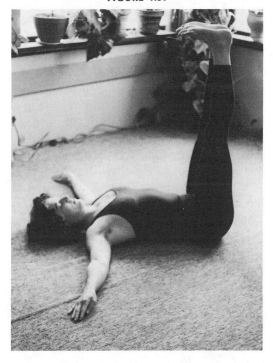

through both waistlines, and pull back and down with the right rib cage and right shoulder. Look to the right (Figure 4.5E). Hold for a few seconds, inhale, return to the position shown in Fig. 4.5-D, and repeat to the other side.

Inhale, bring both legs straight up, and stretch through the heels (Figure 4.5F).

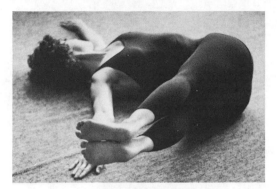

FIGURE 4.5G

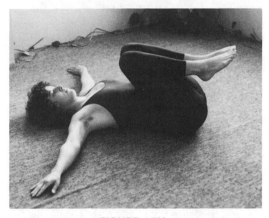

FIGURE 4.5H

Deep, slow, rhythmic breathing is an important element of the sitting twists. Each inhale should bring about a lift and expansion of the chest, and each exhale a rotation of the rib cage. Before the trunk can rotate freely, the spinal column must be elongated. To attain a lift through the trunk of the body, imagine a rope is attached to the center of your head, lifting you upward. As you lift through the rib cage, spine and chest, let the shoulders drop down.

To do the twist shown in Figure 4.6A, begin in a seated position, both legs extended straight out on the floor. Bend the right knee, and place the right foot to the inside of the left knee. Lift upwards through the spinal column (imagine a rope is attached to the center of

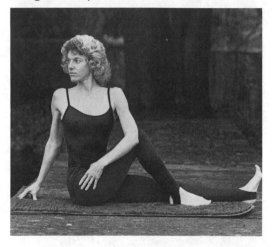

FIGURE 4.6A

Exhale, slowly lower the legs to the right side, pull back and down with the left rib cage and left shoulder, and look to the left hand, keeping the feet and right thigh off the floor (Figure 4.5G). Work for a few seconds, breathing deeply. Exhale, bend the knees, and then bring them to the chest.

Breath deeply for a few seconds with the knees to the chest, (Figure 4.5H), then inhale and straighten the legs up (Figure 4.5F). Repeat the lowering of the legs to the other side, and repeat to both sides once again.

Sitting Twists Benefits of doing the sitting twists include relief of muscular backaches, stimulation of the internal organs, increased flexibility of the spinal column, and increased lung capacity.

your head, lifting you up), twist to the right, and place the right fingertips on the floor behind the back. Bring the left arm to the outside of the right leg as shown in Figure 4.6A. (If this arm position is difficult for you, use your left hand against the knee for leverage.) Keep the abdomen drawn in, take a deep inhale, expand the chest, lift through the top of the head, then exhale and twist the rib cage further to the right. Keep the right elbow slightly bent, drop the right shoulder, look to the right, and continue lifting with each inhale and twisting with each exhale. Work in the pose for ten to 20 seconds and repeat to the other side.

To do the twist shown in 4.6B, begin in a seated position with both knees bent, feet approximately 24 inches from the hips and also 24 inches apart from each other. Drop both knees to the right onto the floor, twist the torso toward the right, placing the right hand onto the floor about 18 inches from the right hip and the left hand to the outside of the right knee, as shown in Figure 4.6B. Lift the chest, drop the shoulders, lean out over the right hand, and twist toward the right. Pull the lower ribs and chest out, breathe softly, and continue to twist for ten to 20 seconds. (You can vary the angle of the torso by bending both elbows and dropping the chest toward the floor, maintaining extension through the spine and rotation of the ribs.) Repeat to the other side.

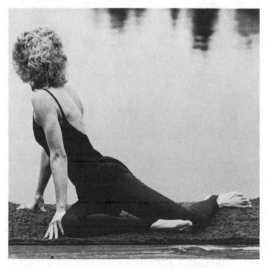

FIGURE 4.6B

Shoulder-Looseners An excellent way to loosen the upper back, shoulders, arms, and chest before moving onto the more difficult yoga postures is to stretch the arms back and forth with the use of a strap. For those who have problems associated with tight shoulder-joint areas, such as bursitis, these

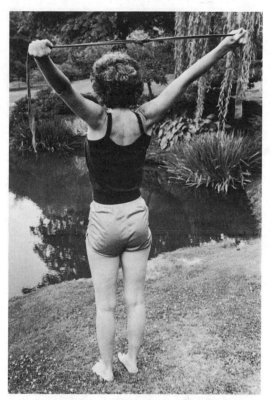

FIGURE 4.7A

shoulder-looseners provide an effective means of lessening and alleviating the problem. Use a strap that is at least as long as the span of the arms.

Begin with the hands stretched out to the sides above the head and the strap stretched tautly. Drop the shoulders and draw the shoulder blades in toward the spine. Tuck the pelvis and pull the navel in, as shown in Figure 4.7A.

Pull the left arm down, stretch up through the right arm, and pull it back (Figure 4.7B). Release, stretch the left arm straight up, and pull the right arm down. Go back and forth between these two positions several times. Then return to the position shown in Figure 4.7A.

To bring both hands down slowly with a taut strap, you may need to shorten the distance between the hands on the strap.

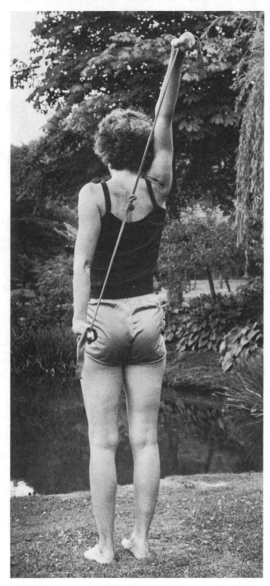

FIGURE 4.7B

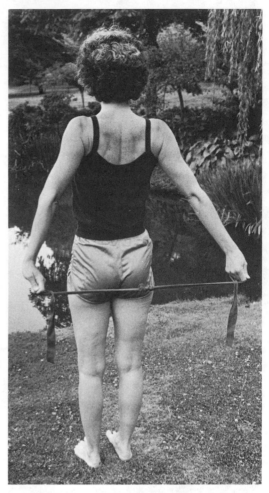

FIGURE 4.7C

From the position shown in Figure 4.7A, slowly lower the arms behind the back, contracting the shoulder-blade muscles, tucking the pelvis, and lifting the chest (Figure 4.7C). Go back and forth between these two positions several times. Then return to Figure 4.7A and repeat the entire series of shoulder looseners once again.

Forward Bar Stretch This can be used either as a preparatory yoga posture or as a tension-relieving stretch at various times during the day. It can be done using a counter or tabletop as well as a bar. It helps to loosen the shoulder joints and opens the chest for deeper breathing. It can be held for long or short periods.

Position the body so that the feet are placed underneath the hips, the wrists rest on whatever surface is being used, and the arms and spine stretch to their utmost (Figure 4.8). Lift through the back of the legs, tilt the pelvis upward, pull back and away from the hands

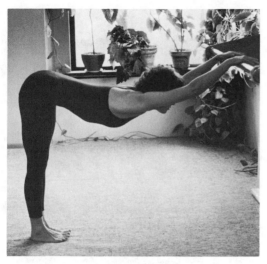

FIGURE 4.8

with the bottom, relax the shoulders, and let the chest drop. Breathe deeply and work in the pose for ten seconds to one minute.

Downward-Facing Dog Stretch In the dog stretch blood pours into the brain, the shoulder joint is opened, and the chest expands, allowing a deeper, fuller breath. The whole backside of the body is stretched in this posture, thus increasing the blood circulation throughout the body. This posture can be held for ten seconds to one minute.

FIGURE 4.9

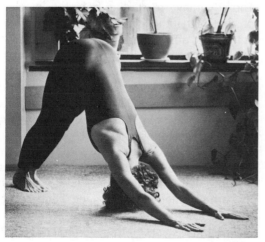

The key to doing the downward-facing dog stretch (Figure 4.9) is to lift the buttocks high into the air, as this brings about a deep fold between the thighs and abdomen. In the beginning of the pose, a deeper fold can be attained by lifting the heels as high as possible.

Dog Stretch—from Standing Position

The advantage to starting from the standing rather than the kneeling position is that walking down the wall works more strongly on opening the shoulder joint.

Place the feet about one foot from the wall, extend the arms up, place the hands on the wall and the buttocks over the feet (Figure 4.10A). Walk the fingers up the wall, breathe deeply and slowly, and let the chest move toward the wall. Use the exhale to let go of tightness.

FIGURE 4.10A

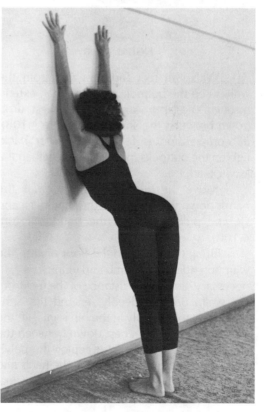

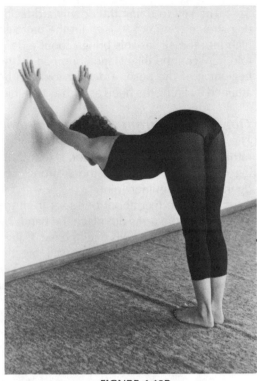

FIGURE 4.10B

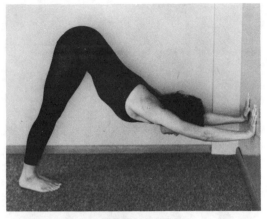

FIGURE 4.10C

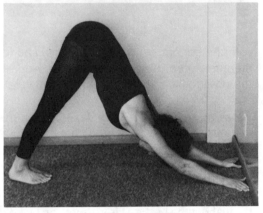

FIGURE 4.10D

Walk the feet further away from the wall. Keep the buttocks over the feet, extend through the arms, and let the chest drop down between the shoulders (Figure 4.10B). (If compression is felt in the lower back, tighten the buttocks muscles and lengthen the lower back.)

Move the feet back further, walk the hands down the wall, relax the shoulders, and lift and pull back with the bottom (Figure 4.10C).

Bring the hands to the floor next to the wall, spreading the thumb and index finger. (If necessary, adjust the distance of the feet from the wall.) Breathe deeply, extend the arms and trunk, fold deeply at the hip joints, lift the heels, and drop the chest down between the shoulders (Figure 4.10D). Keeping the pelvis tilted up, stretch down through the heels and try to bring them to the floor. Work in the final pose for ten to 20 seconds.

Dog Stretch—from Kneeling Position
The advantage to starting from the kneeling position is that the lift of the buttocks, the fold at the hips, and the stretch of the lower spine can occur more naturally here than from the standing position.

Place the knees under the hips and hands on the floor in line with the shoulders. Spread the thumbs and index fingers apart and place them against the wall (Figure 4.11A).

Let the lower back sway, hook the toes under, pull the shoulders back, and straighten the arms (inner elbows facing each other, outer elbows facing out) (Figure 4.11B).

Lift the knees off the floor and move the

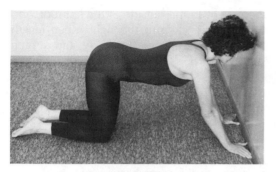

FIGURE 4.11A

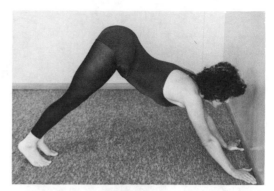

FIGURE 4.11C

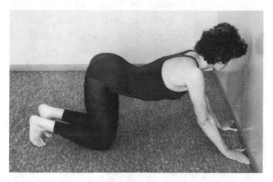

FIGURE 4.11B

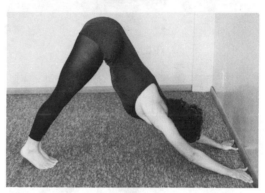

FIGURE 4.11D

buttocks upward. Extend through the arms and back, bring the weight toward the heels, and fold deeply at the hips. Look toward the wall (Figure 4.11C).

Drop the chest down between the shoulder joints, move the shoulder blades in toward each other. Let the head hang, stretch throughout the entire backside of the body, and breathe slowly and deeply (Figure 4.11D). Work in the final pose for ten to 30 seconds.

Modified Dog The benefits of the modified dog are similar to those of the downward-facing dog. With the feet spread apart, however, it is easier to tilt the pelvis upward and thus to flatten the back. The modified dog also loosens the hip socket, stretches the inner thigh muscles, and develops the arches of the feet.

Bring the feet three to four feet apart with the heels one to two inches away from the wall and the feet parallel to each other. Bring the hands around three feet in front of the hips, roll to the outer edges of the feet while keeping the base of the big toes on the floor, lift the kneecaps, lift the buttocks up the wall, and fold deeply at the hips. Stretch through the arms and let the chest drop toward the floor (Figure 4.12). Blood will freely flow down toward the head, stimulating the brain and the pituitary gland. Breathe deeply and work in the pose for ten to 30 seconds.

Hip-Loosener The hip-looseners are excellent movements for bringing flexibility to the hip sockets and pelvic and lower back areas. They stretch the outer and inner thigh muscles, develop the arches of the feet, loosen the shoulders, stretch the arms, and free the rib-cage area of tension.

Place the feet three to four feet apart

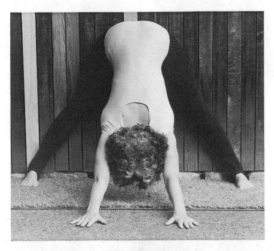

FIGURE 4.12

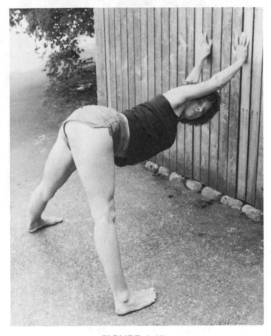

FIGURE 4.13

the weight to the outside of the left foot, and twist the rib cage to the right. Keep length through the trunk of the body and stretch strongly through both arms. Repeat to the other side. Shift back and forth between the two sides a number of times, pausing for a short while at each end of the swing, exhaling to each side, and inhaling to the center.

Standing Rotation The standing rotation posture has the same basic effects as the hip loosener just shown, with the added benefit of increased loosening of the waist, lower-back, rib-cage, upper-back, and chest areas of the body. It also helps one develop awareness of the muscles between the shoulder blades.

Begin with the feet around three feet apart and parallel, with the weight to the out-

FIGURE 4.14

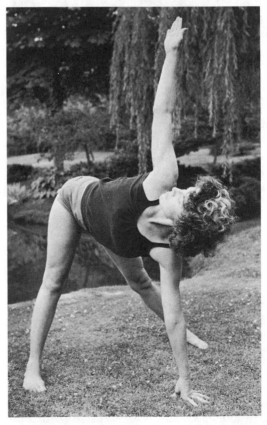

and the hips above the line of the feet. Place the hands against a wall (or hang them over a bar or tabletop). Roll to the outer edges of the feet, tilt the pelvis upward, and stretch through the arms and the spine. As shown in Figure 4.13, shift the weight to the right, lift the right hip, pull back with the left hip, keep side of the feet and the knees lifted. Keeping the hips above the line of the feet, fold forward at the hips, and bring the fingertips of the left hand to the floor about two feet in front of the toes, centered between the feet. Shift the weight to the right, lift the right hip, pull the left hip back, roll to the outside of the left foot, stretch straight out with the spine, keep the head above the left hand, and stretch vertically up with the right arm. Pull both shoulder blades in toward the spine, lengthen the back of the neck, and look up to the right hand as you twist further. Work in the pose (Figure 4.14) for a few seconds and repeat to the other side. Do each side twice. Exhale as you twist to each side and inhale back to the center.

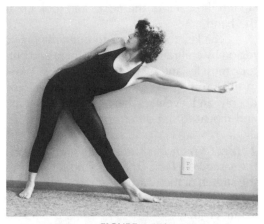

FIGURE 4.15A

Triangle Triangle builds strength and stamina, tones and firms the legs and buttocks muscles, opens the pelvic region, and stretches the inner thighs and waistline. Bringing the back and hips against a wall can be a helpful way to learn the pose.

Place the feet about 40 inches apart. To achieve good alignment, turn the left foot out 90 degrees, placing the heel of the left foot in a straight line with the arch of the right foot, and turn the right foot slightly in toward the left. Roll the weight to the outside of the right foot and turn the knee clockwise until it faces forward, turn the left knee counterclockwise and face the center of the knee over the third toe; contract the buttocks and outer thigh muscles to do this (Figure 4.15A).

There must be a folding in at the left hip joint as the trunk lengthens laterally. The right hip shifts to the right as the left hip folds in deeply. The kneecaps should lift by contraction of the thigh muscles. Stretch the left arm out; imagine that someone has taken hold of your hand and is pulling it in an attempt to lengthen the trunk of your body.

Figure 4.15B shows the final triangle pose, done to the opposite side from that de-

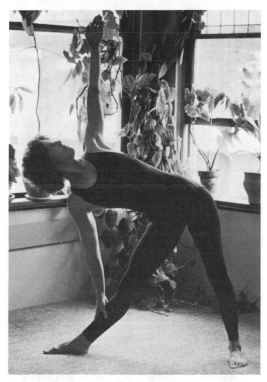

FIGURE 4.15B

scribed in Figure 4.15A. Linda has brought the bottom hand to the front shin and stretched the top arm vertically up. While in the triangle position, extend the arms from the shoulders, pull the top shoulder away from the ear, draw the top shoulder blade in toward the spine, stretch the back of the neck, and look up at the hand.

The key to triangle is to open the pelvic region by contracting the outer-thigh and buttock muscles and by tucking the pelvis. Work in this position 20 to 30 seconds, breathing deeply and evenly. Then inhale, come up, and repeat to the other side.

Lateral Stretch The lateral stretch offers the same benefits as triangle, and it increases the stretch of the waistline and rotation of the rib cage. It is a good pose for loosening the shoulder joints.

Place the feet the same as described for triangle. Lift the kneecaps and direct them out over the third toe. Squeeze the buttocks muscles, extend the torso laterally, and bring the left hand to a bar or countertop and the right hand behind the back to the inner left thigh (Figure 4.16). Extend through the spine and rotate the chest toward the ceiling. Basically, the work is the same as in triangle. Work in the pose for ten to 20 seconds, breathing deeply and evenly. Release and repeat the same movements to the other side.

FIGURE 4.16

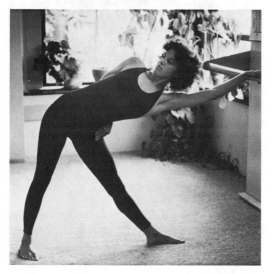

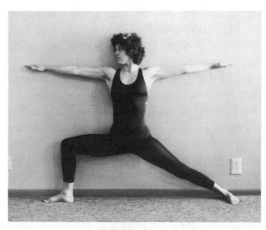

FIGURE 4.17

Warrior The warrior pose builds strength, stamina, and endurance. It tones and firms the legs and buttocks muscles, loosens the hip joints, frees the pelvic-girdle region, lengthens the spine, and tones the abdominal, upper-back, and arm muscles.

Place the feet four to five feet apart with the heel of the left foot touching the wall and the outside of the right foot about two inches from the wall and parallel to it. Bend the right knee and direct it over the third toe. Ideally, the knee should be bent to a 90-degree angle (Figure 4.17). Roll the weight to the outer edge of the left foot, keep the left knee turned out, lift the left inner thigh, and tuck the pelvis strongly under. Draw in and up with the navel, contract the abdominal and buttocks muscles, and extend out through the arms. Drop the shoulders down and back by pulling the shoulder blades in toward the spine, and extend through the back of the neck as you look to the right hand. Inhale slowly and deeply; concentrate on lengthening through the spine and extending out through the legs, arms, and neck. Exhale slowly and deeply, using the exhale to release any muscles that should relax. Work in this pose for 20 to 30 seconds and repeat to the other side.

Extended Warrior The extended warrior has the same benefits as of warrior and also stretches the lateral side of the body and helps to loosen the muscles of the rib-cage area.

From warrior position, extend the trunk out over the right thigh, drop the right elbow to the knee, and stretch the left arm over the head with the palm facing down. Press the elbow against the inner knee, twist through the trunk of the body, and try to bring the left shoulder to the wall (Figure 4.18). Draw the left shoulder blade in toward the spine, rotate the chest toward the ceiling, extend the neck, and elongate through the entire left side of the body on an inhale. Exhale, contract the buttocks muscles, tuck the pelvis under, and open the hips. Work for 20 to 30 seconds and repeat to the other side.

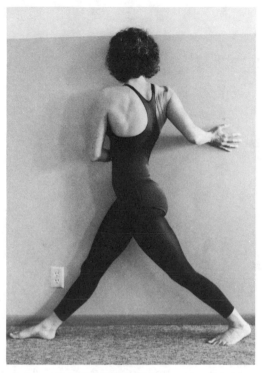

FIGURE 4.19A

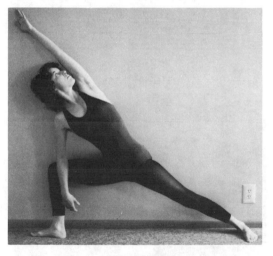

FIGURE 4.18

Standing Twist The standing twist tones the leg, buttocks, abdominal, and upper-back muscles; frees the rib cage for rotational movement and a deeper, fuller breath; and relieves tension throughout the back.

Stand up straight with the back to the wall and the feet three to six inches from the wall and four feet apart. Turn the feet toward the right and twist the torso toward the wall. Draw in the navel, tuck the pelvis, and lift through the spine as the hands are brought to the wall (Figure 4.19A). Keep the left hip square with the right hip.

Bend the right knee, lift the left kneecap, and drive the left hip down toward the floor, keeping the hips level to each other. The left heel should come off the floor, but continue to stretch firmly through the back of the left ankle. Bring the right knee toward a 90-degree angle, contract the left buttock in order to tuck the pelvis, and rotate the rib cage around to the right with the aid of a strong contraction of the right shoulder-blade muscles. Drop both shoulders, lengthen the back of the neck, and look over the right shoulder, as shown in Figure 4.19B. Work in the pose for ten to 20 seconds and repeat to the other side.

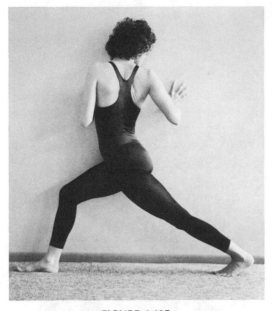

FIGURE 4.19B

Sun Salutation (Shortened Version)

The sun salutation is based on the movements of the cat–cow; it is a series of counterbalancing movements from arching backward to stretching forward. The sun salutation is performed in a dancelike manner that brings harmony to the body, mind, and spirit. It brings flexibility to the spine, stretches the front and backside of the body, loosens all the main joints, and stimulates the internal body.

Standing straight, place the hands in a prayer position at the chest, and breathe slowly and deeply (Figure 4.20A).

Inhale, raise the arms with the thumbs clasped, pull the shoulders down away from the ears, and stretch straight up through the entire body (Figure 4.20B). Squeeze the shoulder blades toward the spine, contract the buttocks muscles, pull the hands back, and arch slightly backward.

Exhale, bend forward, folding at the hip joints, and place the hands next to the feet (Figure 4.20C). (If the hamstrings are too tight to do this, bend the knees.)

Bring the left foot about four feet behind

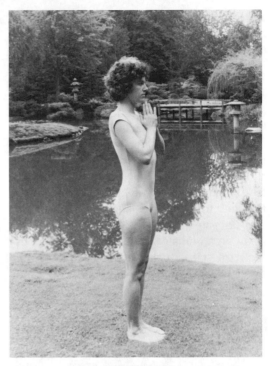

FIGURE 4.20A
FIGURE 4.20B

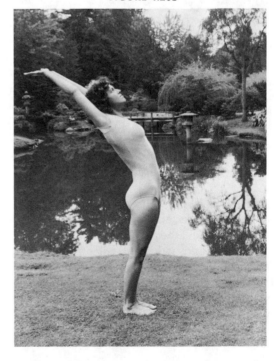

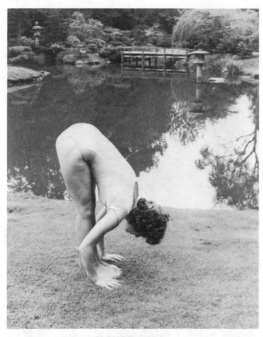

FIGURE 4.20C

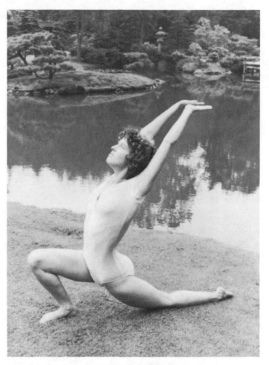

FIGURE 4.20E

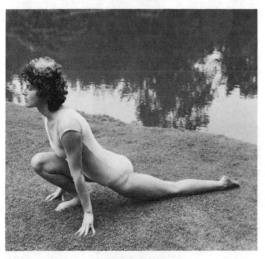

FIGURE 4.20D

you with the knee to the floor, and drop down with the hips, as you stretch the spine (Figure 4.20D).

Inhale, reach the arms up, drop the shoulders, and pull the shoulder blades in toward the spine. Draw in the navel, contract the left buttock muscles, and drive the hips down, as you look up to the ceiling (Figure 4.20E).

Exhale, bring the hands to the floor in line with the right foot shoulder-width apart, as in Figure 4.20D. Inhale, hook the left toes under, and bring the right foot back alongside the left foot. Push the weight back toward the feet and extend through the arms and trunk. Lift the hips high and fold deeply at the hips. Drop the chest down toward the floor (Figure 4.20F).

Exhale, bring the left foot between the hands, and bring the right knee to the floor. Inhale, stretch up through the arms, pull the shoulder blades in toward the spine, drop the shoulders down from the ears, and look up (Figure 4.20G). Draw in the navel, contract the right buttock muscles, and drive the hips down. Exhale and bring the hands to the floor in line with the left foot about shoulder-width apart.

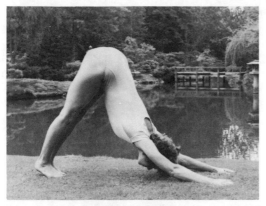

FIGURE 4.20F

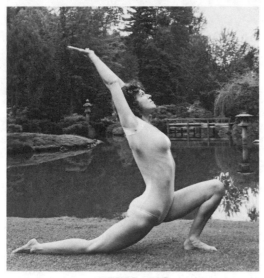

FIGURE 4.20G

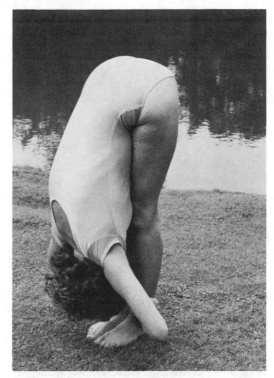

FIGURE 4.20H

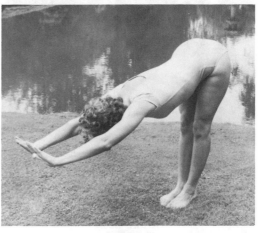

FIGURE 4.20-I

Inhale and bring the right foot up to the left. Exhale deeply, lengthen the spine, and flatten the back. Stretch the abdomen out over the thighs, take hold of the back of the calves at the ankles, and pull the chest toward the legs (Figure 4.20H).

Release the hands from the legs and stretch the arms out, flattening the back (Figure 4.20-I). Inhale to a standing position, keeping the legs straight and the kneecaps lifting.

Exhale, bring the hands to prayer position, close the eyes, breathe deeply, and go within (Figure 4.20J). Feel a string attached to the top of the head lifting you upward. Relax the shoulders, jaw, and forehead, expand the chest, and lengthen the lower back. Feel the flow between the body, breath, and mind. Remain in this pose five to ten seconds and then repeat the sun salutation once more.

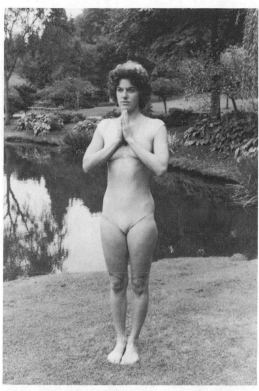

FIGURE 4.20J

Dancer's Pose The dancer's pose improves internal balance, strengthens and stretches the leg muscles, and opens the chest for deeper breathing.

Standing straight, focus the eyes on an object straight ahead. Take hold of the right foot with the right hand. Tuck the pelvic girdle under, draw the shoulder blades in toward each other, try to feel a lengthening through the spinal column, and stretch the left arm up (Figure 4.21A).

The front thigh muscle of the standing leg should contract and lift. Squeeze the right buttock, pull the navel in, and lengthen the lower back. The hips and chest should both face squarely forward. Stretch through the trunk and begin to lean forward (Figure 4.21B).

Continue to lean forward. Keep the eyes focused straight ahead, pull back with the right foot, and keep the chest facing forward (Figure 4.21C). Breathe steadily and deeply. Work for ten to 15 seconds. (The upward-stretching hand can be placed on a wall to help keep your balance.)

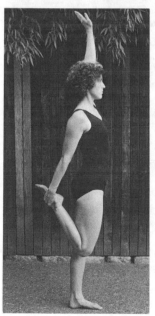

FIGURE 4.21A

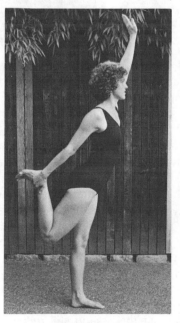

FIGURE 4.21B

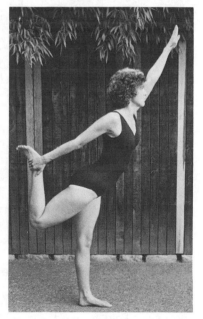

FIGURE 4.21C

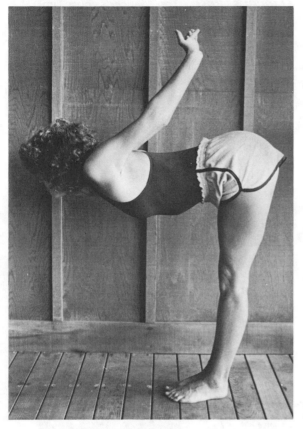

FIGURE 4.22A

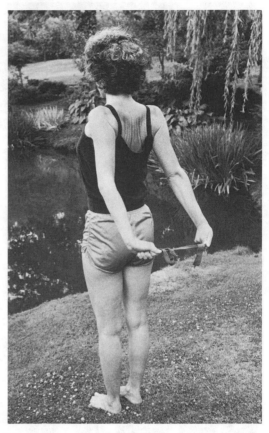

FIGURE 4.22B

Forward Stretches Benefits to be gained from doing forward stretches include (1) increased blood flow through the arms, legs, and back, (2) elongation of the spine and hamstring muscles, so the nerve energy can flow without hindrance, (3) relaxation and calming of the mind, and (4) improved digestion.

Standing Stand straight, interweave the fingers behind the back, turn the palms toward the buttocks, and stretch the arms and open the chest by pulling down through the straightened arms. (An alternative is to make a fist with one hand, embrace it with the other, and then pull the hands down toward the floor.) Fold forward at the hips, lift the kneecaps, and stretch out through the spine

by extending forward with the chest. Lift up through the back of the legs, tilt the pelvis upward, lift the hands, and stretch through the arms (Figure 4.22A). Work for ten to 20 seconds.

A second alternative arm position for the posture shown in Figure 4.22A involves the use of a strap. Clasp the hands onto the strap one inch to one foot apart, rotate the shoulder joint back and down, and turn the inner elbow and inner wrist outward (Figure 4.22B). Fold forward as described in Figure 4.22A.

Figure 4.22C shows an excellent way to slowly stretch the hamstring, buttocks, and back muscles. It is one that you can relax into and still receive many benefits. Exhale, fold forward, clasp the hands onto the elbows,

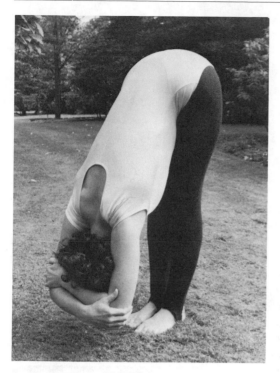

FIGURE 4.22C

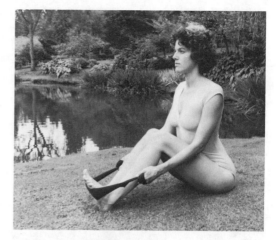

FIGURE 4.23A

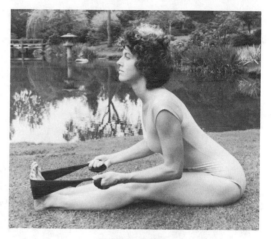

FIGURE 4.23B

and stretch the arms out behind the head. Extend through the legs and torso, then breathe deeply and relax. Let go into the pose for ten seconds to one minute.

Sitting   With the use of a strap around the bottom of the feet, bend the knees, expand the chest, pull the shoulders back and down, elongate through the spine, and slowly straighten the legs (Figure 4.23A). Adjust the distance of the strap in order to maintain a straight spine.

This is a very effective way for a person with tight hamstring muscles to work toward proper body alignment in a sitting forward stretch.

To stretch the hamstring muscles fully, bring the back of the knees to the floor and stretch through the heels of the feet. Using the same action through the upper body as discussed in Figure 4.23A, lift the chest and move it toward the feet (Figure 4.23B). Work

in the pose for ten seconds to one minute. Breathe deeply; use the exhale to stretch further forward, and the inhale to expand the chest.

Slow-Motion Firming   The flowing motion of this series of movements strengthens and tones the abdominal and thigh muscles; stretches the calf, hamstring, buttocks, and back muscles; increases circulation throughout the body; and moves the breath, body, and mind into a harmonious flow.

Sitting straight, place both hands behind the buttocks with the legs outstretched, push

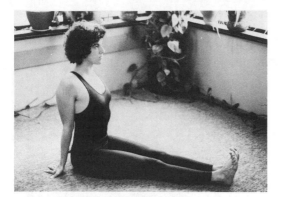

FIGURE 4.24A

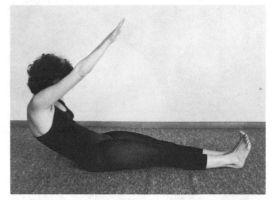

FIGURE 4.24C

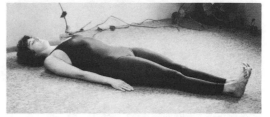

FIGURE 4.24D

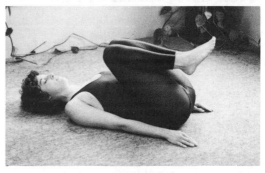

FIGURE 4.24E

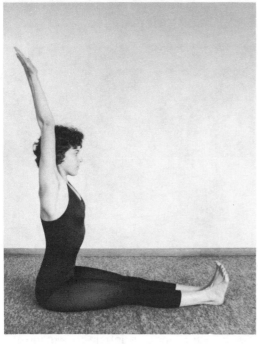

FIGURE 4.24B

the hands down, and lift through the spinal column (Figure 4.24A).

Begin with a deep, slow inhale and stretch the arms up over the head (Figure 4.24B). Continue stretching and lifting vertically upward through the spinal column and arms, and stretch out through the legs.

Exhale, begin rounding the back, contract the buttocks muscles, bring the chin to the chest, and lower the back to the floor very

slowly, one vertebra at a time, keeping the chin to the chest until the very end (Figure 4.24C). Bring the hands to the thighs as you come down.

Rest onto the floor, bringing the arms next to the body with the palms face down (Figure 4.24D).

Inhale and bend the knees to the chest (Figure 4.24E).

Continuing the inhale, stretch the legs straight up in a flowing motion, and stretch through the heels (Figure 4.24F).

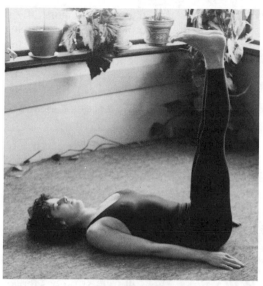

FIGURE 4.24F

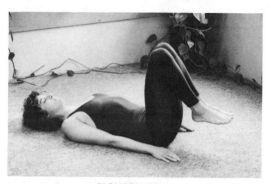

FIGURE 4.24H

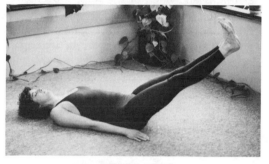

FIGURE 4.24G

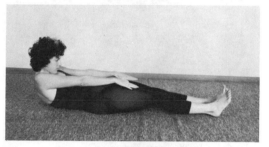

FIGURE 4.24-I

Press the lower back down onto the floor, exhale, and slowly begin to lower the straightened legs to a 45-degree angle (Figure 4.24G). Relax the shoulder, neck, and jaw muscles.

Continuing to exhale, bend the knees and bring the feet to the floor close to the bottom (Figure 4.24H). Slide the feet out and rest onto the floor.

Inhale, bring the chin to the chest and hands to the thighs, and very slowly come to a sitting position with a rounded back until the spine is vertical (Figure 4.24-I). Keep the heels on the floor while coming up.

Lift the chest, drop the shoulders back and down, and continue to inhale as you

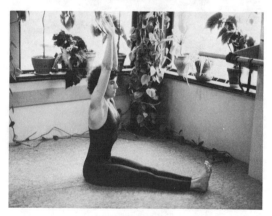

FIGURE 4.24J

stretch upward through the trunk and arms (Figure 4.24J). Keep the legs firm and point the toes upward.

Exhale deeply, reach the arms out, move the chest toward the feet, and stretch the stomach out over the thighs (Figure 4.24K).

Bring the hands to the feet, stretch through the legs, and lengthen the spine

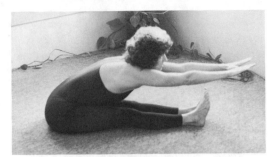

FIGURE 4.24K

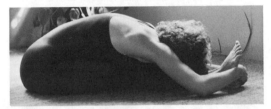

FIGURE 4.24L

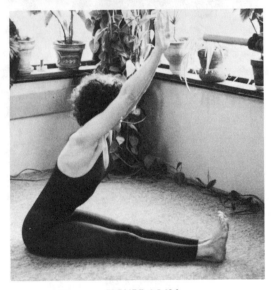

FIGURE 4.24M

(Figure 4.24L). Breathe deeply in this pose for a few seconds.

Inhale, stretch up through the trunk and the arms, and come to a sitting position (Figure 4.24M). Exhale, round the back, and slowly uncurl the back to the floor, as shown in Figure 4.24C. Repeat this entire series of movements twice more.

Half Boat The half boat (Figure 4.25) strengthens the abdominal area. While lying on the back, clasp the fingers behind the head, and lift the head and feet about one foot off the floor. Rest the head in the hands, let the elbows fall open, and stretch through the legs. Hold for ten to 20 seconds, rest, and repeat two more times.

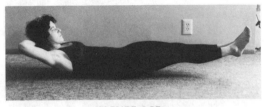

FIGURE 4.25

Wall Splits The wall splits stretches the inner thighs and back of the legs, loosens the hip socket, and allows the back to relax. Lie on the back with the bottom against the wall and the legs straight up. Spread the legs apart slowly, stretch through the heels, pull the chin down toward the chest, and allow gravity to spread the legs wider apart (Figure 4.26). You may want to massage the inner thigh muscles to release tightness. Hold for ten to 30 seconds and come out of it very slowly.

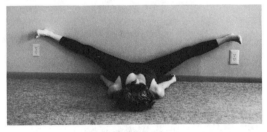

FIGURE 4.26

Bridge The bridge pose loosens the shoulder joints, stretches the arm, leg, and neck muscles, strengthens and tones the buttocks and leg muscles, brings flexibility to the spine, and awakens the upper-back muscles.

Begin on the back, bend the knees, place the feet hip distance apart and parallel to each other, and bring the heels close to the

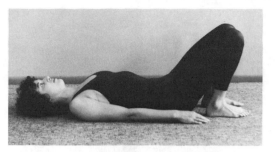

FIGURE 4.27A

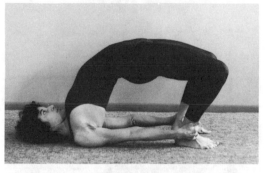

FIGURE 4.27B

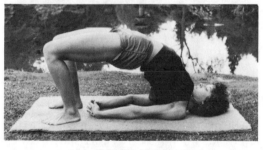

FIGURE 4.27C

the shoulder blades, lift the chest, and relax the neck and shoulder-joint muscles. Work in the pose for five to ten seconds, unfold down slowly one vertebra at a time, tucking the pelvis until the end, rest, and repeat twice more.

If it is not possible to hold the ankles with the heels down, as shown in Figure 4.27B, then interweave the fingers and push the straightened arms down (Figure 4.27C). Beginning from Figure 4.27A, lift the hips, clasp the fingers, stretch through the arms, and follow the instructions given for Figure 4.27B.

Knees to Chest The knees-to-chest pose helps to stretch the lower-back muscles and spine and is a necessary counterbalance to the back-arching poses, such as bridge and bow.

Lie on the back, bring the knees to the chest, hold the knees, and gently squeeze (Figure 4.28). Lengthen the back of the neck and focus on breathing deeply and slowly. This pose can be held for short or long periods.

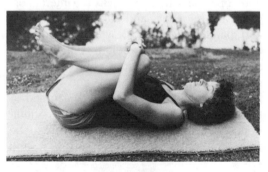

FIGURE 4.28

bottom (Figure 4.27A). Lengthen the lower back by squeezing the buttocks muscles and pushing the lower back down onto the floor. Pull the shoulders away from the ears, stretch the arms down along the sides of the body, and lengthen the back of the neck.

Lift the hips and take hold of the ankles; tuck the pelvis under strongly by squeezing the buttocks muscles and lengthening the lower back. Push the heels down onto the floor, keeping the feet parallel; try to keep the knees close together as you lift the hips higher (Figure 4.27B). Contract the muscles between

Bow The bow pose stretches the front side of the body, loosens the shoulders, awakens the upper-back muscles, stretches the arms, and is very invigorating for all the major systems of the body.

Lying on the stomach, bend the knees and bring them eighteen to twenty-four inches apart. Take hold of the flexed ankles,

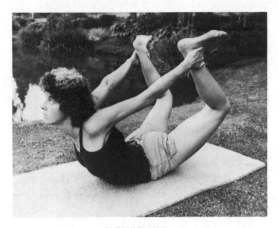

FIGURE 4.29

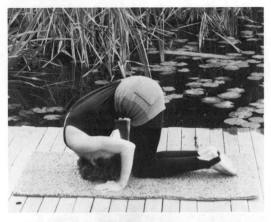

FIGURE 4.30A

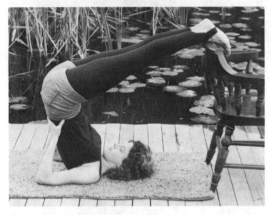

FIGURE 4.30B

contract the bottom, push the hips to the floor, and lift the chest and knees. Pull back with the ankles, draw the shoulders back and down, expand the chest, and look up (Figure 4.29). Work in the pose for five to ten seconds.

Shoulderstand Preparations (Hare and Tranquility Poses)

The preparations for shoulderstand loosen and stretch the neck and upper-back muscles, relax the internal organs, and stimulate and balance the thyroid and parathyroid glands, which control the body's metabolism. In addition, practicing the shoulderstand preparations calms the mind, soothes the nervous system, and helps the body and mind slowly grow accustomed to the feeling of the inverted postures. (Shoulderstand for the beginning student can be found in Chapter 6, Figures 6.16A, B, C, and D.

Hare Pose

Hare pose stretches the neck and upper-back muscles to the utmost, helping to align the neck vertebrae and relieve neck tension. Begin on all fours, place the top of the head on the floor, and walk the knees in toward the forehead. Bring the hands next to the head and press down with the hands to keep the weight off the top of the head (Figure 4.30A). Exhale deeply and roll to the back of

the head; inhale deeply and come back to the forehead. Round the back as shown when doing hare pose. Move back and forth from the forehead to the back of the head several times, then rest in prayer pose (Figure 4.31A).

Tranquility Pose I

Tranquility pose I is a good preparation for shoulderstand, as it slowly loosens the neck muscles, stretches the spine, and moves you toward the completed shoulderstand. If you have been mentally active, this is an excellent pose for calming the mind. If you have been on your feet a lot, it is very beneficial for the feet and legs. Begin on the back and lift the legs, buttocks, and lower back off the floor. Straighten the legs at an angle from the floor, as shown in Figure 4.30B. Place the hands on the lower back and the elbows shoulder-width apart. Resting the feet on a chair table or ledge helps you relax into the pose more deeply, but the body can be placed in the same position without the prop. Breathe deeply and relax the neck, jaw, and eye muscles. Stay in the pose for 30 seconds to two minutes.

Tranquility Pose II Bringing the knees to the forehead (tranquility pose II) increases the stretching of the neck muscles and has a more stimulating effect upon the thyroid and parathyroid glands than does tranquility pose I. From Figure 4.30B, bend the knees and bring them to the forehead or temples, as in Figure 4.30C. Breathe deeply and relax the neck and jaw muscles. Stay in the pose for 30 seconds to one minute. To come down straighten the arms, palms down, and slowly roll down, vertebra by vertebra, until you rest on your back.

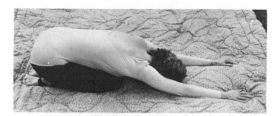

FIGURE 4.31A

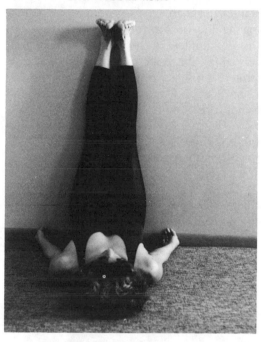

FIGURE 4.31B

FIGURE 4.31C

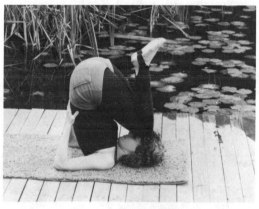

FIGURE 4.30C

Rest Positions Prayer pose is an excellent rest position to perform periodically throughout a yoga workout. It is especially good to do after backward-arching or twisting postures, as it stretches the lower-back muscles quite nicely. To move into prayer pose, sit onto the heels, lengthen the abdomen, rest the abdomen on the thighs, and stretch the arms out past the head (Figure 4.31A). This is also a good position in which to massage the shoul-

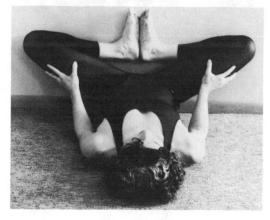

der and neck muscles. Once in the pose, focus on deep, slow, rhythmic breathing and relax the body for 20 seconds to two minutes.

The pose shown in Figure 4.31B is a good rest position. It relieves lower-back aches and helps to reduce a swayback problem by lengthening the lumbar vertebrae. If you have been doing prolonged sitting or standing, it is an excellent position for reversing the flow of blood and relieving pressure in the legs and feet. It can be held for long periods. Bring the bottom next to the wall and stretch the legs up against it. Lengthen the spine and back muscles, rest the arms and hands, and then rest the entire body.

Figure 4.31C shows a rest position that loosens the hip sockets, stretches the inner thighs, and lengthens the back muscles.

From the position shown in Figure 4.31B, bend the knees, bring the bottoms of the feet together, and push the knees toward the wall. Relax the shoulders, neck, jaw, and forehead. Lengthen the back of the neck and breathe slowly and deeply, letting go of tightness in the hip, pelvic, and leg areas.

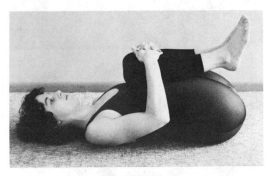

FIGURE 4.31D

Rest on the back, holding the knees toward the chest (Figure 4.31D). This lengthens the lower-back muscles and feels wonderful at the end of a yoga workout. A very soft rocking action helps to soothe the nervous system. This posture is a good preparation for corpse pose, which follows.

Corpse Pose   It is good to end a yoga session with corpse pose. Lying on your back after the stretching and contracting exercises of Hatha Yoga gives you an opportunity to notice the benefits of the practice. Corpse pose allows you to withdraw from the external world and focus on the internal body processes. The goal is to attune to your innermost being as you let the muscles relax more and more. Three to ten minutes is the recommended amount of time to be in corpse pose at the end of a yoga workout.

To prepare for corpse pose, lie on your back and align the body by lengthening the lower back and neck muscles. While lying on your back, bend the knees, place the feet flat on the floor, tuck the pelvis, and bring the chin toward the chest. Then slowly straighten the legs down, bring the feet 12 to 30 inches apart from each other, and let the toes drop out to the sides (Figure 4.32). Place the arms comfortably away from the body with the palms face up and the shoulders rolled back and down. Once the body is in good alignment, focus on deep, slow, rhythmic breathing. The breath is the key to relaxing in corpse pose. During the first three minutes or so of corpse position, the main focus of attention should be upon deep, slow, rhythmic inhalations and exhalations.

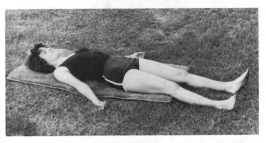

FIGURE 4.32

A good breathing exercise would go as follows: on the inhale, draw energy inward and become aware of the expansion of energy within the lungs. As you exhale, bring awareness to the muscular system and let the muscles relax. Go through the various muscle groups of the body. You can add a retention of the breath after the inhale, but it is important to direct the energy toward tension areas on the exhale. After a number of rounds of this type of focused breathing, shift awareness and begin to feel the pulsation of blood and nerve energy through the body. Keep the breath rhythmic but begin to breathe a finer and lighter breath. Draw the blood and nerve energy into the chest cavity on the inhale and send the blood and nerve energy throughout the body on the exhale. Begin to feel the intricate network of arteries, veins, and nerves inside your body. Find the peace within by letting the body and the mind relax more and more.

To come out of corpse pose, take a few deep, slow breaths, wiggle the fingers and the toes, then stretch the arms up past the ears and the legs down, and yawn a couple of times. Roll over to one side and gracefully come out renewed and recharged.

MASSAGE

Hatha Yoga and massage are techniques that help to awaken a new understanding of oneself. Combined, they work toward increasing one's awareness of the body, mind, emotions, and spirit.

Learning how to relax the muscles of the body is essential to the alleviation of physical, emotional, and mental stress. As the muscles are freed of some of their tightness, the body will be able to move toward greater flexibility in the yoga postures. Massage aids the release of muscular tension, and this helps the practice of yoga to proceed with much less resistance. Massage points out the particular areas of the body where we are holding the greatest amount of tightness. More important, however, massage can give us the actual experience of how to let go of this tension. We frequently use massage at the classes taught at the Hatha Yoga Center in Seattle. It is especially healing to end a yoga workout with massage, though massage can also be done at the beginning or in the middle of a set of yoga postures.

The head, neck, shoulders, back, abdomen, and feet are the most common places that need massage. Massage is not difficult to learn, and there are many different techniques that can be used. Basically, the work consists of rubbing, kneading, stroking, or squeezing the muscle fibers with your fingertips, thumbs, knuckles, palms, or heels of the hands. It is best to work lightly until your partner has become accustomed to your strokes. Slowly increase the amount of pressure. Try out different pressures, speeds, and strokes to let your hands do most of the "thinking" and feeling.

It is important to stay conscious of the alignment of your own body while giving another a massage. The actual work should be primarily spontaneous, but you should have basic strokes in mind. The person receiving the massage should take careful notice of the parts of his or her body that are holding excess tension. The following photographs show the common positions for massage.

Back Massage

The back is an area of the body where deep pressure can usually be applied safely. The techniques of kneading, stroking (long or short strokes), rubbing and squeezing knotted muscles can be done all over the back. In Figure 4.33 Linda is working deeply along the sides of my entire spine with her thumbs.

Neck Massage

It is very common for people to experience neck pain or headaches because of tight neck muscles. One side of the neck is usually

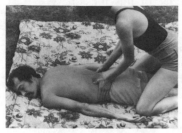

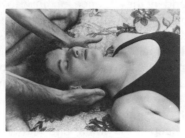

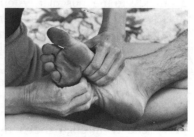

FIGURE 4.33	**FIGURE 4.34**	**FIGURE 4.35**

tighter than the other and should be given more attention than the less tense side. Balancing the neck muscles is very important to help keep neck vertebrae in alignment. In Figure 4.34, I stroke along the backside of Linda's neck muscles with my finger tips. As I find knots, I slowly and carefully try to smooth the knotted areas out.

Foot Massage

Massaging the feet, as shown in Figure 4.35, helps to relax and energize the entire body. As the muscles in the feet are massaged, the nerve endings corresponding to all parts of the body are affected. Deep pressure can be used to release tight areas in the soles of the feet. The tops, bottoms, outsides, and toes of the feet should all be worked on. Foot massage can be done with another person or on yourself. Do not neglect the alignment of your body while massaging another or while massaging yourself.

YOGA ROUTINES

routine 1.
Simplified routine for those with back problems.

- Knees-to-chest *(Fig. 4.28).*
- Floor twists *(Figs. 4.5A–H).*
- Knees-to-chest *(Fig. 4.28).*
- Slow-motion firming *(Figs. 4.24A–M).*

- Standing twist *(Figs. 4.19A and B).*
- Hip-loosener *(Fig. 4.13).*
- Standing rotation *(Fig. 4.14).*
- Standing forward stretch *(Fig. 4.22C).*
- Prayer pose *(Fig. 4.31A).*
- Rest positions *(Figs. 4.31B and C).*

routine 2.
Easy, calming routine.

- Cat–cow *(Figs. 4.1A and B).*
- Bent-knee shoulder-loosener *(Fig. 4.4).*
- Prayer pose *(Fig. 4.31A).*
- Cat–cow *(Figs. 4.1A and B).*
- Hare pose *(Fig. 4.30A).*
- Pose of the child *(Fig. 4.3).*
- Dog stretch *(Figs. 4.11A–D).*
- Sitting twist *(Fig. 4.6B).*
- Slow-motion firming *(Figs. 4.24A–M).*
- Knees-to-chest *(Fig. 4.28).*
- Tranquility pose I *(Fig. 4.30B).*
- Tranquility pose II *(Fig. 4.30C).*
- Corpse pose *(Fig. 4.32).*

routine 3.
Good for those with back problems.

- Forward bar stretch *(Fig. 4.8).*
- Shoulder-looseners *(Figs. 4.7A–C).*
- Standing forward stretches *(Figs. 4.22A–C).*

- Dog stretch (from kneeling position) *(Figs. 4.11A–D)*.
- Floor twists *(Figs. 4.5A–H)*.
- Bridge *(Figs. 4.27A–C)*.
- Knees-to-chest *(Fig. 4.28)*.
- Cat–cow (Figs. 4.1A and B).
- Sun salutation *(Figs. 4.20A–J)*.
- Dancers' pose *(Figs. 4.21A–C)*.
- Hip-loosener *(Fig 4.13)*.
- Standing rotation *(Fig. 4.14)*.
- Modified dog *(Fig. 4.12)*.
- Pose of the child *(Fig. 4.3)*.
- Corpse pose *(Fig. 4.32)*.

routine 4.
Good daytime or evening routine.

- Cat–cow *(Figs. 4.1A and B)*.
- Cat stretch *(Figs. 4.2A–D)*.
- Bent-knee shoulder-loosener *(Fig. 4.4)*.
- Dog stretch (from standing position) *(Figs. 4.10A–D)*.
- Dog stretch (from kneeling position) *(Figs. 4.11A–D)*.
- Hare pose *(Fig. 4.30A)*.
- Lateral stretch *(Fig. 4.16)*.
- Triangle *(Figs. 4.15A and B)*.
- Standing twist *(Figs. 4.19A and B)*.
- Rest positions *(Figs. 4.31A–D)*.
- Slow-motion firming *(Figs. 4.24A–M)*.
- Wall splits *(Fig. 4.26)*.
- Rest position *(Fig. 4.31C)*.
- Corpse pose *(Fig. 4.32)*.

routine 5.
Good energizing routine.

- Sun salutation *(Figs. 4.20A–J)*.
- Triangle *(Figs. 4.15A and B)*.

- Warrior *(Fig. 4.17)*.
- Extended warrior *(Fig. 4.18)*.
- Standing twist *(Figs. 4.19A and B)*.
- Sitting twists *(Figs. 4.6A and B)*.
- Pose of the child *(Fig 4.3)*.
- Cat–Cow *(Figs. 4.1A and B)*.
- Bow *(Fig. 4.29)*.
- Dog stretch (from kneeling position) *(Figs. 4.11A–D)*.
- Bridge *(Figs. 4.27A–C)*.
- Knees-to-chest *(Fig. 4.28)*.
- Half boat *(Fig. 4.25)*.
- Sitting forward stretches *(Figs. 4.23A and B)*.
- Corpse pose *(Fig. 4.32)*.

routine 6.
Good routine for building strength and stamina, breaking up tension, and unwinding.

- Shoulder-looseners *(Figs. 4.7A–C)*.
- Forward bar stretch *(Fig. 4.8)*.
- Hip-loosener *(Fig. 4.13)*.
- Standing rotation *(Fig. 4.14)*.
- Sun salutation *(Figs. 4.20A–J)*.
- Dancers' pose *(Figs. 4.21A–C)*.
- Triangle *(Figs. 4.15A and B)*.
- Warrior *(Fig. 4.17)*.
- Extended warrior *(Fig. 4.18)*.
- Standing forward stretch *(Fig. 4.22C)*.
- Prayer pose *(Fig. 4.31A)*.
- Bent-knee shoulder-loosener *(Fig. 4.4)*.
- Bow *(Fig. 4.29)*.
- Floor twists *(Figs. 4.5A–H)*.
- Slow-motion firming *(Figs. 4.24A–M)*.
- Corpse pose *(Fig. 4.32)*.

IV

WORKBOOK FOR THE BEGINNING, INTERMEDIATE, AND ADVANCED STUDENT OF YOGA

Comprehensive coverage of the yoga postures is given in Chapters 5 through 9. All the postures in these five chapters are classified as beginning, intermediate, or advanced. A single asterisk next to the Figure number indicates that the posture is one that beginners can work on; two asterisks indicate an intermediate-level posture, and three asterisks an advanced posture.

The graduated series of exercises yoga offers gives a practical way of achieving physical, mental, and emotional balance. However, to attain balance we must work on all the main groups of yoga asanas: these are standing postures (Chapter 5), inverted postures (Chapter 6), twists (Chapter 7), backbends (Chapter 8), and forward stretches (Chapter 9). By performing a well-rounded set of yoga postures, we can discharge the built-up frustrations of the aggressive, assertive, and competitive aspects of our being. At the same time, we can awaken the more yielding, receptive, and passive parts of our being. The left and right hemispheres of the brain, corresponding to the rational and intuitive aspects of the mind, can find harmony through the practice of a full range of yoga asanas.

It is recommended that the beginning student of yoga devote fifteen minutes to one hour a day to concentrated asana practice, the intermediate student at least one hour a day, and the advanced student one to two hours a day. The quality of practice, however, is much more important than the quantity.

Sixteen sample routines are given in the appendix. Most of these routines are aimed toward the beginning student who has had some experience and toward the intermediate student. A few sample routines are given for the flexible student of yoga. I recommend that all students use these routines as a takeoff point for individually created sets.

Yoga is a joy to do with another or with a group. Most of the partner postures shown in Chapters 5 through 9 are recommended for the beginning, intermediate, and advanced student. For the majority of students who come to the classes I lead, partner work is the most popular work done. Please do not disregard the partner adjustments shown in Chapters 5 through 9 because you are unfamiliar with the yoga postures. We gain tremendous awareness of the way the human body works by working with another.

The intermediate and advanced student should continue to work on the postures that are marked with only one asterisk. A single asterisk does not imply the pose will be easy to perform correctly; rather, it is one that the beginning, intermediate, and advanced student all should work on.

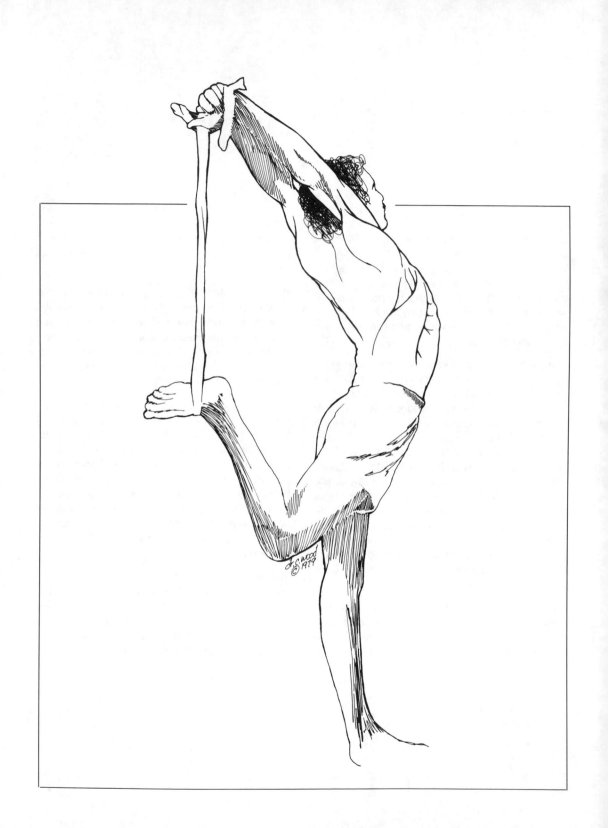

FIVE

standing postures

ATTITUDE FOR STANDING POSTURES

Yoga is the path of mastery. If you are to become your own master, your mind must control your body and your will must control your mind. Correct performance of the standing postures helps you to discipline your body and mind in a very positive way. The standing postures are the most physically taxing of all the main groups of yoga asanas. You must take charge of your body to do the standing postures correctly. As you train the body in these postures, the power of the will most definitely grows, and this increase of will-power quite naturally carries over into other facets of daily life.

While in the standing postures, work the body hard, but do not overstrain. Think of yoga as a dance. Do the dance with precision and with determination, but also with grace. Let the energy move from the center of your body outward. Attune yourself to the rhythm of the universe as you do your yoga practice.

The standing postures are extremely difficult asanas to perform correctly. Upon them, the beginning and intermediate student

should spend a great amount of Hatha Yoga practice time. You should work toward perfection in the standing postures because they form the foundation for the rest of the main groups of yoga asanas.

The standing postures bring strength, good body alignment, and flexibility to the entire body. Strong muscles develop because the whole muscular system is used in a very demanding way. The standing postures also bring a true sense of stability and strength to the mind. Out of this well-grounded base, the body and the mind can move toward greater flexibility in the other yoga asanas.

The main physical benefits resulting from the performance of the standing postures will be listed individually with each posture, except for those of the standing forward stretches, which will be presented in the introductory discussion. As a whole, the standing postures can greatly improve the efficiency of the muscular, circulatory, respiratory, digestive, eliminative, reproductive, endocrine, and nervous systems of the body.

When practicing the standing postures, you may be confronted by considerable amounts of pain. There are three areas of the body that you must guard carefully: the neck, the lumbar vertebrae, and the knees.

1. As a general rule, try to keep the neck as passive as possible and the back of the neck as long as possible while doing the standing postures.

2. The broad guideline for the lumbar spinal region (lower spine) is to try to lengthen and straighten it. Do not overarch the lumbar vertebrae while doing any of the standing postures!

3. The knee is a very delicate joint, but the standing postures, if done correctly, are the best possible exercises for building strength in the muscles and ligaments surrounding it. It is the quadriceps group of muscles (frontside thigh muscles) that must be strenghtened to help weak knees.

Special caution must be taken whenever you bend the knee. Make sure it is directed over the center of the foot as you bend it. Be careful to avoid twisting the knee; the knee is a hinge joint constructed to fold, but not to twist. Realize that whenever the knee is turned, the movement should originate from the hip joint. The knee opens to one side or the other only because rotation in the hip socket first moves the femur (thigh bone) in a particular direction. The knee joint, being at the bottom end of the femur, moves as a re-sult of the rotational movement taking place in the ball-and-socket hip joint. (The head of the femur is the ball; the acetabulum of the pelvis is the socket.) Figure 5.1A shows the construction of the hip joint.

A guiding principle of the standing postures is to find your center, which is your spinal column, and the energy that moves along the spine. From the center of your being, you should move outward: so the arms are moved from between the shoulder blades, and the legs are moved from the pelvic area.

Movement in the standing postures is to be circular and fluid, rather than sharp and abrupt. Whenever you move the arms, think of the movement as a rotational one that originates in the ball-and-socket shoulder joint, the main muscles that control the movement being located between the shoulder blades. Whenever you move the legs, think of the rotational movement as being one that originates in the ball-and-socket hip joint, the main muscles that control the movement being located in the buttocks area. Figure 5.1B shows the construction of the shoulder joint.

As a general rule, while in any of the standing postures you should continually make subtle adjustments to improve the pose. As soon as you feel you can go no further in a pose, breathe deeply and slowly. Focusing on your breath will provide a concentration

FIGURE 5.1A

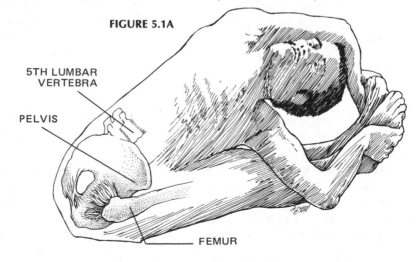

5TH LUMBAR VERTEBRA

PELVIS

FEMUR

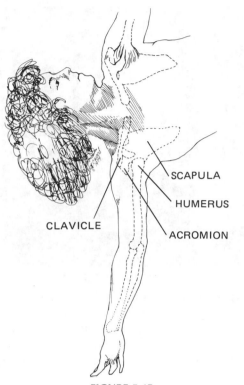

SCAPULA

HUMERUS

CLAVICLE

ACROMION

FIGURE 5.1B

technique that allows you to mindfully move beyond whatever pain is holding you back. Thus, you will be enabled to go a little further into the pose, to stretch or twist a little more. If you do not focus on a deep, slow breath, most likely you will come away from the posture more frazzled than integrated. The breath is the key, and you should keep trying to move the body to its limits only by moving with the breath. As a general rule, the exhale is the time to make the greatest progress in the standing postures, and the inhale is the time to draw energy in and lengthen the spine.

It will become very obvious to you that the two sides of the body are not symmetrical. You will find that one leg stretches more easily than the other, one side of the back twists more easily than the other, one hip joint is more flexible than the opposite, and one shoulder joint is looser than the other. Still, it is best to do both sides an equal number of times unless you are terribly unbalanced, since balance will come with daily practice over the course of time. If you do find a huge imbalance between the sides, it is a good practice to do the weaker side (the side that is most difficult to do) twice and the strong side only once. This rule may be applied throughout the yoga postures.

Let us now look at the standing postures.

Standing Postures

Standing-Posture Warmup The sequence in Figures 5.2A–C is an excellent warmup for the standing postures. It brings flexibility to the spine, loosens the shoulder and hip joints, frees the rib-cage area for rotational movement, relaxes the eyes, improves the efficiency of the internal organs of digestion, elimination, and reproduction, and improves circulation throughout the body. It can be done in a fast or slow rhythm for short or long periods.

Position the feet shoulder-width apart and begin swinging the torso and arms from side to side. Keep the legs straight as the arms, head, and eyes are carried by the movement of the torso. The movement can be done very gently or fairly vigorously. Swing from side to side for thirty seconds to one minute.

Classical Sun Salutation

The classical sun salutation is a beautiful series of movements that loosen and energize the entire body. It is one of the most highly recommended sets of postures for the beginning, intermediate, and advanced student of yoga. The classical sun salutation increases the circulation of blood throughout the body, stretches the arm and leg muscles, loosens the spine, helps develop fullness of breath, helps loosen all the main joints of the body, increases the efficiency of the nervous, digestive, eliminative, reproductive, and endocrine systems, and generally serves as a tonic for the body, mind, and soul. It should be performed as a moving meditation.

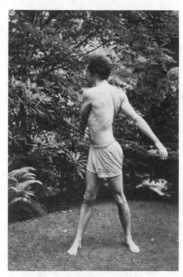

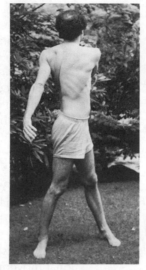

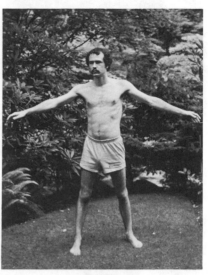

FIGURE 5.2A*   **FIGURE 5.2B***   **FIGURE 5.2C***

The classical sun salutation is done in a slow-motion fashion, with a fluid movement from one posture to another. Emphasis in each movement should be placed on the breath. Many variations can be performed as offshoots of the main postures; the particular sun salutation presented here can serve as a springboard for your own creatively inspired yoga dance.

The classical sun salutation is often used as a warmup for further yoga work; however, it can be done in the middle or at the end of a yoga session. The full series of movements can be performed from one to ten times; two is the recommended number on a day-to-day basis.

Usually, the sun salutation is performed with one movement per breath. While you are in some of the forward-stretching or back-arching poses, you can breathe deeply and hold the pose for a couple of breaths. The rapidity of the movements depends on the effect you are seeking.

By both moving the body rhythmically and by flowing with the breath, you can get the body and the mind working in unison. The classical sun salutation helps to balance the assertive and receptive parts of our being.

It is especially recommended as a morning salutation to the sun, which gives us life. Not only should the divinity of the light of the external sun be honored, but also the divinity of the light that radiates from your own heart center.

Begin by standing upright with the feet together; lift the leg and abdominal muscles, lengthen the spine vertically upward, tuck the pelvis under, lift and expand the chest cavity, lengthen the back of the neck, and close the eyes. Bring the palms of the hands together at the center of the chest with the thumbs touching the chest bone and the elbows lifted gently (Figure 5.3A). Go within and focus on the breath and the alignment of the body.

Open the eyes, spread the toes, plant the feet, lift through the leg muscles, contract the buttocks muscles, and stretch the arms up past the ears, interweaving the thumbs. (Interweaving the thumbs is optional; some people feel more comfortable with the hands shoulder-width apart.) Inhale deeply, lift the chest as high as possible, continue contracting the buttocks muscles and tucking the pelvis, and arch the spine gracefully backward. Try to minimize the arch of the lower back and maximize the arch of the upper back. Do this arching movement slowly and carefully. Bring the arms behind the ears through the strong contraction of the shoulder-blade muscles (Figure 5.3B). Squeeze the buttocks muscles tightly throughout this back arch.

Exhale and slowly stretch the spine and arms forward. Keep reaching out and bring the weight forward onto the balls of the feet (Figure 5.3C). As you fold forward, tilt the pelvis upward by lifting the hips, and bring the hands onto the floor next to the feet. Exhale totally, lift through the back of the legs, stretch through the spine, and let the head hang down (Figure 5.3D).

Inhale and bring the right (or left) foot back, about four feet behind the left foot, and hook under the toes of the right foot. Stretch through the back of the right leg and lift the right kneecap. Release the hands from the floor and stretch the arms up next to the ears. Drop the shoulders down and back, contract the right buttocks muscles, and arch the spine gracefully back by contracting the shoulder-blade muscles (Figure 5.3E). Expand the chest and stretch through the heel of the right foot, drive the right hip down, and tuck the pelvis. Make sure the left knee is directed over the center of the left foot, lift through the spine, stretch through the arms, bringing them behind the ears, draw the abdominal muscles in, and look upward. Exhale, bring the hands down to the floor next to the left foot, shoulder-width apart.

Inhale, bring the left foot back next to the right foot, and come into dog stretch. Lift the hips as high as possible, tilt the pelvis upward, stretch up through the arms and spine, and down toward the floor with the heels. Draw the upper-back muscles in toward the spine, stretch up through the spine, expand and drop the chest, and relax the neck (Figure 5.3F).

From dog stretch, lift the head and look between the hands. Exhale, tighten the buttocks muscles, tuck the pelvis, and slowly lower the hips and chest toward the floor until the chest is over the arms. Form a straight line with the legs and torso by gently drawing in the abdominal muscles and by squeezing the buttocks muscles. Push the straightened arms against the floor and look down toward the floor while passing onto the next pose (Figure 5.3G).

Inhale, contract the buttocks muscles very strongly, and bring the hips toward the floor, keeping the legs off the floor. Pull the chest through the arms, arch the spine, expand the chest cavity, arch the neck, and look upward. Lift the knees by tightening the quadriceps muscles, stretch through the back of the legs, and draw the shoulders back and down by contracting the shoulder-blade muscles. Keep the arms straight and the upper arms touching the rib cage (Figure 5.3H). Continue the strong contractive work of the buttocks muscles, and expand the chest.

Exhale and return to the position shown in Figure 5.3G (push-up position). Inhale, lift the hips high into the air, and come back to dog stretch. Try to flatten the back muscles by

FIGURE 5.3A   **FIGURE 5.3B***

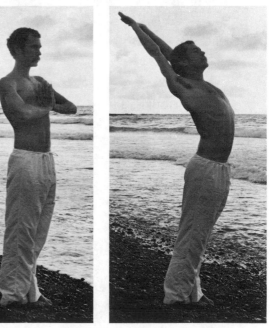

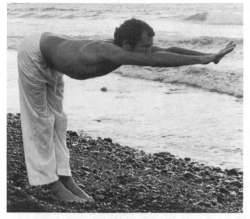

FIGURE 5.3C*

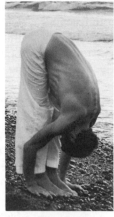

FIGURE 5.3D*

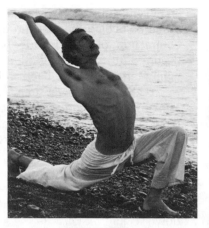

FIGURE 5.3E*

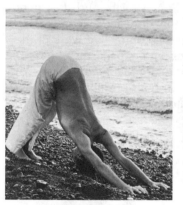

FIGURE 5.3F*

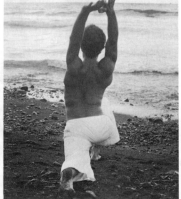

FIGURE 5.3G*

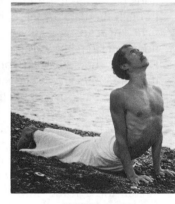

FIGURE 5.3H*

FIGURE 5.3-I*

FIGURE 5.3J*

FIGURE 5.3K*

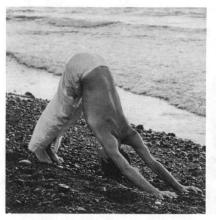

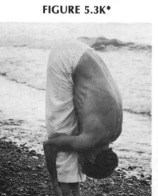

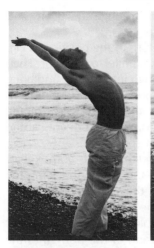
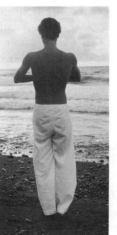

FIGURE 5.3L*   **FIGURE 5.3M***

lifting the bottom high into the air and by dropping the rib cage toward the floor (Figure 5.3-I). Stretch through the entire backside of the body, and try to attain a deep fold in the frontside of the hip socket.

Exhale, bend the right knee, and bring the right foot between the hands (opposite foot forward, as in Figure 5.3E). Inhale, lift the left kneecap, and stretch through the heel of the left foot, keeping the toes hooked under. Contract the left buttocks muscles, take the hands off the floor, and stretch the arms up past the ears. Make sure the right knee is directed over the center of the right foot. Inhale more deeply, contract the upper-back muscles, and arch the spine gracefully backward. Lift the chest, bring the arms behind the ears, drop the shoulders down and back, stretch the arms, and look upward (Figure 5.3J).

Exhale, bring both hands next to the right foot, lift the bottom, bend the left knee, and bring the left foot forward next to the right one. Exhale further, hold the back of the ankles, lift through the back of the legs, shift the weight toward the ball of the toes, and stretch the spine and back muscles to the utmost. Let the head hang (Figure 5.3K).

Now bring the hands forward in front of the feet, inhale, and slowly raise the torso and the arms (similar to the way you went down in Figure 5.3C). As you come up to a vertical position, inhale more deeply, contract the buttocks muscles, stretch the spine and arms straight up, and look straight ahead. Tuck the pelvis under very strongly, contract the shoulder-blade muscles, drop the shoulders down and back, stretch the arms, and gracefully arch the spine backward (Figure 5.3L).

Exhale and slowly return to the standing prayer position (Figure 5.3M). Tuck the pelvis under, stand evenly on both feet, bring the palms to the chest, gently lift the elbows, expand the chest, relax the shoulders, and lift up through the legs and spine. Close the eyes; feel the effects of the first round of the sun salutation. Repeat the set again.

Modern-Day Sun Salutation

The modern-day sun salutation is more vigorous and abrupt than the classical sun salutation. Here you move from one position to another in quicker bursts. Both a shortened and a slightly longer version of the modern-day salutation will be presented; both work on strength, endurance, and flexibility. The modern-day sun salutation has physical benefits similar to those of the classical salutation. It increases the circulation of blood throughout the body, helps all the major systems to function more efficiently, and has a very energizing effect upon the body and the mind.

Doing a number of rounds of the modern-day salutation will increase the heart rate. For those who seek an aerobic type of exercise, this series of movements is excellent. The shortened version can be performed anywhere from two to twenty times in succession, one after the other. I recommend that the shortened version be done two to four times as a warmup for further yoga work and that the longer version be done once. The longer one is geared more for the intermediate and advanced student.

Even though certain of the movements are done quickly, there must be short pauses in which one stretches or arches the body in a very conscious way. The inhalations and exhalations will occur with greater rapidity than in the classical sun salutation, but they should be deep, thorough, and rhythmic just the same.

Many of the modern sun-salutation positions are the same as those in the classical sun salutation, and the discussion will be shortened for these positions. Refer back to the classical salutation for greater explanation. I do recommend practice of both these salutations.

Shortened Version Stand straight and bring the palms together at the center of the chest. Close the eyes and center yourself by focusing on the breath and on straight alignment of the body (Figure 5.4A).

Inhale, stretch the arms up, squeeze the buttocks muscles, tuck the pelvis, contract the shoulder blades, and arch gracefully back (Figure 5.4B).

Exhale, stretch the arms out, and bring the hands next to the feet (Figure 5.4C). Stretch up through the back of the legs and down through the spine.

Now bend the knees, squat down, and bring the knees to the chest. Exhale further and gracefully jump the feet four feet back from the hands with the toes hooked under. Straighten the body and tuck the pelvis by contracting the buttocks muscles and lifting the abdominal muscles. Stretch through the back of the legs to bring the body parallel to the floor. Slowly lower the torso and leg close to the floor, but do not let them touch it. Push down with the hands and keep the bent elbows next to the ribs (Figure 5.4D). All of this is done on the exhale.

Inhale, arch the spine back, pull the chest through the arms, contract the buttocks muscles very strongly, and pull the shoulders back and down. Keep the kneecaps lifted and off the floor, stretch through the heels, and look upward (Figure 5.4E).

Exhale and return to the position in Fig. 5.4D, with the body parallel to the floor. Then inhale, lift the hips high into the air, and bring the body to the dog-stretch position (Figure 5.4F). Stretch through the backside of the legs, torso, and arms, and fold deeply at the front side of the hip socket.

From dog stretch, bend both knees, bring them close to the chest, and jump the feet forward until they rest between the hands. Do this on the exhale. Lift the bottom, straighten the legs, fold the torso forward, and straighten the backside of the body into the standing forward-stretch position. Bring the hands back and let the head hang (Figure 5.4G).

Inhale and slowly come up to a vertical position, stretching the arms straight up. Then slowly arch back, contracting the buttocks and shoulder-blade muscles, bring the straightened arms behind the ears, and look up (Figure 5.4H).

Exhale and return to the vertical standing position with the hands in prayer position (Figure 5.4-I). Repeat the series several times.

FIGURE 5.4A*   FIGURE 5.4B*

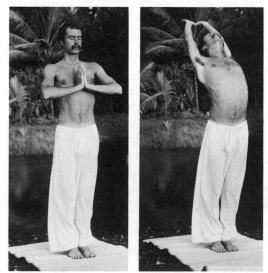

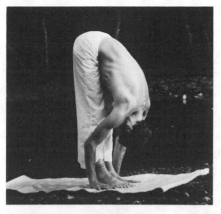

FIGURE 5.4C*

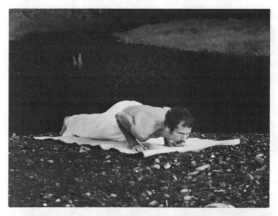

FIGURE 5.4D*

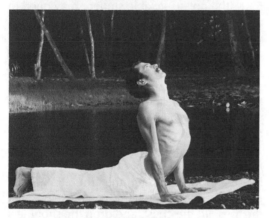

FIGURE 5.4E*

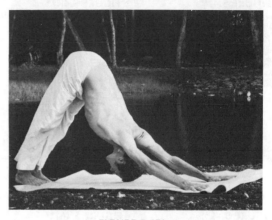

FIGURE 5.4F*

FIGURE 5.4G*　　　　**FIGURE 5.4H***　　　　**FIGURE 5.4-I***

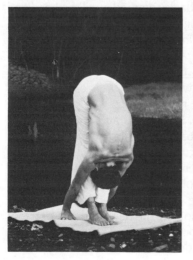

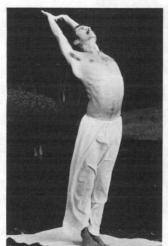

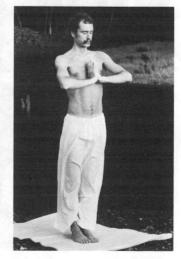

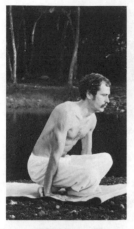

FIGURE 5.4J**

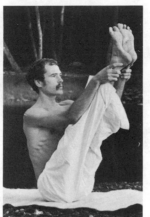

FIGURE 5.4K**

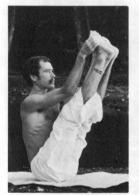

FIGURE 5.4L**

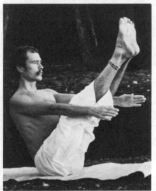

FIGURE 5.4M**

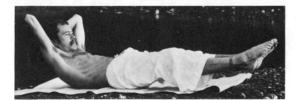

FIGURE 5.4N**

FIGURE 5.4-O**

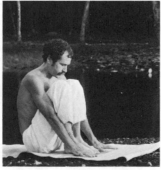

Lengthened Version The lengthened version of the modern-day sun salutation is the same as the shorter version up through Figure 5.4F. To do the longer version, continue from the downward-facing dog-stretch position, shown in Figure 5.4F, and shift the weight forward onto both hands by bringing the chest forward over the hands. Then exhale, push the hands down strongly, and swing the legs through the straightened arms.

From Figure 5.4J, continue to exhale, gently lower the bottom to the floor next to the hands, then lift and straighten the legs and take hold of the ankles as shown in Figure 5.4K (the not-so-flexible student may need to take hold of the back of the knees). The advanced student can take hold of the outside of the feet, as shown in Figure 5.4L. Whatever the hand placement, lift the chest and straighten the legs. Try to bring the chest close to the legs by pulling the upper-back muscles in toward the spine. Try to get as far forward as possible onto the sitting bones.

Release the legs, but in doing so try to maintain the same position with the legs, head, and torso. Stretch the arms straight out next to the legs, stretch through the legs, point the toes, lift the chest, and drop the shoulders (Figure 5.4M). This is called the full boat pose.

Inhale, round the spine, and slowly drop the legs and back (rounded) until the head and feet are brought approximately one foot from the floor. Bring the hands to the back of the head, interweave the fingers, drop the elbows, point the toes, look at the feet, and hold for a few seconds. This is called the half boat pose (Figure 5.4N).

Exhale, lift the legs and chest, and take hold of the back of the legs or feet again, as shown in Figures 5.4K and 5.4L. Release the hands and return to the position shown if Figure 5.4M (full boat). From here inhale and return to the position shown in Figure 5.4N (half boat), holding the head and feet one foot above the floor. Exhale and return to full boat. Inhale back down until the head and feet are one foot above the floor (half boat). Exhale up once again to full boat.

Continuing to exhale, bend the knees and bring the heels down onto the floor next to the pubis (Figure 5.4-0). Take a quick inhale, then exhale, lift the hips, straighten the legs, and come into the standing forward stretch, as shown in Figures 5.4C and 5.4G. Inhale, slowly stand up, stretch up through the arms, and then arch back as in Figures 5.4B and 5.4H. To complete the round, exhale and return to the standing prayer position. Repeat the series once again.

Bar Postures

Full-Body Warmup If you have access to a bar, this is a wonderful warmup that prepares the body for further yoga work. The movements create flexibility through the entire spine, accelerate the blood flow throughout the body, and loosen all the key joints in the body including the ankle, knee, hip, sacroiliac, shoulder, elbow, and wrist joints.

Begin with the feet about one foot away from a vertical line of the bar, hold the bar, and pull the hips back. Inhale deeply and stretch the arms, the spine, and the legs to the utmost. Tilt the pelvis upward to attain a deep fold in the front side of the hip socket and pull the buttocks away from the bar (Figure 5.5A).

Exhale, lift the heels, bend the knees, and bring the chest against the thighs with the head down. Stretch through the arms and lower spine area, and push down the ball of the toes (Figure 5.5B).

Inhale and return to the position shown in Figure 5.5A by pulling the hips back and straightening the legs. Try to tilt the pelvis upward and fold deeply in at the hips. Stretch the arms, the spine, and the legs to the utmost. Look toward the hands (Figure 5.5C).

Exhale, squeeze the buttocks muscles, and tuck the pelvis strongly. Contract the shoulder-blade muscles, lift the chest high, and arch gracefully backward (Figure 5.5D).

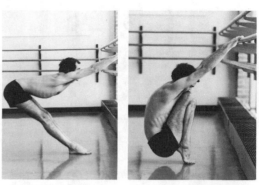

FIGURE 5.5A*   FIGURE 5.5B*

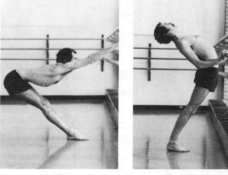

FIGURE 5.5C*   FIGURE 5.5D*

(If there is compression in the lower back, lift the heels to help lessen the arch of the lower back.) Come back to Figure 5.5A and repeat the full-body warmup two to five more times.

Triangle Preparation The key value of the triangle preparation is that it stretches the lateral trunk muscles and the waistline area to the utmost. The benefits to the legs include

FIGURE 5.6*

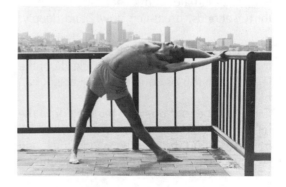

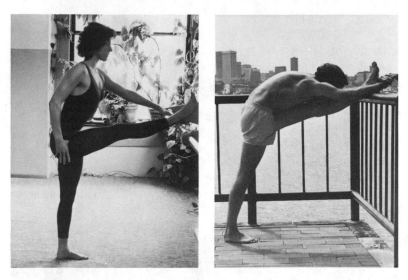

FIGURE 5.7A (FAR LEFT)*

FIGURE 5.7B (LEFT)**

development of stronger foot arches, strengthening and loosening of the ankle joints, and toning of the quadriceps, inner thighs, outer thighs, and buttocks muscles. It also loosens the shoulder joints and lower rib-cage areas and aids the digestive, eliminative, and reproductive organs.

Place the feet 36 to 42 inches apart and position the body as shown in (Figure 5.6). As in triangle, the knees must be turned in opposite directions to bring them over the line of the third toe through the contraction of the buttocks muscles. To help relieve stress on the knee, lift the kneecap by contracting the quadriceps muscles. Hold the bar with the hands slightly in front of the legs, stretch the arms and waist area, contract the buttocks muscles, and roll the rib cage under further with each exhale. Work each side for ten to thirty seconds, breathing slowly and deeply.

Leg Stretch on Bar   This is a good posture for those with tightness in the backside of the legs. A tabletop or counter of any height can be used.

Lift one foot onto the bar, and drop the hip of the outstretched leg. Square the hips forward, lift up through the standing leg, and stretch through the leg on the bar. Lean for-

ward, lift the chest, and lengthen the spinal cord. To help drop the hip of the top leg, you can push the hand or thumb into the fold of the hip joint, as shown in Figure 5.7A. Bring the other hand forward onto the bar if possible. Work each side for ten seconds to one minute.

Continuing from the posture shown in Figure 5.7A, exhale and stretch the abdomen and chest out over the outstretched leg. Drop the hip of the outstretched leg and keep the toes of that foot pointed straight up. Hold the foot with both hands and pull forward (Figure 5.7B). Work each side of the pose for ten to twenty seconds, stretching out further on the exhale and holding the extra stretch gained on the inhale.

Twisting Leg Stretch with Bar   This twisting leg-stretch posture helps to loosen the back muscles, especially those of the upper back. It also stretches and tones the leg muscles, increases your breathing capacity by stretching the chest muscles, stimulates the internal organs of digestion and elimination, and helps to realign the spine.

Continuing from the position shown in Figure 5.7B, hold the bar to the outside of the foot with the opposite hand and twist the rib

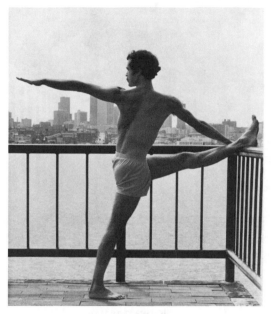

FIGURE 5.8A**

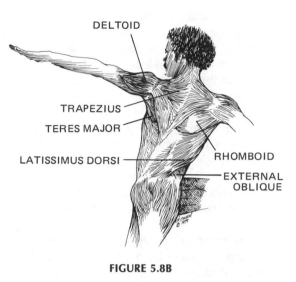

DELTOID

TRAPEZIUS

TERES MAJOR

LATISSIMUS DORSI

RHOMBOID

EXTERNAL OBLIQUE

FIGURE 5.8B

cage toward the outstretched back arm. Drop the hip of the outstretched leg, lift vertically up through the standing leg and spine, and try to turn the lower rib cage and chest more than 90 degrees. Draw the back shoulder blade in toward the spine and reach straight back with the arm. Lift through the back of the neck and look over the shoulder (Figure 5.8A). Work each side of the pose, twisting further with each deep exhale and holding the twist with each deep inhale.

Figure 5.8B illustrates the muscular system of the back while in action. To do the twisting leg stretch, the muscles in the left upper back must contract strongly; the middle portion of the trapezius, the rhomboideus major, and the latissimus dorsi must be pulled in toward the spine. These same muscles must stretch on the right side of the back. The top part of the trapezius and deltoid muscles of the left shoulder area should relax as much as possible, as this allows the shoulder to rotate back and down and the chest to turn further.

Hip-Opener with Bar This posture stretches the inner leg muscles, tones the leg

FIGURE 5.9*

and buttocks muscles, loosens the hip joints, and helps to develop better arches in the feet.

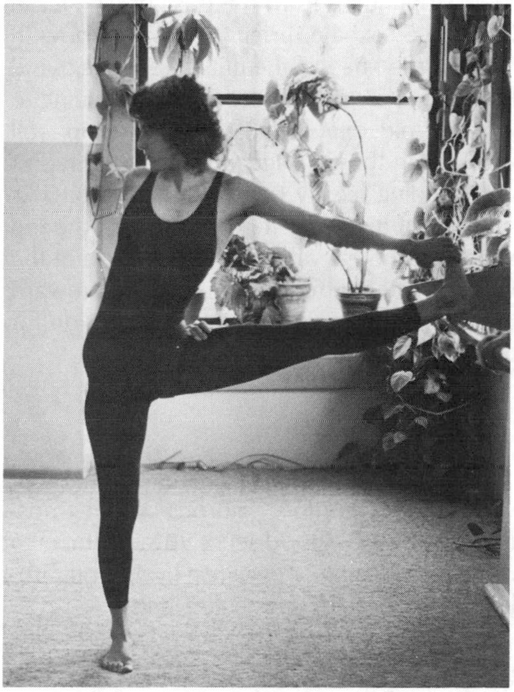

Study Figure 5.9 and note the position

of the legs and feet. Begin by opening the hip of one leg and placing the foot on a bar or tabletop. Contract the outer buttocks muscles of both the standing leg and the outstretched leg. Turn the knees in opposite directions, roll under with the buttocks of the outstretched leg, and pull back the hip of the standing leg. Lift the kneecap of the standing leg and straighten the spine by lifting the chest. As demonstrated by Linda, one arm can come around the back and hold the thigh of the outstretched leg. Work in the pose for 20 seconds to one minute. Repeat to the other side.

Side Stretch with Bar This posture stretches the inner leg muscles, opens the hip joint, stretches the lateral torso muscles, and loosens the back muscles.

Continuing from the position shown in Figure 5.9, exhale, bring the inside elbow in front of the knee of the outstretched leg, and hold the inner side of the foot. Continuing to exhale, fold deeply in at the front hip, roll under with the rib cage, and open the hip of the standing leg by contracting the buttocks muscles of that side. If possible, bring the top arm over the ear and hold the outside of the foot, as you attempt to turn the chest toward the ceiling (Figure 5.10). Work each side for ten to twenty seconds.

Standing Rotations

The standing rotations serve as an excellent warmup for the more vigorous standing postures. They are a good set of yoga postures to do before jogging or engaging in vigorous athletics. They loosen the entire body.

These postures stretch and tone the leg muscles as well as loosen the hip sockets and the abdominal and back areas (lower, middle, and upper back). The whole body gains better blood circulation through practice of the standing rotations, and the rotational movement of the rib cage serves as a tonic for the

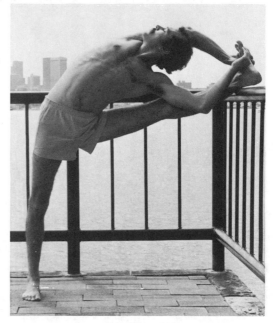

FIGURE 5.10*

organs of digestion, elimination, and reproduction.

In the main series of standing rotations, keep the feet parallel to each other (about three feet apart). Both arms should stretch to the utmost in the standing rotations. To get maximum rotation of the lower back and pelvic area, lift one hip while dropping the opposite hip. This allows the pelvic-girdle and lower-spine areas to loosen. The main rotational movement should occur through the turning of the lower rib-cage and chest areas.

While doing the standing rotations, exhale as you turn the rib cage, and take a few deep, slow breaths while in the pose. Inhale to come out of the rotated position, and exhale as you rotate to the other side. Work each side for five to twenty seconds. These postures can also be done in a slow, dancelike way, moving into the twist with each deep exhale and coming out of the rotation with each deep inhale.

Hip Sway (Warmup for Standing Rotations) The hip sway is a good way to

102

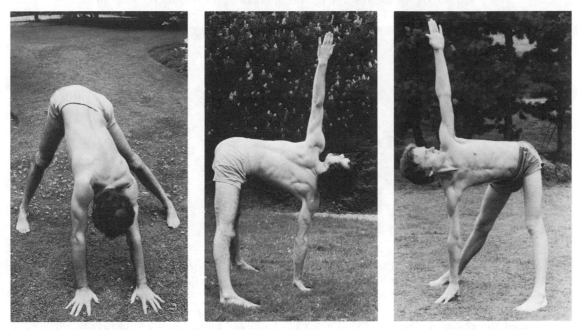

FIGURE 5.11*   FIGURE 5.12*   FIGURE 5.13*

loosen the legs, hip sockets, and lower back before doing the full standing rotation series. While doing the swaying movement, keep the buttocks muscles over the line of the feet and lift the quadriceps muscles (kneecaps). To get into the pose, spread the feet about three feet apart, place both hands on the floor 30 to 36 inches in front of the toes, stretch the arms and spine, and look down between the hands (Figure 5.11). Then lift one hip at a time while turning the other one in. Shift back and forth with the hips. This swaying action can be done over and over again in either a fast or slow rhythm.

Hand in Front of Toes—Head Centered

Pictured in Figure 5.12 is the first hand and head position of the standing rotational series. The hand is placed approximately one foot in front of the line of the toes and the hand and head are centered between the legs. Keep the bottom above the line of the feet while doing the rotational movement. From the position shown in Figure 5.11, bring the right hand in toward the feet, inhale, lift

the chest, stretch the spinal cord straight out, and lift the left hip. Exhale, turn the rib cage to the left, and reach straight up with the left hand. The bottom hand touches the ground gently while the top arm stretches up strongly. As you lift the left hip and rotate the rib cage, keep your weight on the outer edge of the right foot. The shoulder blade of the left arm should be drawn in toward the spine to further the rotational movement of the rib cage. Twist farther with each exhale as you bring the chin toward the left shoulder, keeping length through the back of the neck. Work for five to 20 seconds. Inhale, come out of the twist, and repeat to the other side.

The second hand position is on the floor in line with the toes, and here the hand and head are again centered between the feet (Figure 5.13). This hand position aids the loosening of the lower back more than the first hand position, which more directly aids the loosening of the upper back and shoulder joint. They both loosen the hip joint and leg muscles. In all the standing rotations, the chest will rotate further if the abdominal mus-

103

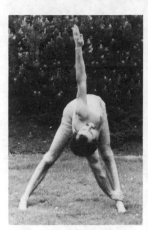
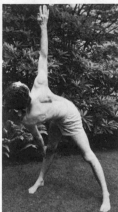
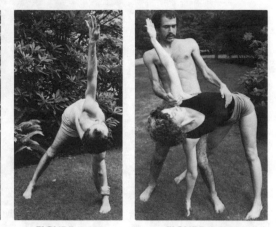

FIGURE 5.14A* **FIGURE 5.14B*** **FIGURE 5.15*** **FIGURE 5.16***

culature pulls the lower rib-cage area across with it. The real key to increased rotational movement is to pull the muscles just below the shoulder blade muscles of the top arm in toward the spine. As shown in Figure 5.13, the midline of the torso, the neck, and the entire spine should stretch out parallel to the floor, and the arms should stretch out opposite to each other and vertical to the floor. Work each side for five to twenty seconds.

Hand Holds Ankle—Head Inside Foot

The next hand and head standing rotational position is to grip the outside of the ankle which you have twisted toward while stretching the head out over the foot. This hand position loosens the middle back more than with the hand on the floor between the feet. As shown in Figure 5.14A, the right hand holds the left ankle, the left arm stretches straight up, the chest expands, and the rib cage turns. Perform the turning action on the exhale. Repeat to the other side after five to twenty seconds of work.

An alternative to the position shown in Figure 5.14A is to push against the outer calf or the outer knee (Figure 5.14B) instead of holding the ankle. This hand position makes the stretch on the inner-thigh muscles and on the back of the legs less stressful and also allows the rotational action of the torso to become the main focus of attention.

Hand Holds Ankle—Head Over the Foot

The final position in the series has the head outside of the foot (in Figure 5.15). This position helps to break up tension in the middle and lower back. In the two standing rotations shown in which the hand is placed on the ankle, the hand grip should be firm and the bottom arm stretched to the utmost as the rib cage is turned. You'll note in Figure 5.15 that the feet have turned slightly in the direction you have twisted toward. Exhale to rotate and make a continual effort to lengthen the spinal cord and lift the chest as you turn further and further. Work in the pose for two to three breaths and repeat to the other side.

Partner Adjustment A partner adjustment feels marvelous with any of the standing rotational hand and head positions. As shown in Figure 5.16, my hip is pushed against the underside of Linda's rib cage in order to aid the rolling under of her rib-cage area. I pull her abdominal muscles and shoulder back with my hands. With help she is able to rotate much further than she could on her own, thus helping to break up deep-rooted back tension. This adjustment should be done to both sides for five to 15 seconds.

Tree Pose The tree is a very basic posture that helps one to develop better balance and better concentration. At a muscular level, it develops the arches of the feet, strengthens the ankle joint, and tones the leg, buttocks, and abdominal muscles. It also helps to straighten the spinal cord and loosens the hip and knee joints.

Stand erect with the feet together, lift through the legs and spine, and breathe deeply. Lift through the right leg, bend the left knee, and bring the left foot to the right inner thigh. Press the foot inward against the inner-thigh muscles. Open the hip of the bent knee, so that the knee comes back, but at the same time keep the hip of the standing leg from turning inward by contracting the outer thigh and buttocks muscles of that leg. The hips should face squarely forward. Contraction of both sides of the buttocks muscles is necessary. Straighten and stretch the arms over the head with the palms together, and elongate through the spine (Figure 5.17A). Focus the eyes on a point straight ahead and hold the pose for ten to 20 seconds, breathing slowly and deeply. Repeat to the other side.

Half-lotus tree pose is much more difficult to perform than the beginners' version shown in Figure 5.17A. In Figure 5.17B, the heel of the bent knee foot rests to the inside of the inner thigh of the standing leg. The bent knee should be drawn down toward the standing knee. Lift through the thigh of the standing leg. Tuck the pelvis under and lift through the spine and arms. You should be steady like a tree in this posture. Look straight ahead and do not let the eyes wander. Work each side for ten to 20 seconds.

Folding Tree The folding tree stretches the spine, back muscles, back of the knee of the standing leg, and the front of the knee of the bent leg. It also loosens the hip sockets and increases the circulation of blood throughout the body.

From the half-lotus tree pose, exhale, fold at the hips, and slowly bring both hands

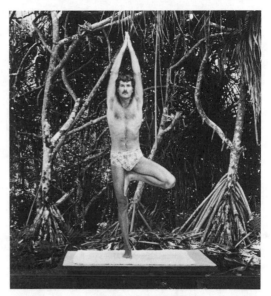

FIGURE 5.17A*

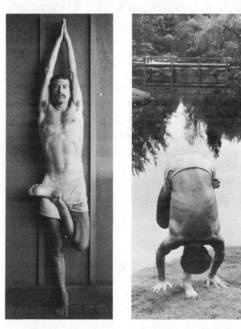

FIGURE 5.17B**   FIGURE 5.18**

to the floor. Stretch the back muscles and spine totally while lifting and straightening the standing leg (Figure 5.18). Once down, the bent knee can be adjusted and brought in close to the standing knee. Hold for five to 10 seconds before coming up slowly on the inhale. Repeat to the other side.

IYENGAR STANDING POSTURES

B.K.S. Iyengar has over the past decade become widely recognized as the foremost authority on Hatha Yoga. He has attained worldwide recognition because his approach is precise, challenging, well grounded in past tradition, and at the same time ever evolving. He insists that his students devote most of their time to the standing postures early in their training.

The next few pages will present some of the standing postures Mr. Iyengar so vehemently emphasizes. These include triangle, warrior I, extended lateral angle, warrior II, warrior III, half moon, rotating triangle, and revolving lateral angle. Certain of the instructions may not coincide with his in all respects. I have not personally studied with Mr. Iyengar, but I have taken numerous workshops from students of his.

The Iyengar standing postures require determined effort to be performed correctly. One must approach them with an attitude of physical and mental strength. Your body will not easily slip into the positions demanded of it in these standing poses, and only by correct body alignment and dedicated practice will you be able to properly perform them.

To move into each of these postures the general instruction is to bring the body to the completed pose on the exhale. You should breathe slowly and deeply in the asana for ten to 30 seconds, once in it. The general rule is then to come out of the pose in the reverse order that you moved into it, on the inhale. The breath is of utmost importance while performing these difficult postures, which demand that the whole body work hard. If you are to gain a sense of renewal from them, the breath must become a main focus of attention while you are working in the Iyengar standing poses.

Triangle

The triangle looks like a simple pose, but it is one of the most difficult of the standing asanas to do correctly. Its benefits are numerous. It develops the arches of the feet, strengthens the ankle joint, increases the circulation of the inner thighs by stretching them, works the quadriceps muscles, tones the outer-thigh and buttocks muscles, stretches the lateral torso muscles, improves digestion and elimination, and strengthens the neck muscles.

To move into the triangle posture, place the feet 36 to 42 inches apart. The heel of the left foot should be in direct line with the center of the arch of the right foot. The left foot turns out 90 degrees, and the right foot turns in slightly. Lift the arches of both feet. Lift the kneecaps and make sure that they are directed over the third toe; this is accomplished through contraction of quadriceps muscles and the outer buttocks muscles of both sides. Exhale, reach out with the left arm, and extend out with the spine. The fold of the front hip can be aided by pushing the left hand into the hip crease. The correct way to move the rib cage in Figure 5.19A is to rotate the left side of it under and roll the right side back as the legs and the buttocks stay solid.

Figure 5.19B shows the completed triangle pose, done to the opposite side from the preparatory posture shown in Figure 5.19A. In triangle the lower hand rests on the front shin bone as the other arm stretches straight up. As the arms reach out in opposite directions, draw the top shoulder blade in toward the spine and keep trying to lengthen the entire torso. Note the triangle formed by the arm, lower rib cage, and front leg.

Once in the pose, continue to open the back hip and roll the rib cage under as you turn the chest toward the ceiling. Try to keep length through the back of the neck as you look up to the outstretched hand. It is difficult to keep the neck vertebrae in alignment, but the neck muscles will become stronger by

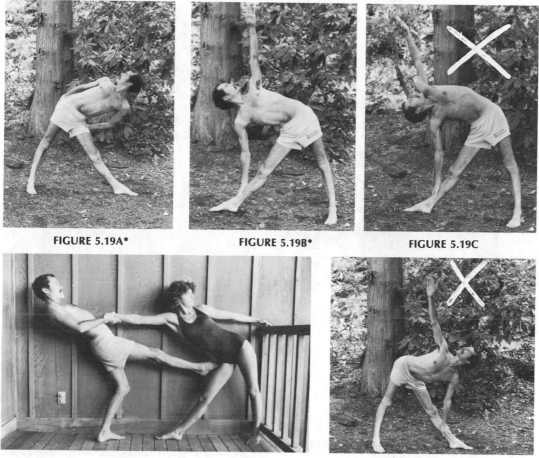

FIGURE 5.19A*   FIGURE 5.19B*   FIGURE 5.19C

FIGURE 5.19D*   FIGURE 5.19E

practicing triangle. Roll the rib cage under and try to turn the chest toward the ceiling with each exhale. Work in the pose for ten to 30 seconds and then repeat to the other side.

Figure 5.19C shows an example of a bad pose. Here the lower ribs are pressing against the hip bone, which causes the spine to bow rather than lengthen. To correct this, bring the bottom hand above the knee, bring the lower right rib-cage area slightly in front of the right hip bone, and extend through the right waist area. Folding inward at the hip socket rather than at the bottom of the rib cage is crucial in triangle.

The proper way to move into triangle can be understood by viewing the partner work shown in Figure 5.19D. Aided by a push with my foot and a pull with my whole body, Linda gets a deeper fold at the hip and increased elongation of the spine. Once there is a proper fold in the front hip, the hand can drop down to the shin; then Linda can contract her back buttocks muscles and open her back hip.

Figure 5.19E shows a bad pose. Here the mistake is opposite that shown in Figure 5.19C; the back is too swayed and there is a lack of work through the hips and the abdominal area. To eliminate swayback and create more length through the lumbar vertebrae, open the hips by contracting the buttocks muscles, tuck the pelvis, draw the abdominal

FIGURE
5.19F*

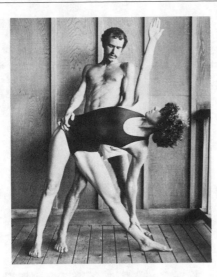

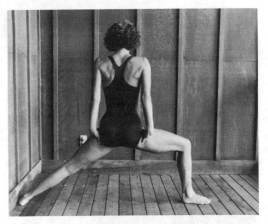

FIGURE 5.20A*

muscles in, and stretch the spine laterally out.

The partner work shown in Figure 5.19F shows how the foregoing can be attained. This is an excellent partner adjustment for triangle. My hip is pushed into Linda's left buttocks muscles to help her to tuck her pelvis under. I use my left hand to open her back (right) hip area by pulling it back. I use my other hand on the bottom side of the rib cage to try to create more length in her lumbar vertebrae and better rotation of her rib cage. Note the work of her feet, thighs, arm, and neck.

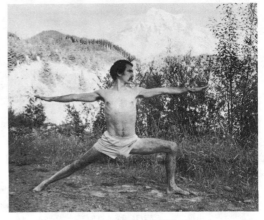

FIGURE 5.20B*

Warrior I

Warrior I is a powerful pose, as it gives you a sense of stability and increases the energy flowing throughout the entire body. It is a very graceful-looking pose, yet it takes a tremendous amount of work to maintain. Warrior I opens the hip joints to the utmost, develops the arches of the feet, tones the buttocks muscles, stretches the inner thigh muscles, strengthens the quadriceps, works the abdominal muscles, loosens the shoulder joints, increases lung capacity by stretching the chest muscles, and increases the circulation of blood throughout the body.

To begin warrior I, spread the feet 48 to 54 inches apart. As shown in Figure 5.20A, the

FIGURE 5.20C

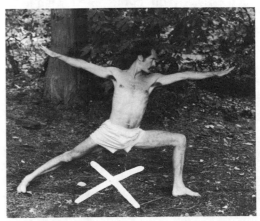

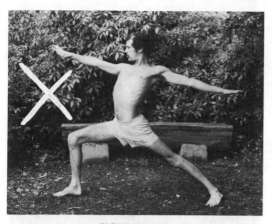

FIGURE 5.20D

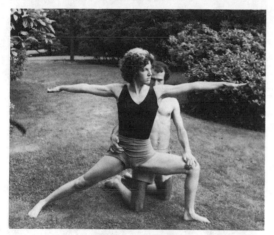

FIGURE 5.20E*

scribed in Figure 5.20A, lift the chest and stretch out through the arms and fingers. Keeping the arms parallel to the floor, look out over the front hand (Figure 5.20B). Keep the shoulders back and down, the back of the neck long, and the abdominal muscles drawn in. Work in the pose for ten to 30 seconds. This may be the most effective of all standing postures for firming up the calf, thigh, and buttocks muscles. Repeat to the other side.

Figure 5.20C shows a warrior pose in which the spine is misaligned. The spine should be lifted vertically in warrior I, and the arms stretched out parallel to the floor.

Warrior I pose done as shown in Figure 5.20D causes lower-back compression. To correct the problem, contract the buttocks muscles, open the back hip, roll the pelvis under, and then draw the lower ribs in through the contractive work of the abdominal muscles.

Figure 5.20E shows a very helpful partner adjustment for warrior I. The incorrect pose shown in Figure 5.20D could result in knee problems, as well as lower-back problems. The front knee should be directed over the center of the front foot; so here I am trying to help Linda open her front hip joint by pushing my hip against her front buttocks and pulling her front knee back. Most importantly, the back hip should open and the knee of the straightened leg should face forward. Here I am helping this to occur by pulling Linda's back hip toward me and helping her tuck her pelvis under. This adjustment allows both of the hip joints to open externally and the knees to safely turn in opposite directions. Then the work is to lift vertically up through the spine and stretch through the arms. (You can perform warrior I against a wall to help you to understand the work of the pose, as shown by Linda in Figure 4.17.)

Extended Lateral Angle

Extended lateral angle has most of the same benefits as warrior I but also helps lengthen

outer edge of the back foot can be placed against a wall. Bend the front (right) knee and make sure it is directed over the center of the right foot. Pull the abdomen in, tuck the pelvis, rotate the quadriceps muscles and knees of both legs outward by contracting the buttocks muscles, and lift the arches of both feet. Keep the hips level and facing forward. Stretch the spine up and out of the seat of the pelvis. Here Linda is using her hands to help tuck under the pelvis.

In the completed warrior I pose, the bent knee forms a 90-degree angle, and the spine is stretched up vertically. Continuing the proper work through the feet, legs, hips, pelvis, buttocks, and abdomen that was de-

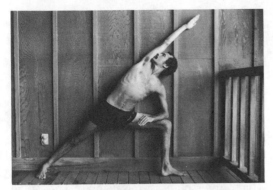

FIGURE 5.21A*

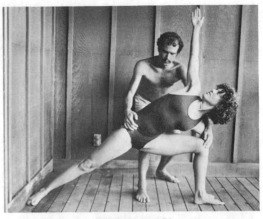

FIGURE 5.21C*

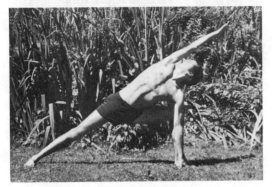

FIGURE 5.21B*

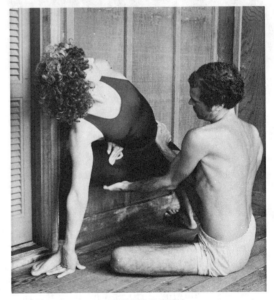

FIGURE 5.21D*

the waist and lateral rib-cage areas. It is excellent for the digestive and eliminative systems; stretching the waist area out gives more room to the internal organs so that they can function more efficiently.

Starting in warrior I against a wall, exhale, extend the torso out over the bent leg, and rest the left elbow on the thigh. Stretch through the outer edge of the back foot, and lift the inner thigh of the back leg. Keep the front knee over the third toe with a little assistance from the elbow (Figure 5.21A). Stretch strongly through the right arm, waist, and leg. Work for ten to 20 seconds, inhale up, and repeat to the other side.

From the position shown in Figure 5.21A, exhale, slide the bottom hand down in front of the shin, and grasp the inner ankle, or bring the hand to the floor as shown in Figure 5.21B. Next push the arm back against the knee, contract the buttocks muscles, open the back hip, and drop down with the hips until the front knee forms a 90-degree angle. Roll to the outer edge of the back foot, tuck the pelvis, and roll the rib cage under with each exhale. Stretch the top arm over the ear. The back leg, the lateral side of the torso, and the top arm should form a perfectly straight line. Do not be static. Upon reaching the final position, try to roll the rib cage under with each exhale by pulling the top shoulder blade in toward the spine and by tucking the pelvis.

Consciously stretch out through the back leg, waist, spine, and top arm with each inhale. The chin should move toward the top shoulder. Work each side for ten to 30 seconds, remembering to breathe deeply and slowly.

Partner work is very helpful for this posture. In Figure 5.21C, I push my right knee into Linda's left gluteus muscles while pulling her right hip and left knee back. Note the position of her back (right) foot; it is very helpful to have the wall to push the outer edge of the foot against. Linda's top arm is stretching straight up, which allows her to pull her top shoulder blade in toward the spine and to flatten the top side of the rib-cage area. I help Linda to move more deeply into the pose for two to four breaths, making the most progress during each exhale.

Another way to teach the body how to properly work in the extended lateral angle is shown in the partner adjustment in Figure 5.21D. Here I am trying to roll Linda's right hip under as she pushes her right knee open with her arm and I push her left hip back with my right hand. Linda has brought her left arm behind her back and is holding the inner thigh of her right leg. This helps her to rotate her upper back properly. Work each side for ten to 20 seconds, making the greatest adjustments each time Linda exhales.

Warrior II

Warrior II loosens and strengthens the shoulder joints, opens the chest, and strengthens the buttocks muscles. It also tones and stretches the calf, quadriceps, outer-thigh, iliopsoas, abdominal, and upper-back muscles. This pose stimulates an increased flow of energy to move throughout the body. Warrior II is a perfect lead-in to warrior III and the revolving lateral-angle pose.

To begin warrior II, spread the feet about four feet apart, inhale, and turn the feet and torso until the chest is square over the front thigh. Squaring the hips is the key to the rotation of the torso. Squeeze the buttocks muscles of the back leg, tuck the pelvis, and stretch the arms upward (Figure 5.22A).

From Figure 5.22A, exhale, bend the front knee, and direct it over the center of the front foot, moving the knee joint toward a 90-degree angle. Continue to squeeze the buttock of the back leg and tuck the pelvis under strongly, pull in and up with the abdominal muscles. Lift the quadriceps muscles of the back leg and stretch through the heel of that leg. In Figure 5.22B, I have the back heel close to the ground, but it is safer on the knee joint to turn the back foot inward, as shown in Figure 5.22C. Rotate your shoulders back and down as you reach upward. Work for ten to 30 seconds in the pose, breathing deeply. Repeat to the other side.

Using a wall is very helpful in the practice of warrior II; pressing the back heel firmly against a wall creates a more solid base to stretch out of (Figure 5.22C). The back leg should be stretched to the utmost, with quadriceps muscles and gluteus muscles of that leg contracting. Work both sides for ten to 30 seconds.

The greatest mistake you can make in warrior II is to overarch the lower spine, as shown in Figure 5.22D. This causes pain in the lumbar vertebrae because of compression of the spinal discs and possible pinching of the nerves. The way to avoid this is to lift the abdominal muscles firmly up and in and squeeze the gluteus muscles of the back leg tightly.

When doing warrior II or any backbend in which the shoulders, arms, elbows, and hands are stretched behind the line of the neck and ears, there is a tendency for the muscles at the top of the shoulders to bunch up. This can create a painful, pinched feeling and must be avoided. In order to rotate the shoulder joint properly, the shoulders should initially drop back and down, and then the arms can be stretched up and pulled back.

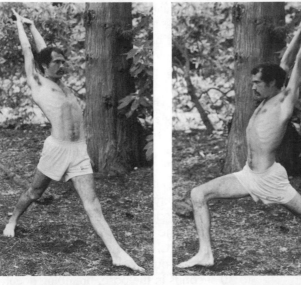

FIGURE 5.22A*   **FIGURE 5.22B***

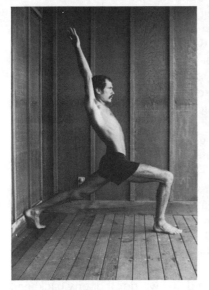

FIGURE 5.22C*

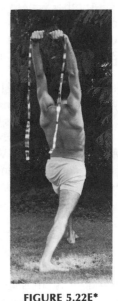

FIGURE 5.22D   **FIGURE 5.22E***

Using a strap helps the upper-back muscles to contract properly, allowing the shoulders to drop back and down (Figure 5.22E). Begin with the hands gripping the strap at shoulder-width apart. The key is to feel as if the shoulder-blade area is brought in toward the spine as you stretch the hands upward. Work each side for ten to 30 seconds.

Warrior III

Warrior III is a real challenge. If done properly, it stretches the whole backside of the body, thus increasing the energy flow throughout. It works the standing leg to the utmost and takes complete concentration for you to maintain your balance. The benefits to

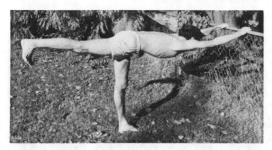

FIGURE 5.23A*

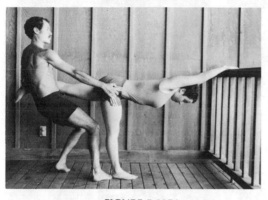

FIGURE 5.23B*

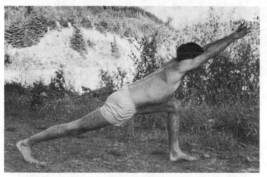

FIGURE 5.23C*

FIGURE 5.23D**

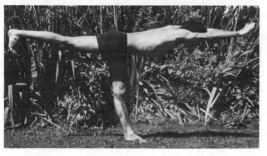

the muscular system are similar to those of warrior I and warrior II.

Warrior III is not too difficult if the wrists rest over a bar or table top, as shown in Figure 5.23A. Rest the wrists on a bar or take hold of it, bring the hips over the feet, lift the right leg until it is parallel to the floor, and stretch through the heel of that foot. Lift up through the standing leg, making sure that the knee is pointing straight forward. Lift up through the hip of the standing leg, level the hips by turning the back-leg hip down, draw the abdominal muscles in, and stretch through the spine and arms. Look toward the hands, breathe deeply, hold for five to ten seconds, and then repeat to the other side.

Partner work is very helpful for warrior III. As one leg is lifted in warrior III, the hips should remain square. In Figure 5.23B, I am pulling the hip of Jennifer's standing leg back and giving her a good stretch throughout the entire body. The stretched-out leg, the torso, and the arms should all be perfectly parallel to the floor. Notice the deep fold in Jennifer's right hip, the length attained through her torso, and the lift through her standing leg. Work each side for ten to 20 seconds.

Warrior III in its advanced stage should be performed in the center of the room following warrior II (Figure 5.22A). From warrior II, exhale and lean out over the bent knee, as shown in Figure 5.23C. Then inhale and slowly straighten the standing leg, bringing the back leg parallel to the floor, as shown in Figure 5.23D. The keys, it is important to remember, are to lift firmly with the quadriceps muscles of the standing leg, square the hips, draw the abdominal muscles up and in, and stretch the arms and the top leg in opposite directions. Make sure that the knee of the standing leg faces forward, that the other knee points down, and that the stretch of the lifted leg carries through the heel and base of the toes. Work in the pose for five to ten seconds and gracefully return to warrior II. Repeat to the other side.

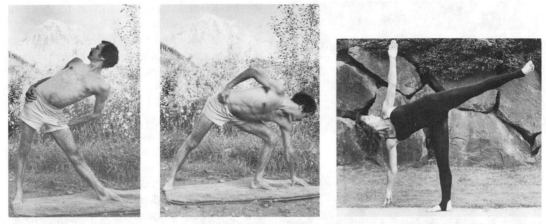

FIGURE 5.24A*   FIGURE 5.24B*   FIGURE 5.24C**

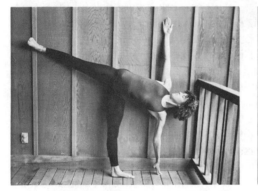 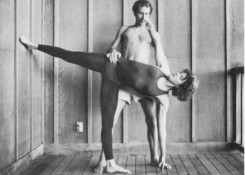

FIGURE 5.24D*   FIGURE 5.24E**

Half Moon

Half moon is a very beautiful pose that can transform both the body and the mind. It is excellent for opening the hips and toning the thigh and buttocks muscles.

Along with the benefits just mentioned, this posture helps to develop the arches in the feet, strengthens the ankles, stretches the calf muscles, trims the outer thighs, frees the rib cage for rotational movement, and opens the chest.

You must be careful to not overstretch the inner-thigh muscles in half moon; it is important to loosen these muscles first. Performing triangle, warrior I, and extended lateral angle before attempting half moon is a good idea.

Study Figures 5.24A and 5.24B carefully. Half moon comes out of triangle pose, Figure 5.24A. From triangle, bend the knee and place the hand two to six inches in front of and to the outside of the front foot, as shown in Figure 5.24B. Then lift one leg, squeeze the buttocks of the standing leg, tuck the pelvis by bringing the bottom over the standing foot, and pull the top hip back. To begin with, you may find it easiest to keep your balance by looking down at the ground. Figure 5.24C shows half moon done to the opposite side from the preparatory poses shown in Figures 5.24A and 5.24B. Once you are in the completed pose, the standing leg should lift strongly as you stretch through the base of the big toe of the lifted leg and lengthen through the spine. Roll the rib cage under until the chest faces forward. Pull the top shoulder away from the ear and stretch out through the arms. Once stability is found, turn the head and fix the gaze in an upward direction. Work in the pose for five to 20 seconds, then bend the knee of the standing leg, inhale, and return to triangle. Repeat to the other side.

The wall is very helpful in doing half moon because it frees you from the concern of a possible fall. Starting in triangle position with the upper back against the wall and the front foot parallel to and two to four inches from it, bend the knee, bring the hand to the floor close to the wall, and move up into the half moon (Figure 5.24D). Work the body in the same manner as just described in Figure 5.24C; try to bring the buttock of the standing leg away from the wall and the other buttock toward the wall. If it is difficult to bring the bottom hand to the floor, it can be placed on a block of wood or thick book three to six inches in height.

Another way to use the wall is shown here by Linda. Partners can be very effective for this pose. In Figure 5.24E, I am trying to open Linda's hips by pushing my hip into her left buttock and pulling her right hip back with my right hand. I am helping Linda to lengthen the lower back with my left hand as she rotates her rib cage.

Rotating Triangle

Rotating triangle is a difficult pose. The intense stretch of the front leg muscles is the major drawback that stops many people from performing it correctly; however, the benefits are numerous. It tones the leg muscles, loosens the hip joints, relieves back tension, and frees the rib cage for rotational movement.

This posture is a superb aid to the functioning of the stomach, liver, gallbladder, intestines, pancreas, kidneys, and adrenal glands.

Begin by bringing the feet about three feet apart (slightly closer than for the straight triangle). Inhale and turn the right foot out 90 degrees and the left foot in 60 degrees. Exhale, lift through the front leg, and fold deeply into the front hip as the left arm reaches straight out (Figure 5.25A).

From Figure 5.25A, continue to exhale and stretch out with the spine as the left hand comes to the floor (Figure 5.25B). Most people will find their balance better if they keep the bottom hand in front of and to the inside of the front leg as the other arm stretches straight up and the head and chest turn. The key to doing the rotating triangle is to keep weight on the heel of the back foot as the spine stretches and the rib cage rolls under. Work in the pose ten to 20 seconds. Inhale to come up slowly, exhale, and repeat to the other side.

The wall is a great aid for the rotating triangle. In Figure 5.25C, the chest has been brought next to the wall as the top arm stretches up against it. To set up the pose, begin with the back to the wall and the feet about three feet apart, with the left heel an inch from the wall and the right foot turned out 90 degrees; the right heel should be in line with the center of the arch of the left foot. Then reach out with the left hand, as in Figure 5.25A, and stretch the right arm back along the wall. Exhale and slowly come down to the position shown in Figure 5.25C, stretching back with the left heel, reaching up with the right arm, lifting up with the inside hip, and rotating the rib cage, chest, and neck as much as possible. Work each side for ten to 20 seconds.

A second way to use the wall in the rotating triangle is to bring the back against it. Begin by facing the wall, bring the toes of the right foot one inch or less from the wall and the heel of the left foot in line with the arch

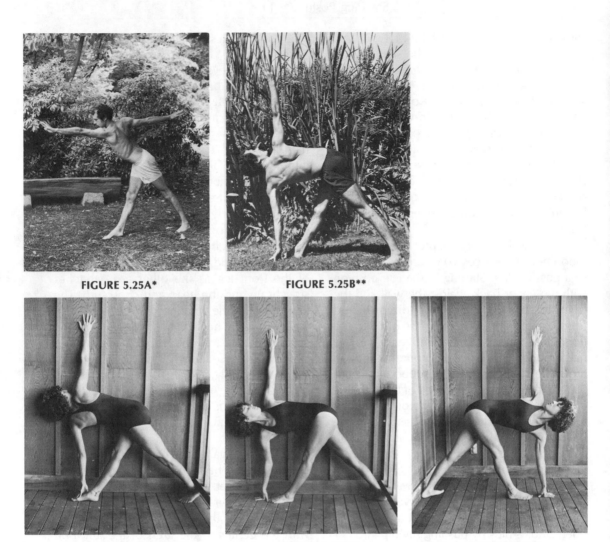

FIGURE 5.25A*   FIGURE 5.25B**

FIGURE 5.25C*   FIGURE 5.25D*   FIGURE 5.25E*

of the right foot and turned out 90 degrees, as shown in Figure 5.25D. While still upright, turn the torso until the back flattens against the wall. Reach out with the right arm and back with the left arm. Slowly descend down to rotating triangle on the exhale. Work each side for ten to 20 seconds, breathing deeply during the pose.

To help keep the back heel down in rotating triangle, the wall can be used in a third way, as shown in Figure 5.25E. Pushing the heel back against the corner of the floor allows proper work in the back leg to occur. The arch of the back foot should lift. The stretch of the front leg stops many people. To help here, instead of bringing the hand to the floor, use a thick block of wood placed on the floor to rest the hand on. Work each side ten to 20 seconds.

Revolving Lateral-Angle Pose

Revolving lateral-angle pose is excellent for toning the thigh and buttocks muscles and breaking up upper-back tension. It is also su-

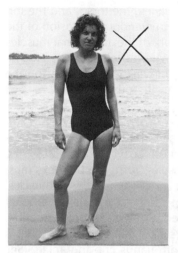

FIGURE 5.26A

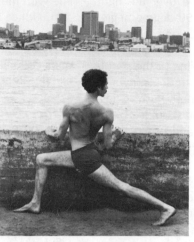

FIGURE 5.26B*

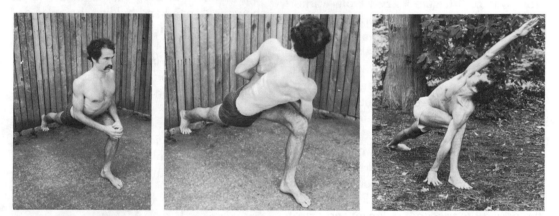

FIGURE 5.26C*   FIGURE 5.26D*   FIGURE 5.26E***

perb for the eliminative and digestive systems. If you are prone to constipation, poor digestion, or liver weakness, you should do this prose daily. I highly recommend the use of a wall or bar while working on the posture, especially for the relief of backaches.

Many people develop the habit of throwing out the hip of the standing leg, causing the lower spine to be pulled in the direction the hip has gone, as shown in Figure 5.26A. The upper spine must move in the opposite direction in order to compensate. This very common habit often leads to an unbalanced carriage of the body and side-

ways curvature of the spine. The unfortunate result is a backache.

If you have developed the habit shown in Figure 5.26A, the posture shown in Figure 5.26B should be emphasized in your yoga workouts. You should practice twisting away from the hip that you tend to throw out. Begin with the back to the wall, the feet three to five inches from the wall and 48 to 54 inches apart. Inhale, turn the feet and torso 90 degrees to the right, lift the left heel, bend the right knee, contract the left buttocks, and square and level the hips. As you stretch through the left leg and slide it back slightly, direct the right knee over the right ankle and move toward a 90-degree angle. Exhale, rotate the rib cage, and bring the hands to the wall slightly more than shoulder-width apart and below the line of the shoulders. Squeeze the buttocks muscles inward, tuck the pelvis, and lift the chest. Push against the wall, contract the right shoulder blade muscles, lengthen the neck, and look over the right shoulder. Work in the pose for ten to 30 seconds, breathing deeply. Repeat to the other side; then repeat both sides once again.

Pushing the back heel against a wall can be of great help in achieving a solid base for the more advanced revolving lateral-angle twist. The best way to approach the pose is from warrior II (Figure 5.22C). From warrior II, inhale and bring both hands to the left knee, pull against the knee, draw the shoulders back and down, and lift the chest out.

From the position shown in Figure 5.26C, exhale, twist the rib cage to the left, and bring the right elbow outside the left knee. Lift the chest out and rotate the rib cage strongly around. Lift the back knee as the back-leg buttock continues to contract, and keep the base of the big toe of the back foot pressed firmly against the floor in order to help avoid overturning the back hip. Work in the pose for ten seconds or longer and repeat to the other side.

In the most advanced pose, the lower hand comes to the floor and the top arm stretches out over the ear. It is a mistake, however, to bring the hand onto the floor until you feel secure doing the posture as shown in Figure 5.26D. Make sure to press the arm and knee against each other when performing the final version of the revolving lateral-angle pose. In the most advanced version of this pose, the back heel will stay down; however, the heel should lift and the foot should turn in 90 degrees if any knee pain occurs when attempting the back-foot position shown here. The goal of the posture is to form a straight line with the back leg, the torso, and the top arm. Notice the tremendous extension of the body and the work of the abdominal muscles in Figure 5.26E. Work each side for ten seconds or longer, moving into the twist on the exhale. Repeat to the other side.

Dancer's Pose (Both Arms Back)
Dancer's pose loosens the shoulder joints, expands the chest cavity, activates the upper-back muscles, firms the buttocks muscles, and tones and stretches the leg muscles. It is a good pose to help you develop better balance and better powers of concentration.

In the version of dancer's pose shown in Figure 5.27, both hands grip the ankle. (See Figures 4.21A, B, and C for the dancer's pose shown with one hand holding the ankle and the other arm stretching up.) The posture shown here is a bit more difficult to do than the dancer's pose in Chapter 4, but it allows a greater expansion of the chest cavity and a deeper contraction of the upper-back muscles.

To do the pose, stand erect, bend the right knee, lift the foot, flex the raised ankle, take hold of the ankle with both hands, contract the buttocks muscles, and tuck the pel-

FIGURE 5.27*

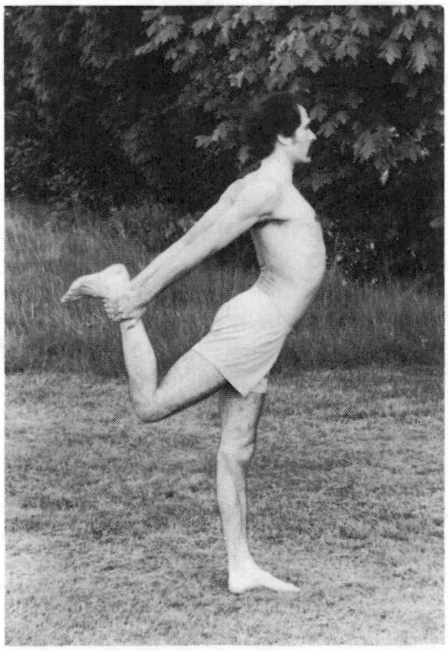

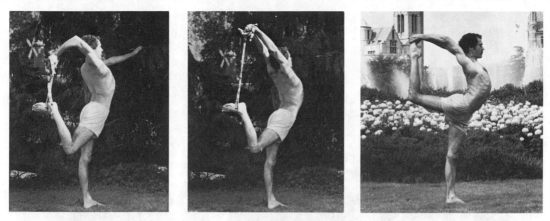

FIGURE 5.28A*   **FIGURE 5.28B****   **FIGURE 5.28C*****

vis. Inhale, lift up through the standing leg, pull the raised foot back, stretch the arms, and open the chest. Look straight ahead and breathe deeply for five to 20 seconds. Repeat to the other side.

King Dancer Pose

King dancer is an elegant pose and its benefits are numerous. It loosens the shoulder joints, improves balance and concentration, strengthens and stretches the leg muscles, tones the gluteus muscles, and increases your breathing capacity.

Pay close attention to working the pelvis and shoulder joint correctly while doing the king dancer pose. Use of a strap is very helpful. Figure 5.28A shows that the elbow is brought in close to the head in the initial rotation of the shoulder. Try to relax the shoulder-joint muscles and squeeze the shoulder blades in before pulling back with the raised foot. Strongly contract the buttocks muscles of the lifted leg; this protects the lower-back area by lengthening the lumbar vertebrae. You should consciously square the hips and tuck the pelvis. Figure 5.28B shows that the upper-back muscles must be drawn inward as both arms are stretched upward. Figure 5.28C shows the final pose without the aid of a strap.

Work each side for five to 15 seconds if you do it without a strap. The posture can be held for ten to 30 seconds with the use of a strap. Do both sides.

Chair Pose   The chair pose strengthens the thigh muscles and helps to straighten swayback. Bend at the knees until the quadriceps muscles have been brought parallel to the floor. Keep the knees together and imagine that you are sitting on a chair (Figure 5.29). Lengthen the spine, draw the abdominal muscles in, and flatten the lower back against the wall. Work in the pose for ten seconds to one minute, breathing slowly and deeply.

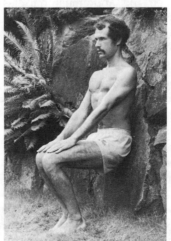

FIGURE 5.29*

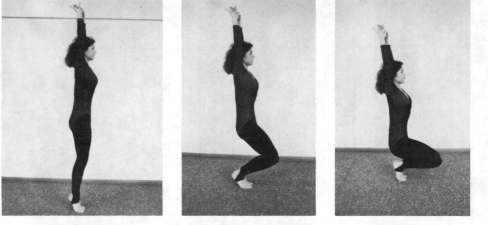

FIGURE 5.30A*   FIGURE 5.30B*   FIGURE 5.30C*

Swayback Exercise   This is a good exercise to do to help correct swayback. It will strengthen the abdominal and quadriceps muscles, loosen the ankle, knee, and hip joints, and develop concentrative and balancing powers. It looks simple, but it is very difficult to maintain a straight spine while descending slowly and coming slowly up.

Bring the feet and legs together, inhale, and raise up onto the ball of the toes. Stretch the arms straight up, draw the abdominal muscles in, and tuck the pelvis under (Figure 5.30A). Exhale and slowly go down by bending at the knees, as shown in Figure 5.30B. Continue to keep the abdominal muscles drawn in, the spine lifted, the knees together, and the arms stretched upward, as you descend until the bottom comes close to the heels. Pause a short while at the bottom of the descent, as in Figure 5.30C. Then inhale, and slowly come up with the abdominal muscles drawn in and the pelvis tucked under to help maintain the straight alignment of the spine. Ascend to the position shown in Figure 5.30A. Practice going down and coming up slowly two or three more times.

Squat Posture   The squat position gives relief to the lower-back muscles and adds more space to the lumbar vertebrae. Practice of it opens the hip socket, loosens the knee joints, breaks up tension in the iliopsoas muscles, develops arches in the feet, and helps the organs of digestion, elimination, and reproduction. Women who are pregnant can find relief from lower-back pain in this posture.

A bar, tabletop, or door handle is a great aid for the squat posture. Begin standing upright with the feet slightly more than shoulder-width apart and parallel to each other. Keep the spine vertical as you go down by drawing in the stomach muscles, dropping the pelvis, lifting the chest, and elongating the back of the neck (Figure 5.31A). Once you are down, try to open the knees and allow the lower-back muscles to elongate. The feet should be parallel while squatting. Remain in the pose for ten seconds to two minutes or longer.

Partner work can be quite helpful in the squat posture. Begin by standing a couple of feet from your partner with the feet spread slightly more than shoulder-width apart, and take hold of your partner's wrist with straightened arms. Both should lean back against the pull of the arms, open the knees, and go down slowly into the squat position with a straight spine (Figure 5.31B). Once down, keep the feet parallel to each other, the heels down, lift the chest, and maintain the pose for a few

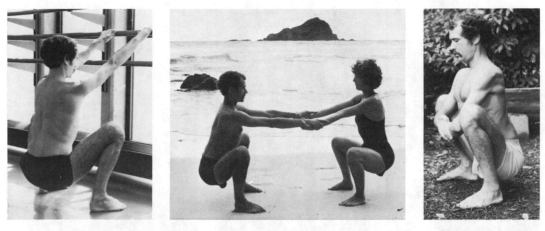

FIGURE 5.31A*   FIGURE 5.31B*   FIGURE 5.31C**

seconds. Try to release the grip of your partner and maintain balance for a brief moment; then rejoin hands and come up slowly.

As you bend your knees, keep the center of the kneecap in line with the center of the foot, if not outside. You may have to lift the heels to do this, although is is best to keep them down as you squat. Once in the squat position, bring the elbows to the inner-knee area and open the hip joint more and more by pushing out with the elbows. Lift and open the chest, draw the upper-back muscles inward, and allow the pelvis to drop close to the floor (Figure 5.31C). The feet should stay parallel to each other, the spine lifted in a vertical direction. Hold this pose anywhere from ten seconds to five minutes.

Standing Forward Stretches

Benefits   The spinal column and the lower-back muscles stretch to the utmost in forward-bending action. A person who sits several hours a day invariably develops a compressed lower back; the back needs to be periodically stretched to relieve stress on the lower-back muscles and to release pressure on the spinal discs. If the spinal discs (the cushions between the individual vertebrae) become overly compressed, the nerves coming out of the spinal cord may be pinched. Forward stretches can increase the length between the vertebrae and can help to relieve backaches.

The most obvious benefit of the forward stretches is increased blood flow into the legs. The legs need to be stretched periodically to bring blood and energy back into them. For the jogger, the forward stretches are an important counterbalance to the shortening of the hamstrings that occurs while jogging. Furthermore, the knee joint and the lumbar vertebrae are compressed while running, and this can lead to serious problems. To avoid this, forward stretches should be done before and after jogging. It is also a good idea to do a few other standing postures before and after jogging as well.

The abdominal area becomes inverted in a forward stretch, which means the internal organs get a deep massage. Squeezing the abdominal muscles against the organs of digestion and elimination helps them to work more efficiently.

The endocrine glands secrete hormones that can only reach their specific target areas through the bloodstream. Forward stretches improve the circulation of blood throughout the body; thus, the endocrine system also begins to work more efficiently. The adrenal

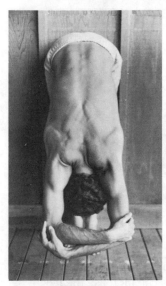

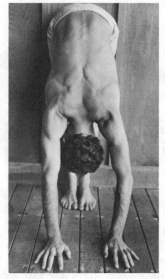

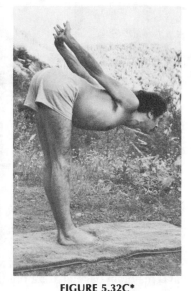

FIGURE 5.32A*   FIGURE 5.32B*   FIGURE 5.32C*

glands are particularly stimulated because of the long stretch across the back muscles. Standing forward stretches will also work directly on the pituitary gland, master gland of the endocrine system, as holding these poses brings increased blood into the pituitary.

Attitude Your attitude in approaching the standing forward stretches should be opposite that of the more vigorous standing postures. You must develop a submissive attitude and allow the leg, buttocks, and lower-back muscles to stretch out passively. The deep fold in the front side of the hip socket is the most active work that occurs in the standing forward stretches, and the main attention should be to tilt the pelvis upward. Allow the whole backside of the leg, from the calf all the way through the buttocks muscles, to stretch out evenly while holding these postures. Do not fight the pain of the stretch at the back of the knees. Let go into the stretch by breathing deeply.

Breath During Forward Stretches Exhale to fold forward and move into a forward stretch. While you're in the pose, you should breathe slowly and steadily. If you want to stretch farther, do so as you exhale. After more elongation is achieved, maintain whatever gain was achieved on the inhale. You can stretch out farther and farther by moving with each exhale. After being in the pose for the desired length of time, inhale and slowly come out of the standing forward stretch. If you have held the forward stretch for more than 20 seconds, be very careful when coming to an upright position, since blood will move out of the brain as you stand.

Resting Forward Stretch This rest position is excellent in between the more vigorous standing postures. It can be done without a wall, but the wall can help you lift the bottom higher. You have a choice of keeping the feet together, as shown in Figure 5.32A, or separating them the width of your hips, or wider. The heels can be anywhere from four inches to one inch away from the wall. The more flexible you are, the closer you can bring them to the wall.

To move into the pose, lift the buttocks up the wall, and keep trying to raise the bottom higher by folding deeper into the hip

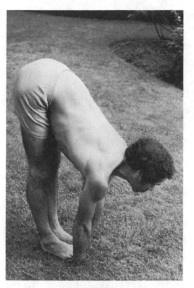

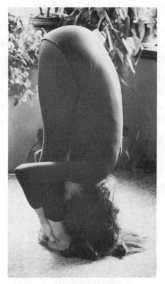

FIGURE 5.33A**   **FIGURE 5.33B****

socket. Keep the folded elbows stretching out behind the line of the ears, as this will aid the flattening of the middle- and upper-back areas. Relax into the pose, breathing steadily and deeply. The longer this pose is held, the greater the flow of blood into the brain. This posture can be held anywhere from ten seconds to three minutes or longer. Holding the pose a long while can elicit a feeling of tranquility.

In Figure 5.32B, the hands rest on the floor a few inches in front of the toes. Keep lifting the buttocks up the wall. As in the previous pose, the heels can be one to four inches from the wall; the feet can be together or apart. This pose can also be held for ten seconds to three minutes or even longer. You can get a true sense of renewal from the postures shown in Figures 5.32A and B.

Begin the pose shown in Figure 5.32C by standing straight. Interweave the fingers behind the back, turn the palms toward the buttocks, and stretch the arms down by moving the heel of the hands toward the floor and rotating the inner elbow out. Then rotate the wrist all the way by stretching through the heels of the hands with the fingers facing out.

The key to maintaining the position is to squeeze the shoulder blades in toward the spine. An alternative is to interweave the fingers and pull the wrists toward the floor. After setting up the arm and hand position, fold forward at the hips, lift the kneecaps, and stretch out through the spine by pulling the chest forward. Continue to lift the hands and stretch the arms. Straightening the arms and reaching up and out with them as you hold the forward stretch helps the upper back to flatten and the spine to straighten. Work in the pose for ten to thirty seconds.

Gaining Leverage in the Forward Stretch
The lower back will get an improper stretch if the upper back is overly rounded in the forward stretches. To straighten the spine, step on the hands, straighten the arms, and look up, as shown in Figure 5.33A. To flatten the upper back, squeeze the shoulder blades inward, pull the expanded chest out and down, and then elongate the entire spine. Work in the pose for 20 to 30 seconds.

Holding the back of the ankles and pulling the elbows in toward each other behind the legs helps you to get good pulling leverage in the standing forward stretch (Figure 5.33B). The hips should continue to lift, and you should persist in trying to fold deeper at the hip socket. Relax the back of the legs, buttocks, and the lower-back muscles and breathe steadily and deeply. Shift the weight toward the ball of the toes rather than the heels and bring the bottom straight above the feet. Feel as if there is an even stretch throughout the whole backside of the legs. The key idea is to lift the legs straight up and stretch the spine straight down. Hold for ten seconds to two minutes.

Forward Stretch (Back Against Wall)

Bringing the back against the wall can help the flexible student get an extra stretch while folding forward. In Figure 5.34, the middle back is flattened against the wall as the folded elbows are extended down toward the floor. The bottom and the legs lift strongly up, as a deep fold in the front of the hip joints occurs and the feet are brought in as close to the wall as is comfortably possible. Hang forward in this pose for ten seconds to two minutes, breathing deeply and relaxing the backside muscles of the body.

FIGURE 5.34*   **FIGURE 5.35****

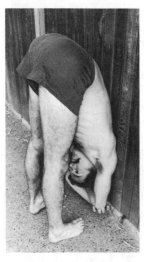
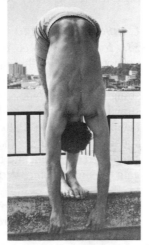

Forward Stretch (With Ledge)

Note the excellent stretch of the spine in Figure 5.35. I have hung my toes over the top of the ledge, hooked my fingers around the bottom of the ledge, and pulled the spine down with the aid of arm leverage. The flexible person has to be creative in finding aids to help his or her postures along. This pose can be worked on for ten seconds to two minutes.

Standing Forward Stretches (Feet Apart)

When the feet are apart, the standing forward stretches loosen the hip sockets for external rotation, stretch the inner-thigh muscles, and develop the arches of the feet as well as providing the benefits previously mentioned for forward stretches in the introduction. Separating the feet makes it easier to lift the bottom and tilt the pelvis upward than when the feet are together. Many people will feel less stress at the back of the knee with the feet apart. You should do both kinds of forward stretches in a workout.

The modified dog posture, as shown in Figure 5.36A, is one of the best of the standing forward stretches for attaining a good even stretch through the whole body. Spread the feet 36 to 54 inches apart, lift the bottom straight up in the air, exhale, fold forward, and stretch the spine and hands out and down. Keep the hips above the line of the feet, grip the ground with the outer edges of the feet, lift the kneecaps, and drop the lower ribs, middle back, and chest. Hold for 20 seconds to one minute or longer, breathing deeply.

From modified dog, grip the outside of the ankles, inhale, expand the chest, and stretch the spine. Keep the middle back dropped by contracting the muscles between the shoulder blades. Looking up helps the middle back to drop. Exhale, and continue to feel the chest muscles expanding as you slowly lower the forehead toward the floor, maintaining the straightness of the spine and the upward tilt of the pelvis (Figure 5.36B). Work in the pose for ten to 20 seconds.

Continuing from Figure 5.36B, drop the

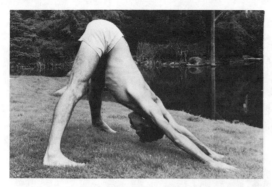

FIGURE 5.36A*

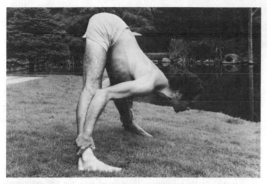

FIGURE 5.36B*

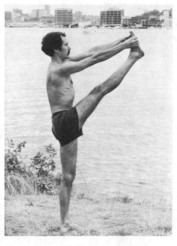

FIGURE 5.37**

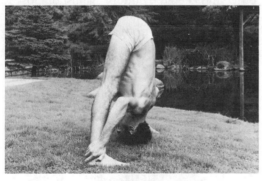

FIGURE 5.36C**

head, lift the buttocks, and stretch the lower back. Notice how straight the back is in Figure 5.36C. This pose will release blocked energy from the back of the legs, hip sockets, inner thighs, pelvic region, and back muscles. If you can, bring the head to the floor and relax in the pose for 20 seconds to one minute. Allow the blood to move into the brain, and breathe deeply.

One-Legged Standing Stretch It is very difficult to maintain straight alignment of the standing leg and spine in the one-legged standing stretch (Figure 5.37) while gaining height with the raised leg and squareness of the hips. The main benefit is that the back of the raised leg is stretched to the utmost.

Grasp the right foot with the right hand, lift and straighten the right leg, and drop the right hip. Then bring the left hand to the foot as well, and lift the straightened leg. (A strap can be used if you cannot hold the leg straight without it.) The standing leg and spine should be perfectly vertical, the shoulders should be dropped, and the chest lifted. Work in the pose for five to 20 seconds. Release slowly and repeat to the other side.

One-Legged Standing Hip Opener
The one-legged standing hip opener stretches and tones the leg muscles, loosens the hip socket, and develops balance and concentration. It is a difficult posture to perform correctly. The work is to take hold of one foot, stretch the leg out to the side, and keep the spine in perfect vertical alignment while standing on the other foot. Ideally, the posture is done in the center of the floor without any aids; however, the lifted foot can be held with

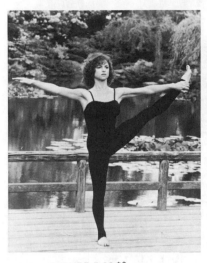

FIGURE 5.38 **

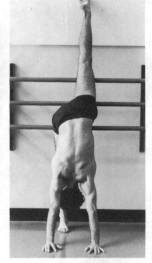

FIGURE 5.39 **

a strap if you cannot reach the foot without this aid. In Figure 5.38, Diann is lifting strongly upward with her standing leg and spine to maintain a vertical line. She is dropping her left hip down, stretching her arms out, and pulling her foot back with her hand. Work in the pose for five to 20 seconds and repeat to the other side.

Standing Front Splits   The standing front splits give a very intense stretch to the back-side of the standing leg, loosen the hip joints and back muscles, and energize the whole body. Begin in a standing forward stretch with the heels together and two to three feet from the wall. Bend one knee and lift the other leg up the wall; straighten both legs, paying most attention to the standing leg. If you can move the standing leg back toward the wall, do so, but make sure that the weight of the torso is carried more by the standing leg than the hands and that the leg is straight. Try to square the hips by lifting strongly with the hip of the standing leg, contracting the outer-thigh muscles of the leg, and turning the upward-stretching leg hip-down. Note the straight line of the spine shown in Figure 5.39. Hold for ten to 20 seconds, breathing deeply.

Standing Side Splits   The standing side splits stretch the inner-thigh muscles to the limit, loosen the hip sockets, and release blocked energy in the pelvic area.

From modified dog stretch (Figure 5.36A), slowly slide the feet away from each other and keep the bottom against or close to the wall. When the inner thighs reach their limit, move away from the wall by pushing down with the hands, and bring the chest down (Figure 5.40). Less stress will be incurred by the inner thigh muscles the further you bring the chest away from the wall. Try it two or three times, but do not hold any portion of the movement for more than a few seconds.

FIGURE 5.40**

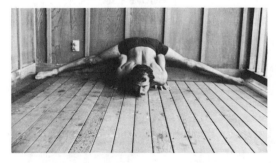

Rhythm of Yoga Movement

We have a choice as to the rhythm in which we perform the Hatha Yoga asanas. We may move in and out of one posture after another in a flowing, dancelike fashion, or we may move through fewer postures and hold them longer. Of course, the particular posture or set of postures chosen to work on will determine to a large extent how long the posture should be held. How long to hold a particular posture is a controversial subject, however, and present-day Hatha Yoga leaders vary widely in what they feel is best.

The main advantage to flowing in and out of many postures, one after the other, is that the joints and muscles loosen without your having to deal with an excessive amount of pain. In contrast, the main advantage of holding a posture for a long time is that the muscular structure is worked on at a much deeper level, so that more profound changes can occur.

I have found that many people feel more comfortable moving in and out of a variety of postures, thereby experiencing a significant increase in blood circulation throughout the body fairly quickly. It seems better in the more advanced stages of asana practice to hold certain postures for long periods. I will next present a set of standing postures that can be performed in a flowing, dancelike manner at the beginning, middle, or end of a yoga workout. This standing-posture dance has a calming effect on the mind and a loosening effect of the entire body. It is geared for the beginning and intermediate student of yoga.

Standing-Posture Dance

The benefits of the standing-posture dance include the following: increased flexibility of the spinal cord; increased stretch and tone to the leg and buttocks muscles; and increased efficiency produced in the respiratory, circulatory, endocrine, digestive, eliminative, and nervous systems.

The feet remain approximately 30 inches apart throughout this set of standing postures; they turn in the direction that the torso has turned. I will present three main arm and hand positions for this dance. In each arm position, first stretch the torso forward over one leg, slowly come up to an erect position, and carefully arch backward; then do the forward stretch and back arch to the other side; finally, stretch forward and arch backward while you are centered between the legs. Before discussing the mechanics of the standing-posture dance, let us take a photographic look at the set. Note: the full routine is shown in the first arm position only.

Positions of Standing-Posture Dance

Figures 5.41A–F show arm position 1 with fingers interwoven and arms outstretched.

Figures 5.42A and B show arm position 2 with elbows held behind the back. Arm position 2 should be done facing right, left, and forward.

An alternative for arm position 2 is shown in Figure 5.42C. This prayer position behind the back is for the flexible student. The palms are together between the shoulder blades and the elbows are pulled back.

Figures 5.43A and B show arm position 3 with elbows held above the head. Arm position 3 should be done facing right, left, and forward.

Breath of Standing-Posture Dance

The exhale and the inhale should both be thorough and complete throughout this series. You should exhale as you stretch forward and inhale as you bring the torso up and gently arch backward. Avoid any jerkiness or abrupt movements while performing the dance. You should merge into the continuous flow of the body and the breath in this moving meditation.

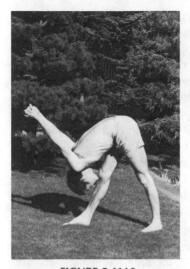

FIGURE 5.41A*

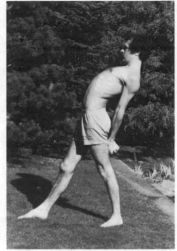

FIGURE 5.41B*

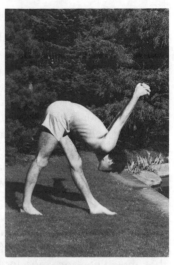

FIGURE 5.41C*

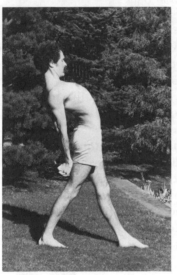

FIGURE 5.41D*

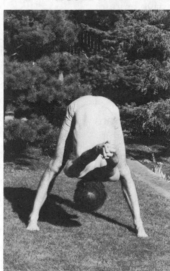

FIGURE 5.41E*

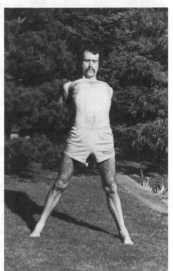

FIGURE 5.41F*

Mechanics of Standing-Posture Dance

Caution must be taken while performing the positions of this set that require you to arch backward. Because of the effect of gravity, blood will flow into the brain area when you bend down in the forward-stretch phase. Standing abruptly from the forward stretch will result in a quick flow of blood out of the brain area and could cause dizziness. You must come up slowly, focusing the eyes straight ahead. The most serious mistake would be to immediately arch the neck back and quickly go into a backbend as soon as you stood up, as fainting could result. The safeguard is to bring the chin down to the chest as you straighten the body, and keep the chin down as you arch the back. You can slowly look up toward the ceiling and let the chin rise slightly near the end of the back arch.

Another important concern while arch-

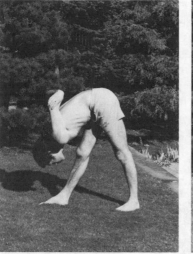

FIGURE 5.42A*

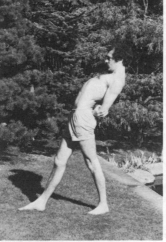

FIGURE 5.42B*

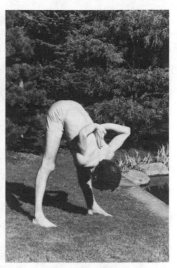

FIGURE 5.42C**

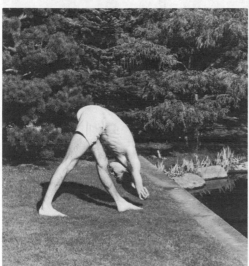

FIGURE 5.43A*

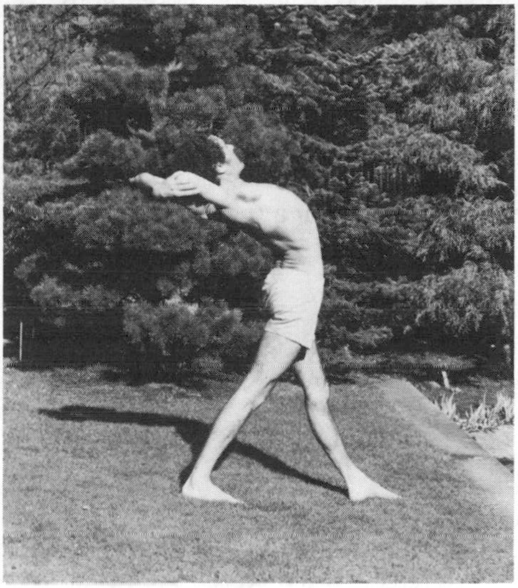

FIGURE 5.43B*

ing backward is the condition of the lumbar vertebrae and the lower-back muscles. We must avoid overarching the lumbar vertebrae if we are to avoid pain in the lower-back area! The safeguard is to tuck the pelvis under as strongly as possible through strong contractive work of the buttocks muscles. While going back, the chest must lift and the shoulder-blade muscles contract forcefully. Try to lengthen the lower back and arch the upper

back. If you cannot go backward without feeling pain in the lower back, simply lift straight upward in an uplifted vertical position after coming up from the forward stretch.

Go back and study the pictures carefully to understand the feet and arm positions. When you are stretching out over the right leg, the right foot turns to the right 90 degrees, and the back foot turns toward the right 60 degrees. The reverse occurs, of course, when you are stretching out over the left leg. Keep the feet parallel to each other as you stretch forward between the legs. The hips are square throughout each of the six main movements.

Do not overstrain in this series! Flow into the dance and loosen up your body painlessly; perform each movement slowly, precisely, and gracefully. Move the body rhythmically with the breath.

Elephant Swing The swaying action of this moving posture resembles that of a swinging elephant trunk. The elephant swing provides a nice way to relax after the standing-posture dance. The gentle movement soothes the nervous system and relieves the lower-back muscles. The movement should be very subtle, soft, and continuous. Begin by holding the elbows above the head, fold forward, stretch the spine, and keep the legs steady by lifting the kneecaps (Figure 5.44). Once the body is brought into motion, the side-to-side sway will quite naturally continue on its own. Do it for a minute or longer, letting the breath take care of itself.

Figure 5.45A shows the warrior I pose (shown in detail in Figures 5.20A–E). Figure 5.45B shows the dancer's pose (shown in detail in Figures 4.21A–C).

The torches and the wall in these photographs are a part of the Paul I. Fagan Memorial located in Hana, Maui, Hawaii.

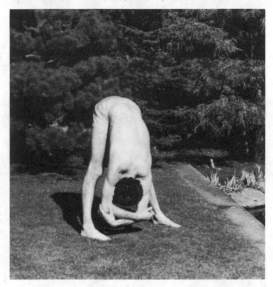

FIGURE 5.44*

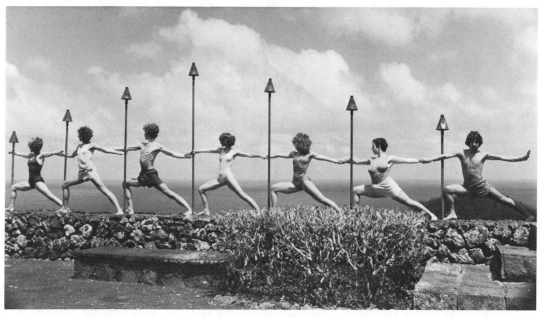

FIGURE 5.45A*

FIGURE 5.45B*

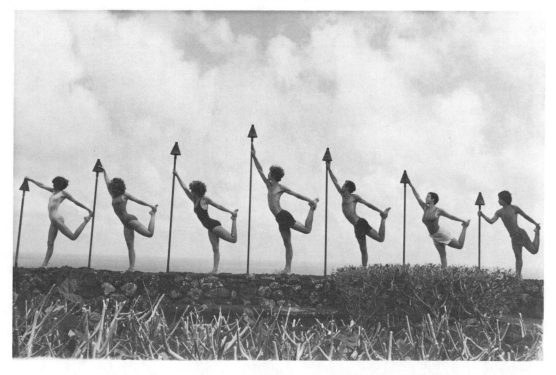

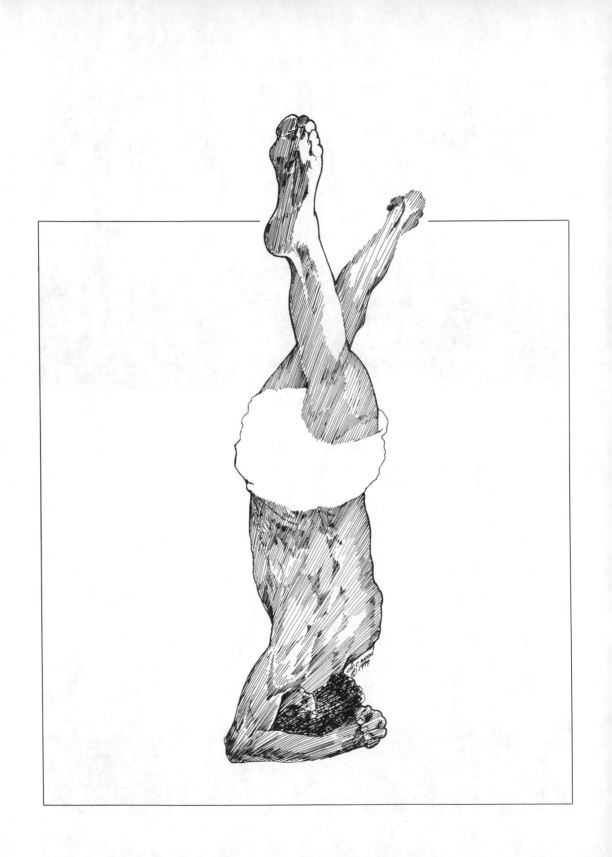

SIX
inverted postures

HEADSTAND

Headstand is said to be the king of the yoga asanas. The muscular, nervous, respiratory, circulatory, endocrine, digestive, eliminative, and reproductive systems all benefit from the practice of the headstand. It is not an overstatement to say that if you stand on your head for a few minutes each day,your whole outlook on life can be improved.

Since the heart is below the brain, the arterial blood that supplies oxygen and cell-building material to the brain tissues must be constantly pumped upward against the force of gravity. One of the greatest benefits of headstand is that it reverses the effect of gravity and brings arterial blood directly to the brain cells, thus rejuvenating one's thinking power.

Hormonal secretion of the endocrine glands becomes more efficient through headstand practice. Situated in the center of the skull is the pituitary gland. This gland, along with the hypothalamus, which is also centered in the skull, helps to control the secretion of hormones by most of the other endocrine glands through a negative-feed-

back system. The thyroid, parathyroid, adrenal, pancreas, and sex glands are all under the control of the pituitary-hypothalamus connection. When you consider that all the body processes are influenced by the chemical secretions of the endocrine system and that the key gland of that system, the pituitary, must have a proper supply of blood to work efficiently, it is no wonder that headstand is the king of the yoga asanas from the standpoint of body chemistry alone.

The person who has digestive and eliminative problems will benefit greatly through headstand practice. Headstand reverses the pull of gravity on the organs of the digestive tract, thus decreasing the tension surrounding them. After the basic headstand posture becomes comfortable, numerous twisting variations can be added that will relieve tension from the abdominal region even more. The headstand and its variations will help a person to overcome problems of constipation, overacidity, hemorrhoids, and disorders of the bladder, kidney, liver, and intestines.

The reproductive system is also aided by doing headstand. Sexual potency can be increased and sexual energy can be rechanneled for physical, mental, and spiritual development. *Headstand helps to regulate the menstrual cycle if done on a daily basis; however, it should be avoided while menstrual flow is heaviest because it could cause a stoppage of the period if held for a long while.*

When we are in an upright position, the venous blood returning to the heart from the abdominal region, pelvic region, and legs must constantly travel upward against gravity. Let us focus specifically on the blood circulation in the legs. Essentially, we have to depend upon the leg muscles that surround the veins to push the blood back to the heart against gravity. Vigorous exercise will greatly increase the venous return of blood, and yet headstand and other inverted postures will do so less stressfully and more directly.

Increased muscular strength is developed in the upper arms, shoulders, upper back, abdominal muscles, buttocks, and thigh muscles through the performance of headstand. Headstand also strengthens the muscles along the spinal cord. This increased muscular strength helps one to maintain better body alignment while sitting and standing. All the main systems of the body function more effectively when the body is held in good alignment.

People who have a dull and forgetful mind can improve the clarity of their thoughts through headstand practice. Possibly even more important is that headstand can help you adopt a more positive outlook toward life. Confronted constantly by life's many demands and duties, you need to find a reliable means of renewal. During headstand, you can become detached from daily problems and get the equivalent of a battery recharge. You can come out of the posture with an elevated psyche and clearer mind. This allows you to function more efficiently and effectively while out and about in the world.

Mechanics of Headstand

How long should you hold headstand? The answer depends on the individual. In the beginning, 20 to 30 seconds is usually a long time. Slowly and carefully you can increase the amount of time the posture is held. After a few years of practice you can work up to holding headstand for 10 to 15 minutes. The longer you maintain the correct pose, the more beneficial, potentially, will be the results.

Headstand must be performed correctly, however, or major problems in the neck and lumbar spine ensue. Many muscles must work to keep the pressure off the neck and to keep the spine and the legs in a completely vertical position. Headstand is not a posture for the novice beginner and must be learned under the guidance of a qualified teacher of yoga. It is not recommended for those with high blood pressure or those with serious eye or ear problems.

The weight of the body should eventually be carried evenly by the elbows, forearms and the head during the performance of headstand. To keep the neck from compressing, the upper arm, shoulder, back, abdominal, buttocks, and leg muscles must all work quite strongly. Basically, the idea is to push the forearms down against the floor while lifting straight up through the rest of the body.

Arching of the lumbar vertebrae must be avoided in order to keep the lower spine from compressing. Length has to be maintained in the lower spine because swayback can cause a serious backache. Straightening of the lower back and tucking of the pelvis occurs mainly through a combined effort of the abdominal and buttocks muscles. To aid the work of the abdominal muscles and the alignment of the spinal cord, the quadriceps muscles (frontside thigh muscles) need to work also. Rather than letting the legs be lax in headstand, the correct procedure is to keep them alive and stretching upward. Actually, the whole body must come to life in head-stand.

All beginning headstand students should use a wall to help their practice of the posture. When doing so, you should be able to lift your head completely off the floor at any point during the headstand. Headstand should not be maintained if more weight is carried by the head than by the arms. In the initial phases of practice of the posture, most weight should be carried by the forearms and elbows.

The variations to headstand are not for the beginning student, owing to the increased difficulty of alignment, lift, and balance. Whenever variations are done, the neck and head should not carry the body's weight, nor should the lumbar vertebrae overarch. The variations of headstand are very challenging and rewarding, but you must have strength and a good sense of body alignment to do them.

Let us now look pictorially at headstand.

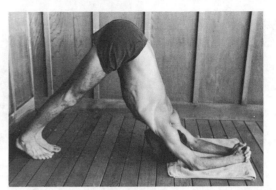

FIGURE 6.1A*

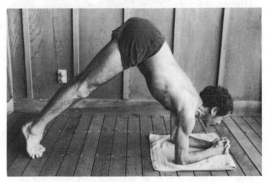

FIGURE 6.1B*

Headstand Preparations

Forearm Dog to Forearm Lift This is a kriya, which means it involves movement from one posture into another. The person moves back and forth between the two postures several times in a fluid way.

The posture shown in Figure 6.1A is the forearm dog stretch with the fingers interwoven. The goal is to loosen up the shoulder joints and bring awareness into the muscles of the upper back.

In the second part of the movement, shown in Figure 6.1B, the head moves forward over the thumbs and the head is kept as high above the thumbs as possible. The forearm lift is good for building shoulder strength.

In the kriya, move to and fro from forearm dog stretch to forearm lift three to six times, pausing for a moment at the end of each swing. The idea is to keep the back straight, the pelvis tilted upward, and the bottom lifted as high as possible throughout the motion. Move into forearm dog stretch on either the in or out breath and into the forearm lift on the opposite. See which works best for you. Rest in prayer pose when done.

Dog Stretch as Headstand Preparation
The dog stretch is one of the best of the headstand preparations. It builds strength in the arms and shoulders, loosens the upper back and shoulders, gives you the feeling of how to lift the hips, and works the leg muscles. The whole body should come alive in dog stretch. Although it is not totally necessary, the wall can be used as a brace to keep the hands from sliding.

Bring the hands shoulder-width apart, spread the thumb and index finger, and place them on the floor next to the wall. Bring the knees under hips, drop the abdomen, and lift

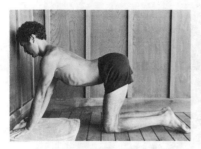

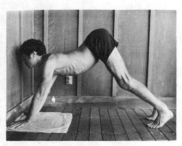

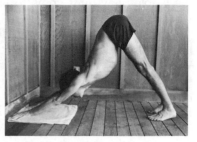

FIGURE 6.2A*   FIGURE 6.2B*   FIGURE 6.2C*

the head up (Figure 6.2A). This is cow position —the abdomen hangs low like a cow's.

Inhale, hook the toes under and lift the pelvis high into the air. Slowly straighten the legs by lifting the bottom higher and higher as you look toward the wall (Figure 6.2B). Staying up on the toes helps the pelvis to tilt upward as you move toward the completed dog pose.

Keep the arms and legs stretched, drop the chest, tilt the pelvis upward, and breathe deeply. If you can flatten out the hump in the upper back, let the head hang down; otherwise, look toward the hands. Stretch up through the spine and down through the heels (Figure 6.2C). This is dog stretch. It can be held anywhere from ten seconds to one minute or longer.

Hand and Arm Position in Headstand
Kneel in front of a blanket or mat. Spread the elbows a forearm's distance apart. The tendency in the beginning is to place the elbows too far apart in headstand; this makes the lift of the shoulders much more difficult than if the elbows are kept forearm distance apart, as shown in Figure 6.3A.

Interweave the fingers, making certain that the elbows are even with each other. The hands form a Gothic arch (Figure 6.3B).

Proper placement of the hands for the beginning headstand student is shown in Figure 6.3C. If you have not done a lot of headstand, move the base of the thumbs down toward the floor, lessening the arch between the hands (but do not bring the base of the

thumbs all the way onto the floor). The beginning student needs a stronger forearm push than does the advanced student.

The shoulders should lift very strongly. As a precaution, beginning headstand students should carry more weight along the elbows and forearms, with only a minimal amount being carried by the head. The neck must be protected at all cost. *If you cannot support most of the weight on the forearms in the early phases of headstand practice, you are not ready for headstand.*

Proper placement of elbows, wrists, and fingers for intermediate and advanced students is shown in Figure 6.3D. The fingers should be interwoven completely, but the grip should be looser and the arch between the base of the thumbs wider than the beginning headstand student's. The very top of the head should rest onto the floor as the back of the head lightly touches between the base of the thumbs.

Headstand with Wall
As mentioned earlier, all beginning headstand students should use a wall when practicing the posture. The interwoven fingers should be placed right next to the wall and should actually touch the wall (Figure 6.4A). To move up into the headstand, the upper back must be drawn inward and the hips must be lifted upward as the feet are walked in toward the wall. Ideally, you should be able to bring the back of the hip bone to the wall as the upper back is drawn away from the wall. Do not put too much pressure on the head as the feet are brought

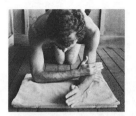

FIGURE 6.3A*

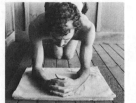

FIGURE 6.3B*

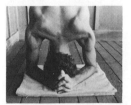

FIGURE 6.3C*

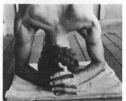

FIGURE 6.3D*

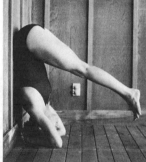

FIGURE 6.4A*

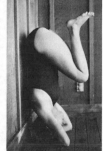

FIGURE 6.4B*

FIGURE 6.4C*

FIGURE 6.4D*

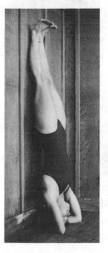

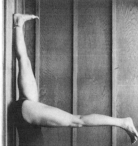

in toward the wall; the forearms must push down and the shoulders, spine, and hips should lift strongly as the feet are taken off the floor.

It is best to try to keep the legs straight while taking the feet off the floor. Until the back muscles have become strong enough to lift the straightened legs, you may need to bend the knees as shown in Figure 6.4B.

It is important to lengthen the lower back through the contraction of the buttocks and abdominal muscles as you stretch up through the spine and legs in the completed headstand against the wall. Notice, in Figure 6.4C, the lift through the shoulders, the openness of Linda's armpit, and the strong work through her legs and feet. The top of the head should rest gently on the floor. If too much weight begins to sink onto the head, bring the weight forward onto the elbows and completely lift the head off the floor for a few seconds. In so doing, make sure to squeeze the buttocks muscles and tuck the pelvis. Work in the pose for 20 seconds to two minutes.

To come down from headstand bring one straightened leg down as slowly as possible until it comes close to the floor (Figure 6.4D); then let the other one follow. Intermediate students should try to lower both straightened legs together in slow-motion fashion.

Headstand with Wall: Common Mistakes

Swayback   The headstand shown in Figure 6.5 would result in a backache in the lumbar vertebrae, owing to pressure that builds up at the arched area of the spine.

Collapsing Shoulders   The fault in Figure 6.6 is that the upper back and shoulders have ceased to lift, which causes compression on the neck vertebrae.

Correction of Problems   Shown in Figure 6.7 is a proper headstand with the aid of

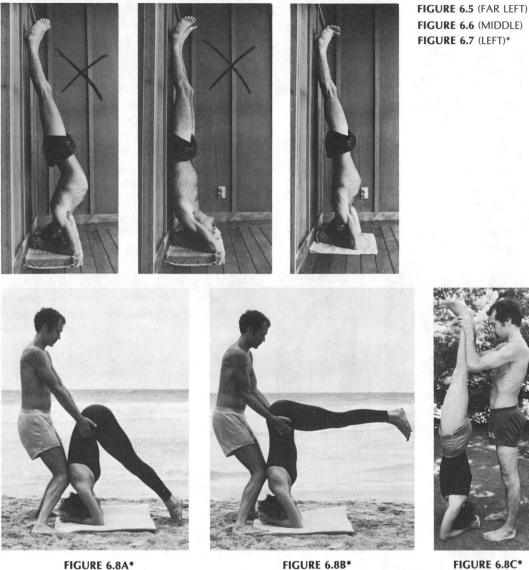

FIGURE 6.5 (FAR LEFT)
FIGURE 6.6 (MIDDLE)
FIGURE 6.7 (LEFT)*

FIGURE 6.8A*   **FIGURE 6.8B***   **FIGURE 6.8C***

the wall. The forearms are pushing down, the shoulders are lifting; the armpits are opening; the abdominal, buttocks, and quadriceps muscles are working to keep the lower spine straight; the thigh and calf muscles are stretching; and the feet are alive. When using the wall, the buttocks should move slightly away from the wall as the gluteus maximus muscles contract. To help the quadriceps muscles work properly, it is best to firmly push through the base of the big toe and then spread the other toes. Work in the pose for 20 seconds to two minutes.

Headstand with Help   After practicing headstand against the wall for a few months, you may want to try it in the center of the room. At first it would be helpful to have the aid of a partner.

In headstand, the upper back must flatten through the contractive work of the shoulder-blade muscles before you are ready to bring the feet up. As shown in Figures 6.8A and B, I am pressing my knees into Linda's upper back and lifting up her hips as she moves her feet in slowly. This helps her to flatten her back so she can press down with her forearms and begin to lift her feet off the floor. She does not kick up into headstand, but slowly walks her feet in until her legs are ready to be lifted to a vertical position through the work of her lower back and hips. Figure 6.8C shows how I can help her to find her balance by lifting up her ankles. As she finds her balance, my hands can come away from her ankles a few inches. Then I help her gain the best possible body alignment through words and touch. After she has worked in headstand for a short while, I help her to come down in the same way as I helped her to go up.

Headstand without Wall

To begin with, headstand should be learned by using a wall. Gradually, as your shoulders become stronger and your balance becomes better, you can take your feet away from the wall. The next step is to bring the hands four to six inches away from the wall and try to come up into and remain in headstand without relying on the wall, but knowing that the wall is still there for security. As you gain confidence, move farther away from the wall and try to hold the basic vertical headstand for increasingly longer periods.

The directions previously given for the practice of headstand when using a wall also apply to the posture without a wall. The goal of headstand is to be perfectly vertical through the legs and through the sacral, lumbar, thoracic, and cervical vertebrae. The most common mistake in the pose is to overarch the lumbar vertebrae; this must be alleviated by contracting the buttocks muscles and drawing the lower ribs in by means of abdominal muscle contraction. Notice the

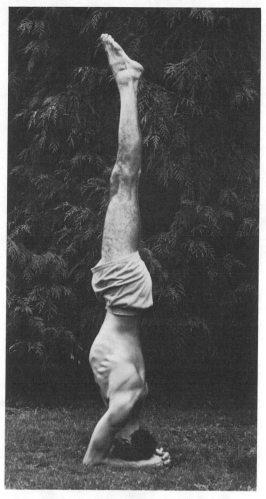

FIGURE 6.9**

work occurring through the body in Figure 6.9. Not by any stretch of the imagination is headstand a passive pose. Once in headstand, breathe deeply and slowly. Maintain the pose as long as you maintain good alignment through the body and strength through the arms and shoulders. Then come down very slowly, with straight legs if possible, and rest in prayer pose.

Headstand Variations

Countless numbers of variations can be performed while you are in headstand. These variations should be learned under the guidance of a competent teacher. It is important to have someone watch the alignment of your body as you move through the different variations. The key is to keep the spinal cord vertically lifted and to keep the weight evenly distributed on both forearms. While doing the headstand variations, it is best to carry more weight on the forearms and elbows than on the head. Do not overarch the lower back or allow the neck vertebrae to compress. If you cannot hold the basic vertical headstand position for at least two minutes, then you are not ready to try the variations.

The headstand variations are usually done in slow-motion fashion. You should move in and out of them in a fluid, graceful way. If they are done correctly, the headstand variations can elicit a wonderful feeling of joy. They are postures that loosen the muscles along the spine, help to relieve lower-back problems, and are tremendously helpful for all the internal organs of digestion, elimination, and reproduction. The variations give you incentive to stay up in the headstand longer, so that all the effects discussed in the opening discussion of headstand are substantially increased.

Headstand Variations with Wall

Vertical Twist The key in the vertical twist, as shown in Figure 6.10, is to stretch straight upward through the spine and legs as the hips twist. The weight should be distributed equally on both forearms as you twist to either side. There should be little weight on the head so that neck and lower-back compression can be avoided. The stomach muscles keep the lower ribs drawn inward, and the buttocks and quadriceps muscles must work strongly as you twist. Work each side a few seconds.

Bent-Knee Twist Starting from the vertical twist shown in Figure 6.10, bend both

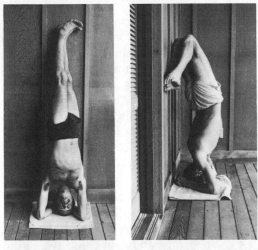

FIGURE 6.10**   FIGURE 6.11**

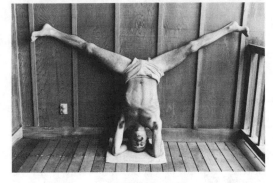

FIGURE 6.12**

knees and squeeze the buttocks muscles very firmly. The hips must both lift straight up as the forearms and elbows push down solidly. The pelvis tucks as you stretch up through your knees, the lower ribs draw in, and the spine and thighs stay as vertical as possible (Figure 6.11). Work each side for a few seconds.

Splits As you spread both legs, keep tucking the pelvis, stretch through the heels of both feet, and then allow gravity to open the legs to the utmost (Figure 6.12). Breathe deeply and try to relax the inner-thigh muscles.

The headstand splits results in a release of energy in the pelvic and inner-thigh areas. Hold for a few seconds.

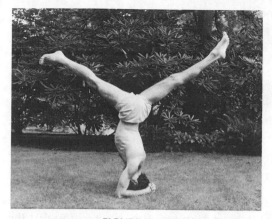

FIGURE 6.13A**

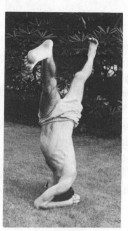

FIGURE 6.13E**

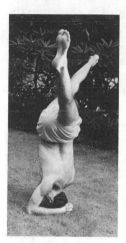

FIGURE 6.13B**

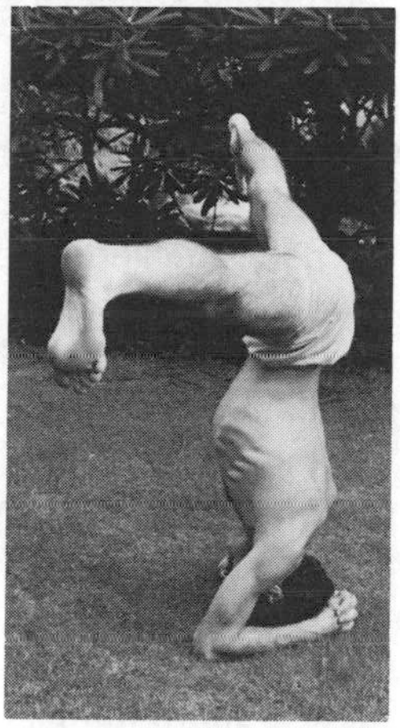

FIGURE 6.13C**

FIGURE 6.13D**

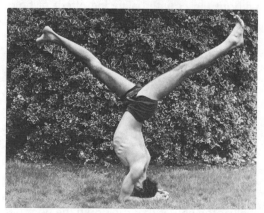

Headstand Variations without the Wall (Twisting Routine) The use of a wall for headstand eventually should be abandoned. The wall is a useful tool, but a much freer feeling is attained by doing headstand without this crutch. When doing headstand in the center of the room, position the forearms and head on a neatly folded blanket or on a padded rug. Make sure to keep a good distance between you and all furniture.

Falling from headstand is inevitable when you first go away from the wall. It is not a serious matter to fall out of headstand if you give in to it. If you are about to fall from headstand, do not stiffen up; rather, let the body loosen and tumble—into a somersault. You must have clear, open space in all directions, as you may need to roll after falling. After you are more experienced with headstand practice, you will become confident that you can perform any of the variations, and falling will not be your concern. Next is shown a flowing headstand routine that uses the twisting scissors and the splits. Study the pictures carefully before attempting this routine. The first few times through, it is important to have someone at your side to guide you through and keep you from falling in an uncontrolled way.

In performing the headstand twisting routine, move slowly and continuously from Figures 6.13A to B to A to C to D to E to D to C to complete one round. Go through the

141

series twice. Keep the breath deep and steady throughout. The weight must be maintained equally on both forearms, and both shoulders must lift throughout the routine. Keep the pelvis tucked and the legs stretching as you move from posture to posture. Study each picture carefully before attempting it. Make sure to have someone watch you and give you corrections until you are certain that you can do it properly without help.

SHOULDERSTAND

Shoulderstand is known as the queen of the yoga asanas. B.K.S. Iyengar recommends that shoulderstand be performed as a followup to headstand, since it provides a perfect counterbalance to headstand. The thyroid and parathyroid glands are directly stimulated in shoulderstand, owing to the inverted position of the body and the neck and head position. You'll recall that it was primarily the pituitary gland that was stimulated by headstand. The mind calms down more in shoulderstand, owing to the head, neck, and body position. The two work together as a unit and should be

practiced together—shoulderstand after headstand.

Although it is important to work the body hard in both poses, a very different attitude is required in approaching each one. You must give into the stretch of the neck muscles and neck vertebrae while practicing shoulderstand and adopt more of a yielding, receptive attitude, whereas in headstand, pushing down hard with the forearms and lifting through the shoulders and the rest of the body becomes the main concern. This is not to say that the whole body should be passive while you are performing shoulderstand. On the contrary, the elbows should be drawn inward, the upper-back muscles should be drawn in toward the spine and lifted very strongly, the buttocks muscles should be contracted, the hips lifted, the pelvis tucked, and the legs stretched upward. Shoulderstand is a difficult posture to maintain because the body must work hard to maintain a good pose, and yet the activity of the mind begins to decrease the longer the posture is held. Your will power is put to test by these two opposing forces.

Shoulderstand can be held for up to ten minutes by the very advanced practitioner, but it is more difficult to hold for this lengthy period than headstand, mainly for the reasons just cited. As a general rule, it is good practice to hold shoulderstand for at least half as long as headstand. It is said that holding headstand without the counterbalancing effect of holding shoulderstand can cause irritability.

A most obvious benefit of shoulderstand is that it stretches and breaks up tension in the muscles that run along the back of the neck. Shortness at the back of the neck causes too much cervical curve and can be the cause of headaches, neckaches, upper-back pain, slipping of vertebrae out of place, and pain or lack of feeling in the arms and hands. As the muscles at the back of the neck stretch, the cervical curve lengthens, and the nerves that emanate from between the neck vertebrae, as well as the nerves that run down the neck, are

FIGURE 6.14

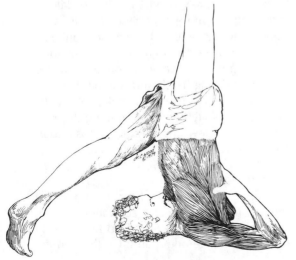

able to function more freely. Shoulderstand also stretches out the muscles on both sides of the neck equally, and this allows the vertebrae to move back into good alignment.

An extremely important benefit of shoulderstand is that the thyroid and parathyroid glands are stimulated to function more efficiently. The thyroid gland controls the body's metabolic rate. The two main hormones secreted by the thyroid gland govern the overall rate at which oxygen is used by the body. Efficient metabolism of carbohydrates and proteins depends directly on the condition of the thyroid gland, as do the normal growth and development of the body, especially the brain.

The parathyroid glands lie close to the thyroid gland and control the metabolism of calcium and phosphate in the body. Normal skeletal and cardiac muscular activity, as well as blood clotting, depend on normal calcium levels in the plasma. Stiffness, cramps, and muscle spasms can result from lack of calcium. Overactivity of the parathyroid glands could result in serious kidney, bone, or muscular problems.

Daily practice of the shoulderstand will stimulate an underactive thyroid or parathyroid gland or both in such a way as to increase hormonal activity. On the other hand, if there is overactivity in either or both of these glands, shoulderstand practice will help to slow down their hormonal secretion. A balanced level of hormonal secretion by the pituitary gland will be attained through shoulderstand and headstand practice in the same regulatory way. The adrenal glands, pancreas, and sex glands will balance their production of hormones through a well-rounded set of standing postures, twists, backbends, forward stretches, and inverted postures.

To be calm and yet full of energy is the goal of yoga practice. Shoulderstand is a posture that helps bring about this desired balance. Some of the other tangible benefits of shoulderstand include a decrease of head-aches, nervousness, hypertension, insomnia, and ulcers as well as an improvement of memory and mental alertness, better assimilation of food, better elimination of indigestible foodstuff, and an increase in sexual vitality along with better control over the sexual energy.

Another key benefit of the shoulderstand is that it greatly aids the venous return of blood from the legs, pelvic region, and abdominal region to the heart by the force of gravity. If the carbon-dioxide-laden blood in the veins gets bogged down in the legs, serious problems can ensue. The same also applies to the organs of reproduction, elimination, and digestion. Menstrual disorders can be helped through the daily practice of shoulderstand, which, however, should not be done during the heaviest days of menstruation.

Mechanics of Shoulderstand for Beginning Students

Shoulderstand must be approached with great caution in order to avoid damage to the neck. A thickly folded blanket or mat, as well as the wall, should be used while practicing shoulderstand in the early stages. If these two aids are used, shoulderstand can be practiced without the help of a qualified teacher. A folded blanket helps to keep the weight off the neck, allowing the neck muscles to stretch out slowly and safely. The weight of the body should be carried more by the elbows, arms, and the back of the head than by the neck. Using a wall helps the upper-back muscles to work strongly. A third aid, the use of a strap, helps to keep the elbows from slipping out too far. The way to use a strap will be discussed later (Figures 6.19A and B); for the moment, we shall focus on the use of a blanket and a wall.

The blanket should be folded two to three inches thick, wider than the shoulders and as long as the arms. You may need two blankets to attain these dimensions. It is important that the shoulders and elbows rest securely on the blanket(s) that you use for shoulderstand.

The shoulders, neck, and head must be precisely placed on the blanket; otherwise, more harm can be done than good. Place the shoulders evenly on the blanket about two inches from the edge. The neck should rest on the edge of the folded blanket, and the back of the head should be on the floor. The shoulders must be parallel to the edge of the blanket. If your shoulders shift so that they hang over the edge of the blanket when you are coming up into shoulderstand, then come back down and shift your position.

Beginner's Shoulderstand Place the folded blanket(s) down, bring the bottom next to the wall, stretch the lower back and neck, and breathe deeply to prepare for shoulderstand. As shown in Figure 6.15A, *the back of the head should rest on the floor with the shoulders evenly placed a couple of inches from the edge of the blanket.*

Bend the knees, bring the soles of the feet to the wall, lift the bottom off the floor, clasp the hands, and straighten the arms. Lift the hips and move the feet up the wall until the knees form a 90-degree angle. Tuck the pelvic girdle under by squeezing the buttocks muscles, push the arms down, bring the top of the chest to the chin, and let the neck muscles passively stretch out (Figure 6.15B). The neck vertebrae should not be on the floor. Work in this pose for five to 20 seconds.

Walk up the wall until the legs straighten. Work the thighs by contracting the quadriceps muscles. To begin with, stretch through the calves by bringing the toes away from the wall with the heels remaining on the wall. Eventually, the toes should be pointed. Tuck the pelvis by contracting the buttocks muscles firmly, and lift through the upper back. Make sure that the shoulders have re-

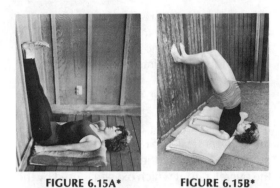

FIGURE 6.15A*   FIGURE 6.15B*

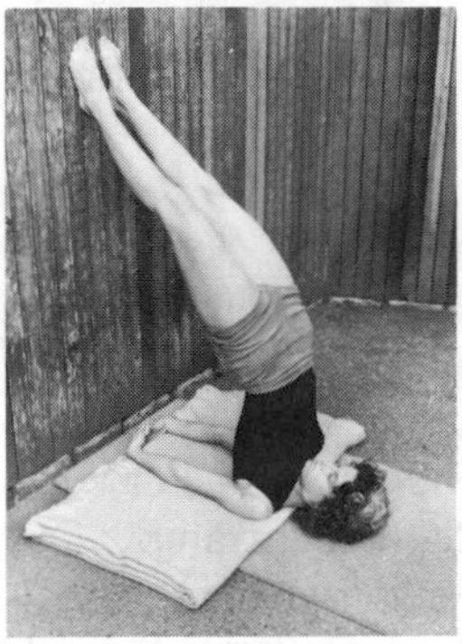

FIGURE 6.15C*   FIGURE 6.15D*

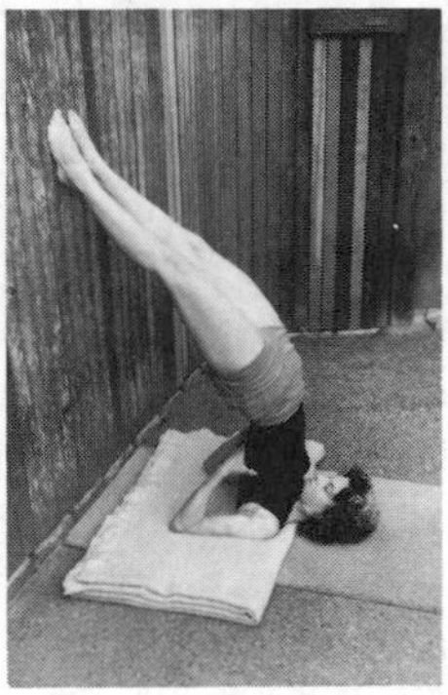

mained on the blanket and the back of the head on the floor (Figure 6.15C). Work for ten to 20 seconds.

From Figure 6.15C, bend the elbows and place the hands on the back with the fingers pointing up. Keeping the elbows as close together as possible, press the upper arms down, relax the neck muscles, lift up through the spine, and work strongly through the buttocks and legs (Figure 6.15D). Hold for 20 to 30 seconds, breathing deeply.

Hare Pose One of the best preparations for shoulderstand is the hare pose, as it stretches the neck and lower-back muscles and awakens the upper-back muscles. Hare is an excellent tension reliever for the neck and shoulder areas and can greatly reduce neck-aches or headaches. This posture loosens the whole upper half of the body.

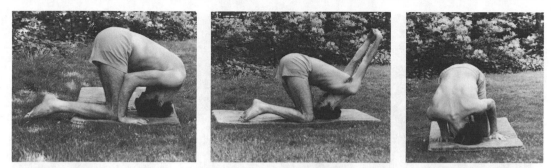

FIGURE 6.16A*   FIGURE 6.16B*   FIGURE 6.17*

To move into hare, place the top of the head on the floor, the hands next to the head shoulder-width apart, roll to the very back of the head, and walk the knees in close to the forehead, as shown in Figure 6.16A. Then interweave the fingers and stretch the straightened arms up, as shown in Figure 6.16B. The completed hare pose can be held for 20 seconds to one minute.

One caution: do not allow the weight of the body to press down onto the head. The shoulders must lift away from the ears so that the head can rest comfortably on the floor and the neck muscles stretch out passively.

Neck Rolls   Neck rolls loosen both sides of the neck and help relieve neck tension. Starting with the position shown in Figure 6.16A, move into the neck rolls by rolling the head in a semicircular fashion (Figure 6.17). Move from one side of the head to the back of the head to the other side of the head; then reverse the semicircular order. Very slowly move from side to side a number of times. As the neck loosens, you can move from side to side a little quicker.

Tranquility Pose   Tranquility pose stretches the neck, spine, leg, and arm muscles and relaxes the mind. It can serve as a preparation for shoulderstand and plough. To do tranquility pose, lie on the back with the palms facing down on the floor next to the bottom, raise the legs and back, and bring the straight-

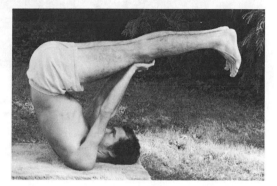

FIGURE 6.18*

ened legs over the head as shown in Figure 6.18. Then bring the hands to the knees, straighten the arms, and let the straightened legs rest onto the hands. Hold the pose for ten to 30 seconds, lifting through the hips while maintaining the posture.

Shoulderstand with Strap   The most difficult work of shoulderstand, if done without a wall, is to keep the elbows from splaying out too far (Figure 6.19A). If the elbows slip outward, the upper back rounds and the weight of the body sinks, causing pressure on the neck when the legs are straightened vertically upward.

With the aid of a strap the elbows can be kept in and the upper back lifted; this will help to take pressure off the neck as the legs are lifted to a vertical position. The loop of the strap should be the length of the forearm, measured from the split between the thumb and index finger to the back of the elbow.

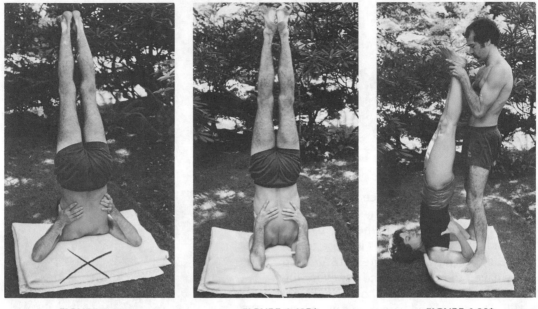

FIGURE 6.19A   FIGURE 6.19B*   FIGURE 6.20*

From the tranquility pose shown in Figure 6.18, slip the already cinched strap up above the elbows, and then lift the legs up into shoulderstand. Push the elbows outward and draw the shoulder blades inward to get more lift with the upper back (Figure 6.19B). Hold for ten seconds to one minute, breathing deeply.

Partner Adjustment   The elbows tend to slip out in shoulderstand, and they must be readjusted periodically. This partner adjustment can feel marvelous to the person being adjusted. In Figure 6.20, I am moving Linda's elbows in with the insteps of my feet as I lift her legs straight up.

Shoulderstand—Final Version   Figure 6.21 shows a well-done shoulderstand. Note the vertical line formed by the back of the legs, the bottom, and the spine. Note the work of the buttocks and quadriceps muscles, the stretch of the calf muscles, and the pressing action through the ball of the toes. The upper-back muscles must continue to be

drawn in toward the spine throughout the pose. Work in shoulderstand for 20 seconds to five minutes, breathing deeply and relaxing the neck muscles.

Shoulderstand Twisting Routine   The shoulderstand twisting routine is best performed in a slow-motion, dancelike manner. You must have some familiarity with shoulderstand before you are ready for this routine, and yet the flexible beginning student could try this series of movements. The benefits of the shoulderstand twisting routine, above and beyond those of the basic shoulderstand, are increased loosening of the neck and upper-back muscles; a deep massage to the internal organs of digestion, elimination, and reproduction; loosening of the lower-back, waist, and lower rib-cage areas; the bringing of increased stretch and awareness to the legs; stimulation of the circulation of blood throughout the body; and the bringing of better hormonal balance to the endocrine glands.

If you try to hold shoulderstand for a long period, you must deal with the resistance

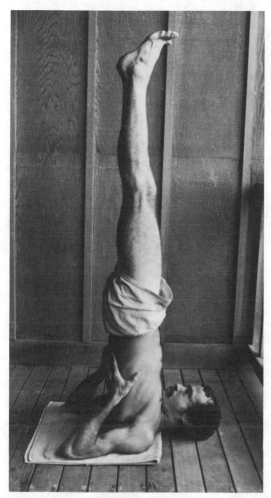

FIGURE 6.21*

and negativity of the mind. The mind does not seem to resist flowing movement in the same manner as it does holding the straight shoulderstand. Moving in and out of many postures gives the mind something interesting to focus on. The shoulderstand twisting routine brings the body and mind to a one-pointed level of concentration. Let us now take a look at the routine.

Vertical Twist (Hands on Back) From basic shoulderstand position, twist the hips to the right; keep the spine and both legs vertical as you stretch upward (Fig. 6.22A). Reach up through the base of the toes.

Leg-Over Twist (Hands on Back) From the position shown in Figure 6.22A, slowly bring the left leg down, as shown in Figure 6.22B. It is important to keep as much length through the left side of the waist as the right, and you accomplish this by lifting the left hip as you bring the left foot toward the floor. It is also important to stretch straight up with the right leg and spine and to not twist the head or neck. Check to see if both elbows touch down equally when you are doing the movement. Pause at the end of the movement, return to the vertical shoulderstand, twist to the left, and then bring the right leg down into the leg-over twist. From the leg-over twist done to the second side, return to the straight shoulderstand position, and then once again move into the vertical twist to the right, as shown in Figure 6.22A.

Bent-Knee Twist (Hands on Back) From the position shown in Figure 6.22A, bend the left knee and bring the knee close to the right temple (Figure 6.22C). The spine and right leg should be lifted vertically upward, and both elbows should touch the floor evenly. Try to keep the lift in the upper back, pause for a moment, and then straighten the bent leg back to the vertical shoulderstand position. Do the vertical twist to the left, bend the right knee, and bring it close to the left temple (bent-knee twist to the second side). Pause briefly with the right knee down, then return to the straight-up-and-down shoulderstand.

Vertical, Leg-Over, and Bent-Knee Twist (Straightened Arms) Next go through the same movements described in Figures 6.22A–C; this time do the movements with the fingers clasped together and the arms straightened (Figures 6.22D–F). You must push down firmly with the whole of both arms; contract the upper-back, buttocks, and thigh muscles; and lift strongly with the back, hips, and legs to initially straighten the spine and legs in the new arm position. Bringing the

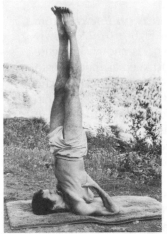

FIGURE 6.22A**

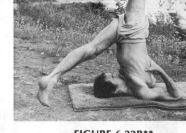

FIGURE 6.22B**

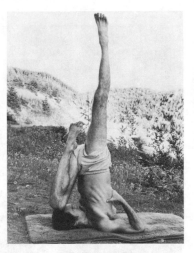

FIGURE 6.22C**

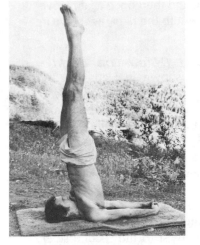

FIGURE 6.22D**

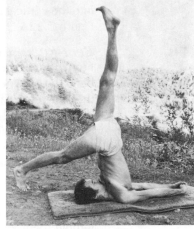

FIGURE 6.22E**

FIGURE 6.22F **

spine and legs to a vertical position with straightened arms and interwoven fingers is a good way to teach the body how to work properly in shoulderstand. Shoulderstand is not a passive pose, as you will see by attempting to hold the position shown in Figure 6.22D.

Doing the twisting variations with straightened arms, rather than keeping the hands on the back brings more awareness to the upper back and arms.

Follow the instructions given in Figures 6.22A–C and complete the shoulderstand twisting routine with the new arm position. After completing the routine, return to the straight vertical shoulderstand position shown in Figure 6.22D and maintain that position for ten seconds to one minute before coming down slowly into the plough posture.

Shoulderstand with Chair The use of a chair is not recommended for the beginning student of shoulderstand. The neck will stretch out quite dramatically if shoulderstand is done with a chair, so this aid should not be used until you have worked a fair amount of

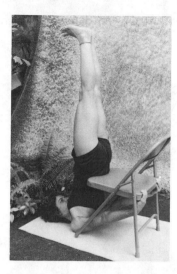

FIGURE 6.23**

time on this pose without a chair. The advantage to using a chair is that the upper back muscles work as they should, straightness of the spine can be maintained fairly easily, and the hips are given a stable support to rest against; this enables you to hold shoulderstand for a long period. When the pose is held for longer periods, the benefits described in the opening discussion are increased.

Shoulderstand with the use of a chair is shown in Figure 6.23. The front edge of the seat of the chair should rest just below the top of the ilium (hip bone); the hands grasp either the back edge of the seat or the back legs of the chair. The arms should be stretched to the utmost, with the upper arms placed to the inside of the front legs of the chair.

To get into the position shown, bring the stretched legs past the head in plough position, take hold of the chair, and slide it into the lower-back area. Go between the front legs of the chair with your arms and take hold of the back legs of the chair. Lift your legs slowly up to a vertical position, and pull the chair in further until the edge of the seat fits tight against your back. Lift strongly through the hips, flex the ankles, stretch up through the inner thighs as well as the outer thighs, and stretch through the inner calves as well as the outer calves. Press through the ball of the big

toes; this will activate a stretch through the front and back sides of the legs. As shown here, bring the hands to the seat of the chair and continue stretching up through the spine and legs. Work in the pose for 20 seconds to five minutes, breathing deeply.

PLOUGH

Plough pose is one of the most highly recommended of the yoga asanas. It stretches the whole backside of the body and increases the flow of blood, oxygen, and nerve energy throughout the body. It greatly helps to calm the mind and helps move you toward a peaceful state of awareness.

Plough produces many of the same benefits as shoulderstand. The main differences are that plough stretches the lower-back and leg muscles more intensely, the abdominal muscles are folded in during plough instead of straightened, and shoulderstand aids the venous return of blood from the legs much more than plough.

Plough pose helps to lengthen the cervical curve of the neck and the lumbar curve of the lower back. We discussed in reference to shoulderstand how lack of space between the vertebrae of the neck can cause many problems; this is also true of the lower-back vertebrae. Pain, numbness, and lack of mobility in the lower back, pelvic girdle, hip joints, legs, feet, and toes can be greatly reduced by doing plough. The lumbar curve and the cervical curve of the spine must be minimized if the nerves coming out from between the vertebrae in these two areas are to function properly.

The muscles of the lower back are usually tighter on one side than the other, as are those of the neck. Plough pose helps to stretch and balance the two sides of the body in these two problem areas. This rebalancing can relieve headaches, neckaches, and back-

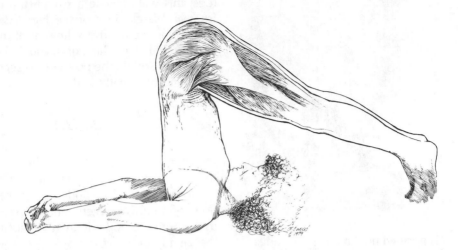

FIGURE 6.24

aches. It helps to make the muscles along the spine and to make the spine itself more supple.

An excellent posture for stretching and toning the arm and leg muscles, plough helps to loosen stiff shoulder, elbow, wrist, finger, ankle, and knee joints. The posture must be thought of as a forward stretch, and length should be maintained through the hamstring and calf muscles. Persons with tightness in the iliopsoas and buttocks muscles will also be aided by the posture.

The organs of digestion, elimination, and reproduction are stimulated to function more efficiently through practice of plough. The abdominal muscles press in against the internal organs during plough; this serves as a massage to these organs. The posture is especially beneficial for those with liver and kidney problems. Menstrual disorders can be helped through daily practice of plough, but like shoulderstand and headstand, this pose should not be performed during days of heaviest blood release in the menstrual cycle.

The endocrine system, composed of the sex glands, pancreas, adrenal, thymus, thyroid, parathyroid, pineal, and pituitary glands, is greatly aided through the practice of plough. The endocrine system, along with the nervous system, affects a person's energy level, physical well-being, emotional stability, mental alertness, and general outlook on life. Plough especially helps to restore the balance of the thyroid and parathyroid secretions. The stretch along the buttocks, lower-back, and middle-back muscles helps to balance the secretion of the sexual and adrenal glands, and the folding of the abdominal muscles stimulates pancreatic secretion. The pituitary gland will be renewed through practice of plough, as blood and oxygen will wash through the brain area.

Plough, like shoulderstand and headstand, must be approached with caution. You must avoid overstretching the neck and lower-back muscles. If aids and muscles are used properly, and if body alignment is good, plough is a posture that the beginning student can work on. It should not be held for more than 30 seconds in the initial stages. The beginning student should not bring the feet all the way to the floor in plough; rather, the feet should rest on chair or on the wall. This is shown by Linda in Figures 6.25A and B.

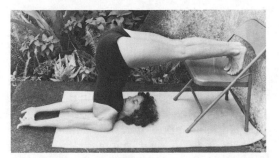

FIGURE 6.25A*

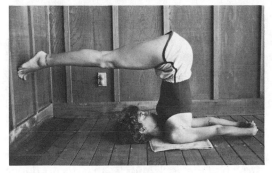

FIGURE 6.25B*

Beginner's Plough What most beginning students fail to realize about plough is that the upper-back muscles (middle trapezius, rhomboideus, and latissimus dorsi muscles) must contract and draw in toward the spine, and the hips must lift strongly to keep the lower back from rounding. A good tool to use is a chair; it helps to take roundedness out of the back and makes it easier for one to lift straight up with the hips and vertically up through the spine. As the hips and spine lift upward, pressure is lessened on the neck and the lower back.

Notice the position of the feet, legs, arms, hands, back, hips, and head in Figure 6.25A. The toes hook under and rest on the seat of the chair, the backs of the legs stretch out, the hips lift vertically upward, and the back of the head and neck rest on the pad or blanket when using a chair. The toes can rest on any part of the seat. Also notice the position of the arms in this photograph; how the fingers are clasped, the palms turned upward,

and the arms stretched out. This allows the shoulders to rotate and loosen, and the upper back to contract in and work in a stronger way. Work in this pose for ten to 30 seconds before slowly coming down and relaxing on your back with the knees to the chest.

Bringing the feet to the wall will aid the lift of the hips and the straightening of the spine. The work here is basically the same as with the chair. Most of the weight should be carried by the shoulders rather than the neck for the beginning plough student; keeping the legs parallel to the floor allows this to happen. Figure 6.25B shows the most commonly used hand position for plough with the arms straightened, the fingers interwoven, the wrists down, and the palms facing the back. Here Linda has a small towel underneath her shoulders, but a thickly folded blanket or two is highly recommended if the feet are brought down to the floor. This pose can be held for 30 seconds or longer, and the work is basically the same as described for Figure 6.25A.

Plough—Final Version Plough can eventually be held for up to five minutes by the advanced student of yoga, but only if a straight spine is maintained the whole time. Plough takes a lot of upper-back work, as well as lifting action through the spine and hips. Increase the amount of time you hold plough very slowly.

Despite the correct use of a double-folded mat under the shoulders, the pose done as shown in Figure 6.26A could result in very serious injuries to the neck and lower back. Walking the feet too far back, compounded by failure to work the upper-back muscles and to lift the hips, causes strain upon the neck and overstretch of the lower-back muscles.

A well-performed plough posture is pictured in Figure 6.26B. Notice the straightness of the spine, the work of the arms and legs, and the grace of the pose. The neck is being stretched, but not strained. With the aid of the

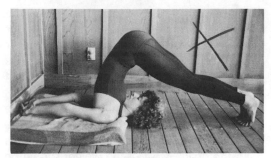

FIGURE 6.26A

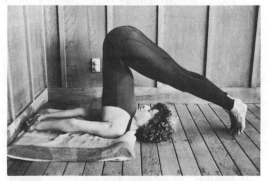

FIGURE 6.26B**

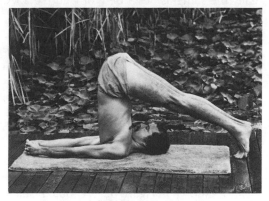

FIGURE 6.26C**

double-folded mat, the neck vertebrae are actually off the floor. The upper arms must push down firmly against the floor as the upper-back muscles contract and lift. The lower back and hips must also lift strongly.

After the neck muscles have stretched out through a fair amount of shoulderstand and plough practice with the aid of a folded blanket underneath the shoulders, plough can

be performed in the center of the room without a blanket (Figure 6.26C). Still, the neck vertebrae themselves should not be squished against the floor. The spine must lift vertically up and the neck muscles be stretched out passively. The deeper the fold in the frontside of the hips, the better the pose. A well-performed plough pose can be maintained from 20 seconds to five minutes, though the lengthy time period is generally not recommended.

Knee-to-Ear Pose The knee-to-ear pose is much easier to do after you have warmed up through numerous other postures. This posture increases the flexibility of the spine and back and serves as a tonic for the internal organs. Unless you are extremely flexible, it should not be held for long periods, because of the roundness of the back and the extreme stretch of the neck muscles that occurs during the performance of the posture.

From plough-splits position, bring the knees down next to the ears (Figure 6.27A). This is a more passive pose than plough and stretches the back and neck muscles more intensely. If this position is too uncomfortable, rest the knees on or close to the forehead or temples.

Three arm positions are commonly used in the knee-to-ear pose. One is with fingers clasped and arms stretched straight behind the back as in basic plough; the second is shown in Figure 6.27A with the hands grasping the feet; the third is shown and described in Figure 6.27B. Whichever hand position you use, hold the posture for ten to 30 seconds.

The hand position recommended in the knee-to-ear pose for the flexible student is to bring the arms around and to the outside of the back of the knees and place the fingers underneath the neck, interweaving them if possible. As shown in Figure 6.27B, once the hands are fixed, the elbows are drawn down toward the floor to aid the stretch of the low-

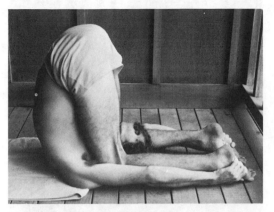

FIGURE 6.27A*

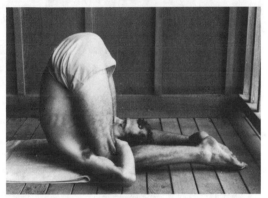

FIGURE 6.27B**

er-back muscles. Breathe deeply and hold the pose for ten to 30 seconds.

Bridge from Shoulderstand

The bridge pose flows nicely out of the shoulderstand. Moving back and forth from bridge to shoulderstand loosens and strengthens the back, leg, and arm muscles, firms the buttocks muscles, stimulates the lower-spine area, loosens the sacroiliac and hip joints, and is very invigorating for all the major systems of the body.

One series of movements that dramatically loosens the lower-back area is to move from shoulderstand to bridge, back up to shoulderstand, over to plough, back up to shoulderstand, and then back to bridge, and

so on. This flowing set can be done either in slow motion or by moving back and forth fairly quickly and can be performed numerous times. Many people have trouble moving from shoulderstand to bridge; this is caused by a lack of work in the buttocks and back muscles, and it results in too much downward pressure upon the wrists and compression in the lower back. A wall can be used as an aid (see Figure 6.28D) if the movement is a difficult one for you.

From shoulderstand, let the hands slide toward the hips, stretch the legs out away from the head, and bend the knees, keeping them fairly close together (Figure 6.28A). At this point, make sure to squeeze the buttocks muscles firmly and tuck the pelvis under forcefully. Try to take the pressure off the wrists not only by lifting and squeezing the buttocks muscles, but by contracting and lifting the upper-back muscles as well.

Continuing from Figure 6.34A, lightly bring the feet to the floor. The motion should be slow and graceful, and the pelvis should be tucked strongly throughout. The feet should touch down like a feather. The elbows and arms are like pillars, which must remain underneath the torso if proper support is to be attained while going down into bridge from shoulderstand (Figure 6.28B). Once down, take a couple of deep breaths, push off the floor with one foot, and follow it with the other to come back up into shoulderstand.

It is easier for most people to bring one foot down at a time than to bring both down together. Bend one knee, bring the foot of the bent leg to the floor, and keep the other leg lifted (Figure 6.28C). The second leg can then follow the first to the floor. Pause in bridge for a short while; then return to shoulderstand position by reversing the action used to go down, lifting one leg up as the other pushes against the floor.

If the wrists carry too much weight when attempting the work shown in Figure 6.28D, use a wall. Position the body far

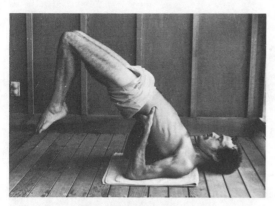

FIGURE 6.28A**

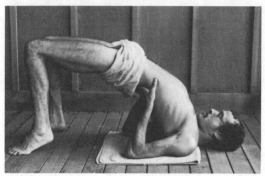

FIGURE 6.28B**

FIGURE 6.28C**

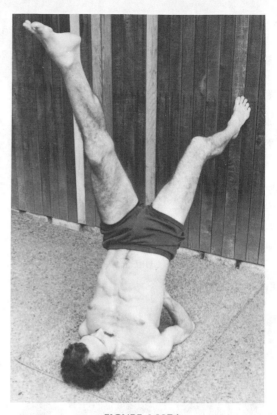

FIGURE 6.28D*

FIGURE 6.28E*

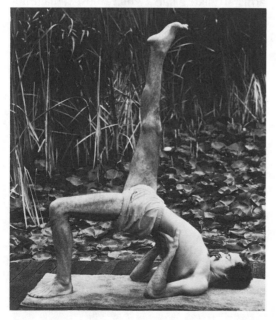

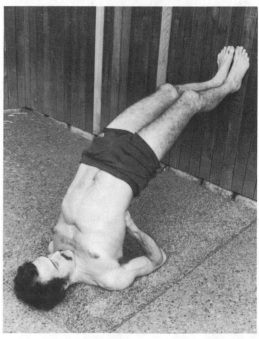

enough from the wall so that the leg has to reach out to touch the wall. Bring one foot to the wall while the other leg lifts (Figure 6.28D).

From the position shown in Figure 6.28D, bring the second foot to the wall and stretch the legs as much as possible. Keep the elbows close together by contracting the upper-back muscles, tuck the pelvis, squeeze the buttocks muscles, breathe deeply, and hold the pose a short while. From the position shown in Fig. 6.28E, push off the wall with one foot and lift back up into shoulderstand. Then repeat the bridge, bringing the other leg to the wall first. Finally, bring both feet to the wall together from shoulderstand position.

FOREARMSTAND

Forearmstand is not an extremely difficult posture to do with the aid of a wall. The benefits of the pose are similar to those of headstand, which is quite a list indeed. Forearmstand will help to build shoulder, arm, and upper-back strength. Practice of the posture will enable you to hold headstand for longer and longer periods. Be very careful not to overarch the lumbar vertebrae while up in forearmstand.

Forearmstand Out of Headstand
From headstand position, push the forearms and elbows down forcibly until the head raises off the floor. Look toward the hands, tuck the pelvis firmly under, and contract the abdominal and quadriceps muscles. Stretch strongly up through the forearms, torso, legs, and balls of the toes. Spread the toes and breathe deeply (Figure 6.29). Hold for ten seconds to one minute.

Ninety-degree Forearmstand with
Wall To loosen the shoulder joints, break up tension in the upper and middle back,

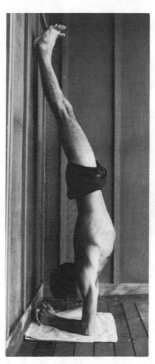

FIGURE 6.29*

build strength in the shoulder and upper-arm muscles, bring blood into the brain, and tone the leg muscles, the 90-degree forearmstand with a wall is highly recommended.

From forearm dog-stretch position with the base of the toes on the floor and the heels on the wall (Figure 6.30A), begin to walk the feet up the wall. Bring the legs to a 90-degree angle, press the feet against the wall, the forearms against the floor, and lift straight up with the spine, as pictured in Figure 6.30B. Move the chest in toward the wall, stretching the armpit and chest muscles. The head should be slightly off the floor, and all weight should be carried by the forearms with the aid of the feet against the wall. It is very important to lift the hips straight upward, getting a deep fold between the torso and the thighs. This upward lift prevents a jamming of the shoulder-joint muscles as the chest is expanded.

This is actually a safer pose than headstand for the beginning student, because no pressure is exerted upon the neck. The 90-degree forearmstand with the wall is an excel-

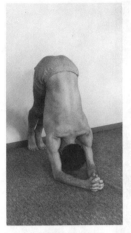

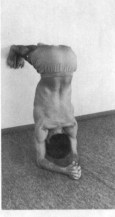

FIGURE 6.30A*   **FIGURE 6.30B***

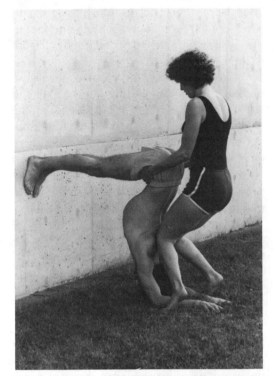

FIGURE 6.31*

lent way to build strength for the performance of headstand. Hold for ten to thirty seconds.

Ninety-degree Forearmstand with Partner

In Figure 6.31, Linda pushes her knees into the muscles between my shoulder blades and lifts may hips strongly upward, dramatically aiding the opening of my shoulder joints and the expansion of my chest cavity. Work in the pose for ten to twenty seconds.

Forearmstand with Strap

Use of a strap will help to keep the elbows from sliding out in forearmstand and bring awareness to the upper-back and shoulder muscles so that a straight upward lift of the body can occur.

The correct placement of the strap is demonstrated in Figure 6.32A. It should be tied in such a way that it keeps the elbows slightly closer than shoulder-distance apart. Ideally, the forearms remain parallel to each other in forearmstand, whether done with or without the wall.

In the final version of forearmstand, the arms, the back, and the legs should form a perfectly straight line in the center of the room. If you are using a strap, once you have found your balance, push out against the strap and lift vertically upward through the whole

FIGURE 6.32B**

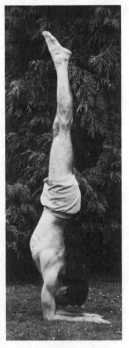

FIGURE 6.32A*

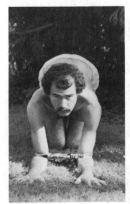

body. Look toward the hands to help maintain balance, but be very careful to keep the abdominal muscles drawn in and the buttocks muscles firmly contracted at the same time. Work in the pose for five seconds to one minute. In Figure 6.32B, the pose is shown without the use of a strap; the same basic instructions apply.

Kicking Up to Forearmstand A wall should be used in the practice of forearmstand until the pose has become fairly easy with its use. Prepare to kick up into forearmstand by walking the feet in toward the wall, lifting the head, and looking toward the wall. Then bring one foot underneath the hips, as shown by Linda in Figure 6.33A. Push off with the front foot and thrust the outstretched leg toward the wall from the position shown. The key to bringing both feet to the wall with the

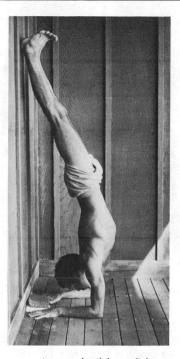

FIGURE 6.33B**

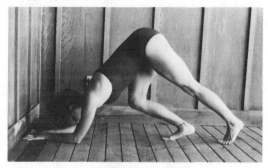

FIGURE 6.33A**

head lifted is to push down strongly with the forearms, lift up with the hips, and follow the thrust of the first leg with an equal thrust from the second one.

Once the feet are against the wall, straighten the legs and stretch through the base of the big toes, lift the shoulders as high as possible, keep the rib cage pulled in, and tuck the pelvis (Figure 6.33B). The abdominal muscles must be drawn in and the gluteus muscles contracted firmly. *Do not compress the lumbar vertebrae and lower-back muscles in forearmstand.* (Note the use of a book as an aid for keeping the hands apart.)

As you build confidence, try to take the feet away from the wall and balance upright. Lift straight up with the shoulders and legs. Do not let the elbows slide out. Hold for 20 seconds to one minute.

HANDSTAND

The handstand is every bit as wonderful as headstand for bringing blood into the brain. It is much safer for the neck than headstand, as no pressure is exerted upon the top of the head or neck. The main disadvantage to handstand is that it is difficult to maintain because it takes a tremendous amount of shoulder, arm, and wrist strength. Added to this is the fact that the lumbar vertebrae tend to overly compress in handstand; thus it becomes obvious that the posture must be approached with caution.

The fear of falling on your head is probably the greatest roadblock to moving up into handstand. However, there is a simple way to

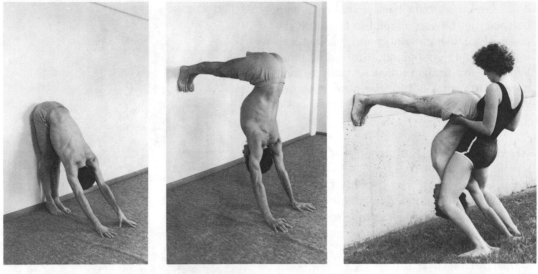

FIGURE 6.34A*   FIGURE 6.34B*   FIGURE 6.34C*

get into handstand that nearly everyone can learn. In Figures 6.35A–D, this easier and safer technique of moving into handstand by walking the feet up the wall is demonstrated. Handstand may be the best of all the hand-balancing poses for stimulating a flow of energy throughout the entire body.

Ninety-degree Handstand with Wall

Handstand with the legs 90 degrees to the wall builds strength in the arms, wrists, and shoulders, loosens the shoulder joints, and is an excellent exercise for flattening the thoracic curve and bringing awareness to the upper-back muscles. It is an effective preparation for backbends as well as handstand.

Begin by doing dog stretch, as shown in Figure 6.34A. Here the hands are placed approximately four feet in front of the toes, shoulder-width apart, the balls of the toes on the floor and the heels against the wall.

Walk the feet up the wall until the legs are parallel to the floor (Figure 6.34B). The most important thing to remember is to not overarch the lumbar vertebrae after the legs and feet have been brought to a 90-degree angle. Avoid compression of the lower-back

muscles by lifting straight up with the hips. Open the shoulder joint and expand the chest by bringing the upper chest toward the wall. Work in the pose 20 seconds to one minute, rest, and repeat.

Partner work is of great value in furthering the benefits of this pose. This adjustment requires the adjuster to do a lot of work. In Figure 6.34C, Linda brings her hands to the fold created by my hips and torso, lifts my hips strongly, and moves my chest toward the wall by pushing her lower abdominal and pelvic areas into my middle-upper back. The straight upward lift of my hips prevents a jamming of the topside shoulder-joint muscles, thus allowing the chest muscles to expand more fully. Work in the pose for 20 to 30 seconds.

Handstand: Walking All the Way up the Wall

Bring the heels close to the wall, the bottom to the wall, and the hands about 30 to 36 inches in front of the toes (Figure 6.35A). Shift the weight onto the hands, bend the knees, and begin to walk the feet up the wall. Push down strongly with the straightened arms.

Bring the spine to a vertical position by

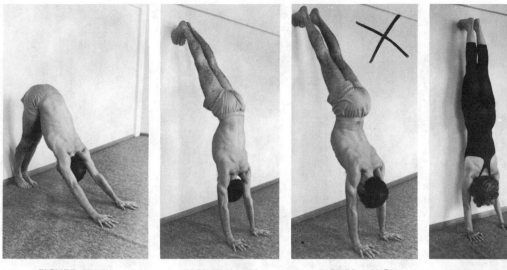

FIGURE 6.35A*   FIGURE 6.35B*   FIGURE 6.35C   FIGURE 6.35D**

walking the feet as high up the wall as possible, lifting the hips straight up, and straightening the legs. The buttocks muscles must contract, the abdominal muscles must be drawn in, the pelvis must tuck, and the lower back must lengthen, as you stretch strongly through the heels of the feet. Let the head hang while the rest of the body lifts up vigorously (Figure 6.35B). Hold for 20 seconds to one minute.

Avoid the mistake of arching the lower back as is illustrated in Figure 6.35C, as it puts terrible pressure onto the lumbar-vertebrae area.

Once you have become accustomed to keeping the spine straight with the hands three feet away from the wall, you are then ready to try walking the hands in toward the wall. When you have brought the hands to their final position two feet to six inches from the wall, contract the gluteus muscles, draw the abdominal muscles in, and stretch straight up through the heels of the feet, as shown in Figure 6.35D. Remain in the pose 20 seconds to one minute. To come out of this version of handstand, walk the hands out, bend the knees, and then slide the feet down.

Kicking Up into Handstand The rules for kicking up into handstand are:

1. Begin in dog stretch, hands just slightly wider than one shoulder-width apart, fingers four inches to one foot from the wall, fingers spread apart, and middle fingers facing the wall.
2. Bring one foot underneath the hips, push down with it, and practice kicking the other leg up toward the wall a few times.
3. Keep the arms straight throughout the kick.
4. To go all the way up into handstand, push against the floor with one foot, thrust the second leg up, and follow with the first leg until both feet touch the wall.

Partner Work in Handstand The handstand shown next is a posture that most people involved in yoga should be able to do within a matter of weeks, provided they have a partner to help lift them. If fear is too great a deterrent, practice walking up the wall, as shown in Figures 6.34A through 6.35B, countless numbers of times before attempting to kick up with the aid of a partner.

Now study the pictures to see how to work with a partner. The person kicking up

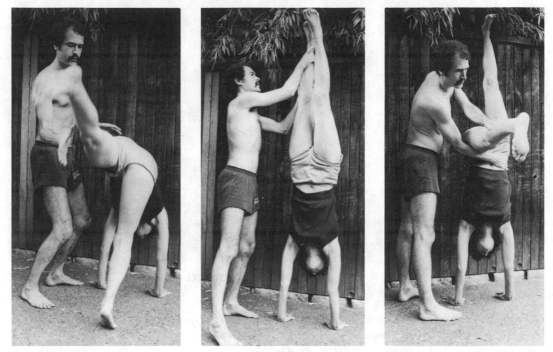

FIGURE 6.36A**   **FIGURE 6.36B****   **FIGURE 6.36C****

into handstand should use the directions just given.

Figure 6.36A shows the initial action; the adjuster simply is in a state of readiness. If one person is not enough support, a partner can stand on each side of the person going up. Even with help, the handstander must use their arms as solid pillars of support and must push down strongly with these straightened arms throughout this partner work. Notice how I am standing to the side of Linda's raised leg, as this will be the leg to initially take hold of.

In Figure 6.36B, I take hold of Linda's straightened leg and move it toward the wall as the other one follows. After both feet are brought to the wall, I next help Linda to achieve a good lift through her body by holding her bottom and lifting her up. This is shown in Figure 6.37C.

In Figure 6.36C, I assist Linda as she lowers one leg at a time. I press my hand against her stomach so that she can come down slowly.

Handstand: Final Pose with Wall
Once up in handstand, the arms, shoulders, upper-back, abdominal, buttocks, and leg muscles must all work strongly. Push the hands down and lift up through the entire body (Figure 6.37A). Hold for ten seconds to one minute, breathing slowly and deeply. Let the head hang loosely.

There is far too much arch in the lower back in the pose shown in Figure 6.37B. Two main actions that would correct this mistake are contracting the gluteus muscles and the abdominal muscles.

The partner correction for the mistake shown in Figure 6.37B is pictured in Figure 6.37C. I am lifting Linda's bottom with my right hand and pressing her rib cage toward

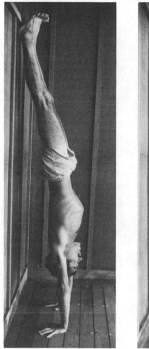

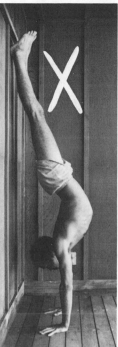

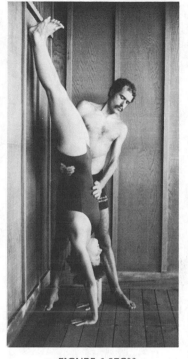

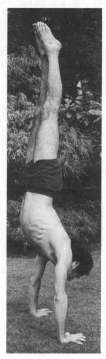

FIGURE 6.37A**   **FIGURE 6.37B**   **FIGURE 6.37C****   **FIGURE 6.38*****

the wall with my left hand. To begin with, it is quite important to work with a partner in handstand, not only to get up, but also to gain good alignment in the pose.

Handstand without Wall Eventually handstand should be done without the aid of a wall. It is a very challenging posture—one that most likely will take countless practice attempts before you find the way to balance in the pose. As shown in Figure 6.38, the body should be close to vertical in handstand. It helps to look down toward the floor and arch the neck, but do not do so at the cost of overarching the lower back.

To come up into the pose, follow the directions given on page 159 for kicking up into handstand, disregarding the directions when the wall is mentioned. Initially to practice handstand away from the wall, a partner should stand behind the handstander to take

hold of the feet and help align the body. Study Figure 6.38 to see the contractive work and lift that must take place in the arm, shoulder, back, buttocks, and leg muscles to hold handstand. Work in the pose for five to 30 seconds.

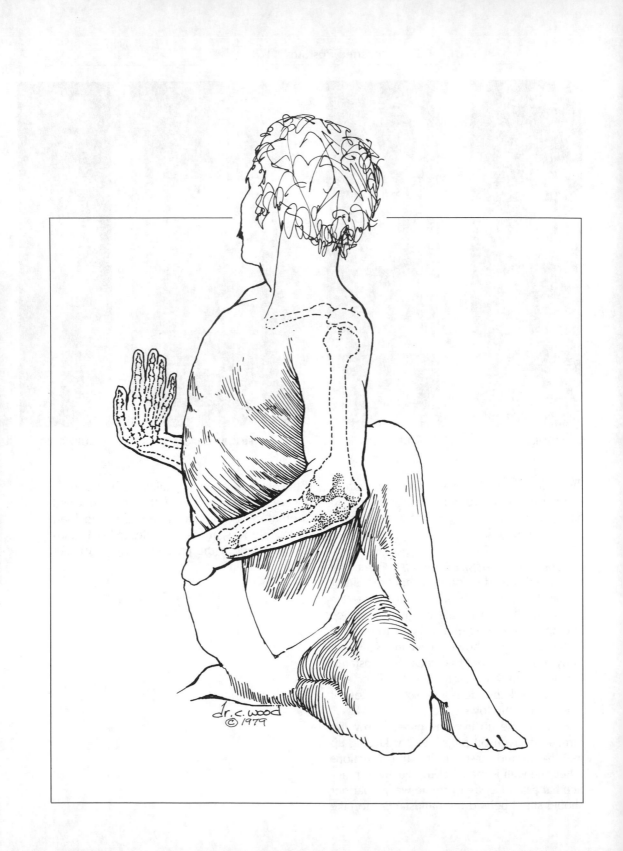

dr. c. wood
© 1979

SEVEN
twists

The most common reason for beginning Hatha Yoga practice is to relieve a backache. Backaches are so common in our society that it is unusual to find someone in the middle years who is not periodically plagued by one. Twists are the most highly recommended yoga postures to help relieve backaches. There are many varieties of twists—some easy to do, some quite difficult. In most cases, a person can find a twist or set of twists that can lessen the pain of a nagging backache fairly quickly.

There are many reasons for a backache to develop, the most common one being a buildup of downward compression upon the muscles of the back and the discs between the vertebrae. The downward force of gravity and the lack of lift of the chest are compounded into tight back muscles. For those who sit the majority of the day, the downward pressure of gravity often ends up focalizing in the lower-back area. Twists can help to relieve tense back muscles and overly compressed spinal discs brought about by the buildup of downward pressure.

Attempting to balance the two sides of the body is a primary concern of yoga practice. Twists can help to bring balance to an unbalanced body faster than any of the other main groups of yoga asanas. People who have a sideways curvature of the spine should do twists often, as should those who suffer from backaches caused by an unbalanced muscular system.

Scoliosis is a frightening word to most people. However, it has been my experience that almost everyone has a slight degree of sideways curvature in the spine. Tight muscles on one side of the back can cause the spine to be pulled in one direction or pushed to the other. Often the spine is forced into a slight S shape by a combination of tight muscles in the upper back on one side and tight muscles in the lower back on the opposite side. Backaches will center in either of the two areas, where the spine curves most to the side.

If tension in the tightest of the back muscles could be broken up, the spine could conceivably be straightened. It has been my experience that minor scoliosis can be controlled, if not eliminated, through the daily practice of yoga. Twists are most helpful in breaking up the tension of tight muscles and in bringing the vertebrae back into alignment.

Another thing that twists can do better

than another kind of posture is to revitalize the internal organs of digestion and elimination. The liver, gall bladder, pancreas, spleen, stomach, intestines, kidneys, and bladder are basically sacs, not muscles. Considering that only the stomach and the intestines have much in the way of independent peristaltic muscular action, it is understandable that the digestive and eliminative systems benefit when the muscles that encase them are stretched, twisted, and folded, which occurs in the various twisting postures.

This is not to say that yoga postures should be done immediately after a meal. On the contrary, at least two hours, preferably three to five hours, should pass after eating an average-size meal and engaging in a strenuous yoga workout. What the yoga asanas, and particularly the twists, can do is help to break up the most difficult-to-digest food substances and to aid in proper elimination.

Another benefit of twists is the reactivating effect they have upon the adrenal glands. Twists increase the blood flow through the adrenal area, which in turn helps to bring the

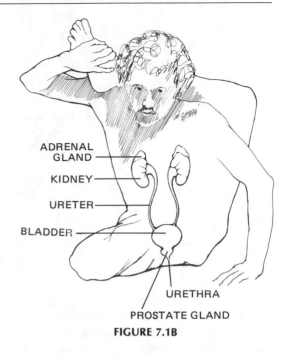

ADRENAL GLAND

KIDNEY

URETER

BLADDER

URETHRA

PROSTATE GLAND

FIGURE 7.1B

adrenals back into harmony with the other endocrine glands. The adrenals have a major influence on the energy level sustained throughout the day. If your energy level is prone to large ups and downs, you should do a few twisting postures each and every day to help the adrenal glands to function on a more even kilter.

TWISTS FOR EVERYONE

There are twists for everyone. Chair twists, shown in Chapter 3, are the simplest of the twisting postures, followed by lower-back twists, shown in this chapter, many of which are most effectively done while lying on the back. Next in line are the sitting floor twists (also contained within this chapter). I have found that the wall can be a tremendous aid to doing twists while sitting upright on the floor.

All of the standing twists are described in Chapter 5. Some of them are fairly easy to

FIGURE 7.1A

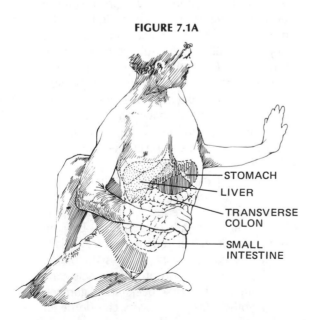

STOMACH

LIVER

TRANSVERSE COLON

SMALL INTESTINE

do, while others are extremely difficult. There are also the headstand, shoulderstand, and arm-balancing twisting postures, all described in Chapter 6. These are, for the most part, fairly difficult postures to perform correctly.

SITTING FLOOR TWISTS

The basic principle of most of the sitting twists is that the rib cage turns away from the suspended position of the hips and knees. For this to occur, the muscles in the upper part of the abdominal area must pull in a direction opposite that in which the muscles in the lower part of the abdomen have moved. This wringing action of the abdominal muscles is the main reason the internal organs are stimulated at such a deep level by the twisting postures.

Whatever twist you are doing, the initial concern should be to elongate the spine before turning the rib cage. Twists are safe only if proper length through the spine is maintained as you turn.

After you have placed the lower half of the body and the spine in their proper positions, the way to move into a twist is to rotate the rib cage on the exhale. Once you are in the final position, the breath should be as deep and slow as possible. Intercostal breathing into the lower part of the rib cage is desirable while working in the twisting poses. Abdominal breathing is usually difficult during an extreme twist, because the upper abdominal muscles should have pulled across with the rotation of the rib cage. When twists are performed properly, they stretch the intercostal muscles very effectively.

You should twist to both sides an equal number of times, provided there is not a huge imbalance between the two sides of your body. If you find that twisting in one direction is far more difficult than twisting the other direction, it would be a good practice to (1) do the more difficult side first, (2) do the eas-

ier side, and (3) go back to the tighter side and do it once more.

Sitting twists can be done any time during a yoga session. You can begin a yoga workout with twists, do them in the middle, or practice them near the end of the asana session. It is a good idea to end each yoga session with a completely symmetrical posture such as plough, forward stretch, or one of the many postures done in a supine position, followed by corpse pose.

Some twists can be held for up to one minute by the more flexible student; however, as a general rule, hold each sitting twist for five to 20 seconds before moving out of the pose. Once in the pose, try to twist farther and farther with each exhale. You should not become static in the twisting postures; rather, you should elongate through the spine with each inhale and continually make adjustments to increase the rotational action with each exhale.

One problem with holding twists is that the neck tires. After reaching the final pose, it is very important to keep the back of the neck as long as possible while bringing the chin down and looking over the shoulder. If the back of the neck is kept long as it turns, with as little cervical curve as possible, the neck muscles will be strengthened by holding the twisting posture.

In sitting twists the tendency is to raise the left shoulder when twisting toward the left and vice versa. This should be avoided, as it creates tension in the shoulder and blocks further twisting action. As you turn, each shoulder should remain an equal height from the floor—or as nearly so as possible. This means that when you are twisting to the left, the left shoulder must drop and the left shoulderblade area contract forcefully as the chest lifts and twists.

Try to expand the upper chest as much as possible in the twisting postures. The lift and expansion of the chest will help you to maintain length through the spine.

Remember, hold the sitting twists shown on the following pages anywhere from five to 20 seconds unless otherwise stated. While turning the rib cage to move into the twist, exhale. Once in the pose, twist farther with each exhale and elongate the spine with each inhale. Move slowly out of the twist and allow the muscles to realign themselves for a few seconds before going on to the other side or on to a new posture.

Now let us take a look at the individual twists.

Outstretched Leg Twists

With Strap With the aid of a strap around the feet and one arm pushing down behind the back, nearly anyone can achieve a fairly good twist, as shown in Figure 7.2. Note the length and straightness of the spine that is being maintained here. Work for five to 20 seconds, slowly release, and repeat to the other side.

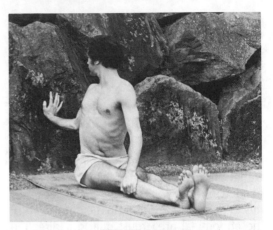

FIGURE 7.3A*

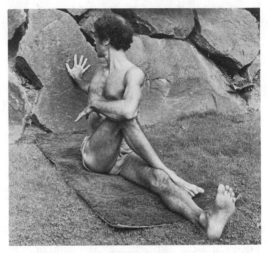

FIGURE 7.3B*

FIGURE 7.3C

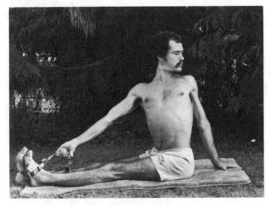

FIGURE 7.2*

With Wall Sit 24 to 30 inches from a wall, stretch your legs out, lift the chest, exhale, and twist to the right. Place the right hand against the wall and the left hand to the outside of the right knee. Draw the right shoulder blade in toward the spine, lift the left lower ribs, and stretch through the base of the toes of both legs, keeping the feet together. Lengthen the back of the neck and look over

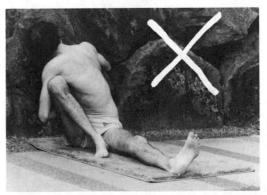

the right shoulder (Figure 7.3A). The placement of the hand against the wall must be carefully positioned slightly lower than the shoulder you have twisted toward and in direct line with the legs. The elbow of the arm toward the wall must be drawn in toward the ribs to free the shoulder joint from jamming. Work each side for five to 20 seconds.

After doing both sides, bend one knee and do the twist shown in Figure 7.3B. Sit about 30 inches from the wall with legs outstretched and bend the right knee, placing the foot to the outside of the left leg. Inhale, lift the chest, exhale, and twist to the right. Bring the right hand against the wall and wrap the left forearm around the right knee (more flexible students can bring their left elbow to the outside of the right knee). Push against the wall with the hand and pull against the knee with the forearm (or push against the knee with the elbow). Lift through the spine with each inhale and use the leverage of pulling (pushing) against the knee to help you twist with each exhale. The right shoulder should rotate back and down, and the right elbow should be drawn down. Do not jam the right shoulder by pushing against the wall before the shoulder has rotated externally (back and down). If your right shoulder feels jammed, pull against the knee with the left arm and lighten the push against the wall. (You may have to move your body another few inches away from the wall before you can get the proper shoulder rotation.) Once the shoulder has externally rotated, allow the right shoulder blade to be drawn inward as you twist. Stretch through the base of the toes of the outstretched leg. Work each side five to 20 seconds.

Twisting with a collapsed spinal column is very harmful; it can pull the spine out of alignment and can strain the lower-back muscles. In Figure 7.3C, the spine is collapsed, the shoulders are hunched, the neck is crooked, and the outstretched leg is slackened. It is through the lift and elongation of the body that twists are done correctly.

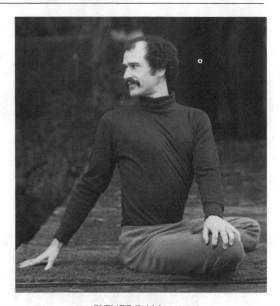

FIGURE 7.4A*

Sitting Twists

To do the posture shown in Figure 7.4A, sit with one heel in front of the pubic area and the other heel in front of the first one. Inhale, lift vertically up through the spine, exhale and twist toward the right, maintaining a lifted spine. As you twist take the fingertips of the right hand down on the ground a foot or so behind the right hip and take hold of the right knee with the left hand. With each inhale, pull against the knee with the hand and lift through the entire spine. With each exhale, push against the floor with the right hand; twist the ribs a little further. Keep your neck long and relaxed as you look over the right shoulder. Work in the post for 20 to 30 seconds; then repeat to the other side.

To prepare for the pose shown in Figure 7.4B, sit with the back approximately 24 to 30 inches from the wall and legs outstretched. Bend both knees and slide the left foot under the right knee; place the foot next to the right hip. Bring the right knee up and slide the right foot to the outside of the left knee. Inhale, pull against the right knee with the left hand or left forearm, twist right, and bring the right hand

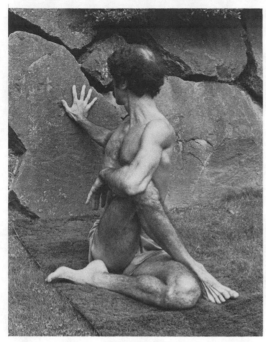

FIGURE 7.4B*

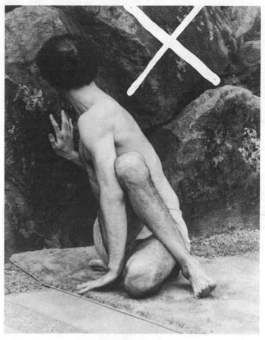

FIGURE 7.4C

to the wall (or the floor, approximately 12 in-ches behind the hips if you are not using a wall for leverage), with the fingers approx-imately shoulder height on the wall. With each inhale, lift through the spine by pulling the left arm against the knee; with each ex-hale, twist the rib cage toward the right. The right elbow is drawn down, the shoulder rotated back and down, and the right shoulder blade drawn inward as you push against the wall.

If your right shoulder feels jammed, then with each inhale pull aginst the knee with the left arm and lighten the push against the wall with the right hand. With each exhale drop the right shoulder and draw the elbow down toward the floor. To help the shoulder rota-tion, the right hand can rotate (thumb above and fingers below—the little finger becoming parallel to the floor). You may need to move further away from the wall to free the shoulder.

Keep the neck long and as relaxed as possible as you look over the right shoulder.

The right sitting bone should remain on the floor as you twist. (If your hip is too tight to allow the right buttock to drop to the floor, it would be best to do the twist shown in Figures 7.3B and 7.4A.)

The twist shown in Figure 7.4B is one of the best twisting postures to gain leverage for maximum rotational movement of the rib cage. After getting into the posture, work for ten to 20 seconds. Then inhale, slowly release the pose, exhale, and repeat to the other side. Do the complete set again. (This twist can be done with the back hand pushing against the floor, fingers pushing down, with the hand ap-proximately 12 to 15 inches behind the hips.)

Figure 7.4C shows a bad pose that results from sitting too close to the wall and from improper work. The back is rounded, the shoulders are tense, the rib cage lacks lift, and the leg and foot are improperly position-ed. To get a proper twist in this posture, you must begin at least two feet from the wall and then work very consciously toward a good alignment.

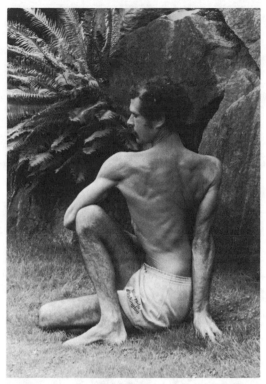

FIGURE 7.5A*

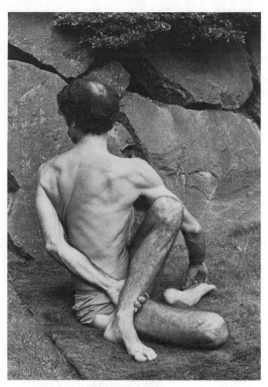

FIGURE 7.5B**

Grasping Ankle If you can get a good lift of the chest and keep the spine straight without the aid of a wall, you are ready to proceed with the pose shown in Figure 7.5A. Use the left elbow against the right knee for leverage, and push the back hand down against the floor. The back hand should be placed next to the bottom to help straighten the spine. Notice the squareness of the shoulders and the work of the upper-back muscles. In all of these twisting postures, you may occasionally wish to look over the front shoulder rather than the back shoulder, as shown here.

From Figure 7.5A, proceed into a more difficult pose by grasping the ankle with the hand that was previously pushing against the floor. (The twist shown in Figure 7.5B is done to the side opposite that shown in Figures 7.4B and 7.5A.) This is a wonderful twist that keeps the lower back from rounding and forces the

right shoulder-blade muscles to work properly. Maintain length through the neck vertebrae as you turn and look over the right shoulder.

The intermediate and advanced student should do this twist daily. Work in the pose for ten to 30 seconds, trying to lift the chest with each inhale and turn farther with each exhale. Repeat to the other side; do the set twice through.

Grasping Wrist From the ankle-grasping twist, you can move into the position demonstrated in Figure 7.6. To do it, set up the ankle-grasping twist to the left, then bring the right arm around the left shinbone and the left arm behind the back, as shown. Take hold of the right wrist with the left hand or vice versa. Taking hold of the left wrist with the right hand can be equally effective in helping you to lift the chest and pull the left shoulder

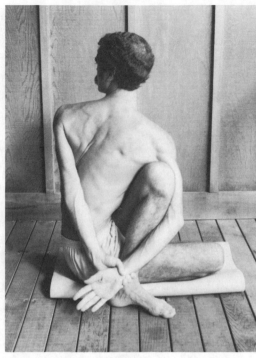

FIGURE 7.6**

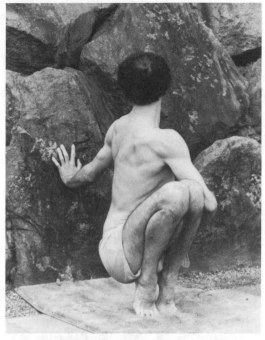

FIGURE 7.7A*
FIGURE 7.7B*

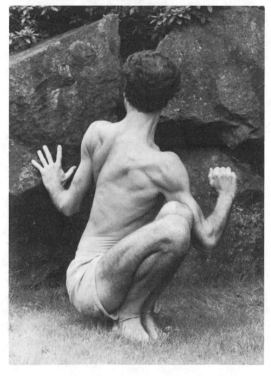

down and in. The key action is that of the right armpit area pushing back against the left knee, the left shoulder area pulling down and in toward the spine as the chest lifts and turns.

    This twist should not be done unless you can do the ankle-grasping twist pictured in Figure 7.5B. The back tends to round in this pose, whereas in Figure 7.5B it is easier to keep the spine vertical. Work in the pose for ten to 20 seconds, repeat to the other side, and then go through the set once again.

Squatting Twist

Beginner's Version Begin with the feet about 30 inches from the wall and the back facing the wall in a squatted position. Inhale, lift the heels, lengthen through the abdomen, exhale, and twist to the left, bringing the outside of the right arm to the outside of the left knee. Bring the left hand to the wall, draw the left shoulder blade in toward the spine, and pull both shoulders back and down as you lengthen through the entire spinal column. The right elbow is bent and the forearm can either face straight up or hold the outside of the left thigh. The knees should stay together. Lengthen the neck and look over the left shoulder (Figure 7.7A). Work each side for ten to 20 seconds.

Figure 7.7B shows the same pose as in Figure 7.7A, except that here, the heels are kept down. Keeping the heels down drops the pelvic girdle lower, allowing the lumbar spine to stretch out a little more as the rib cage is lifted and turned. Notice the straightness of the spine and down-and-back action of the right shoulder as the head turns to look over the shoulder. Work each side five to 20 seconds, breathing deeply in the pose.

Sitting Twists with Partners

Tension in the upper back, shoulder, and neck muscles can be released through deep massage work. The twist done while sitting on a chair or bench, as shown in Figure 7.8A, is a good position in which to massage the muscles between the shoulder blades. As the upper-back tension is released, then the shoulder you are twisting toward can rotate down and back more easily and the neck can lengthen and turn more freely.

Here Linda is stroking deeply along the inner ridge of my right shoulder blade. She is using her knuckles, but the thumbs or fingertips could be used equally effectively. The key to freeing the topside shoulder and the neck muscles for greater movement is to awaken the muscles between the shoulder blades. After she had worked my right upper back for ten seconds to one minute, I would twist to the left and she would work deeply to the inside of the left shoulder-blade area.

In Figure 7.8B, Linda is sitting on her right heel and pushing against her left knee with her right elbow. (This twist was shown in Figure 7.4B.) I help her to twist farther by bringing my right knee into the muscles to the

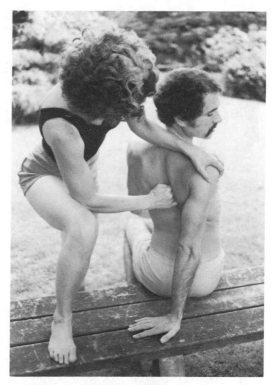

FIGURE 7.8A*

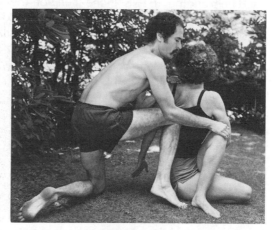

FIGURE 7.8B*

inside of her right shoulder blade, pushing in and up with my knee, pulling her left shoulder back and down with my left hand, and pulling her left knee in with my right hand. Work each side for ten to 20 seconds.

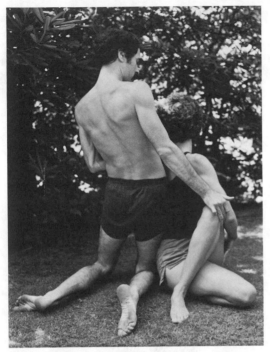

FIGURE 7.8C*

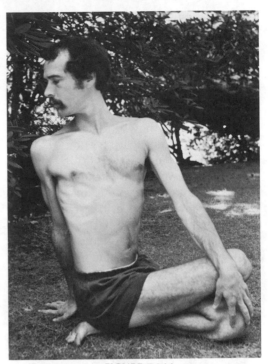

FIGURE 7.9A*
FIGURE 7.9B

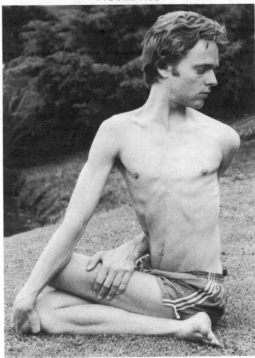

Shown in Figure 7.8C is a slightly less stressful way to work into the upper-back area and help another to twist in the sitting-on-the-heel twist compared with the partner work shown in Figure 7.8B. Here I press my right hip in and up into Linda's middle–upper-back muscles, pull her left shoulder back with my left hand, and pull her left knee back with my right hand. Work each side for ten to 30 seconds. Sometimes the partner adjustment shown in Figure 7.8B works best, whereas at other times the adjustment shown in Figure 7.8C works best.

Heroic Twist   The twists shown in Figures 7.9A and B loosen the shoulder and hip sockets as well as the entire spine, break up tension in the middle- and upper-back muscles, and expand the chest cavity.

Those with tight hips may need to sit on the heel of the foot of the bottom leg rather than between the heels to do this twist. In Figure 7.9A, I sit on the heel of my left foot, cross the right leg over the left leg, bring the heel of the right hand next to the buttocks, and twist to the right. My straightened right arm pushes down to help the lift and twist of the rib cage, and I bring my left hand to the outside of the top knee. As with most twists, you should turn the rib cage and chest farther and farther with each exhale and lift up through the spine with each inhale. Work in the pose for ten to 20 seconds, come out of the twist slowly, and then repeat to the other side.

Sitting between the heels with one knee crossed over the other one, as shown in Figure 7.9B, inhale, lift the chest, exhale, and twist in the direction opposite that of the top knee. To begin with, the back hand pushes down on the floor, as shown in Figure 7.9A. For the flexible student, the back hand can continue to be brought around until it holds first the ankle of the top leg, then the inner thigh of the bottom leg, and finally the outer thigh of the top leg. The other hand goes to the outside of the top knee and holds the bottom knee. Lengthen through the spine and look over the shoulder (Figure 7.9B). Twist a little farther with each exhale for five to 20 seconds and then repeat to the other side. (Figure 7.9B).

Steer Pose In steer pose, the legs resemble steer horns when the pose is viewed from above. Steer pose stretches the outer buttocks muscles as no other posture can. It is a good pose to counter the effect of all the inner-thigh stretching postures so strongly emphasized in yoga.

From Figure 7.9B leg position, bring the feet forward, trying to form a straight line with the two shinbones. Spread the feet as far apart as possible, and try to bring the knees toward the floor. Place the hands behind the bottom, and try to center the body behind the knees (Figure 7.10A).

From Figure 7.10A, place the hands on the ankles, lift the chest out, and slowly stretch the torso forward. Try to rest the chest

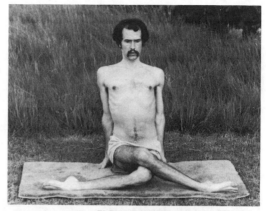

FIGURE 7.10A**

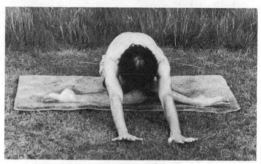

FIGURE 7.10B**

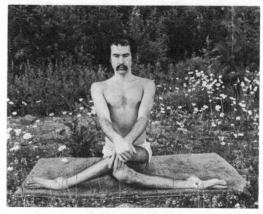

FIGURE 7.10C**

on the top knee, stretch the arms forward, and keep both sitting bones on the floor (Figure 7.10B). Here the outer buttocks muscles are definitely stretched to their limit. Let go into this pose for five to 20 seconds; repeat to the other side.

In the final steer pose, the hands are placed upon the knees and the spine is lifted vertically (Figure 7.10C). Ideally, the two shinbones form a straight line, the bottom knee touches the floor, and the top knee touches the bottom knee. This pose can be held anywhere from ten seconds to one minute. Repeat to the other side.

LOWER-BACK TWISTS

Lower-Back Twist with Bent-Knees

This very simple exercise is one of the greatest lower-back tension relievers of all. It can be done by everyone; it is safe and painless. Do it often! It is also a good warmup for the more difficult lower-back twists.

While lying on the back with the arms stretched out to the sides and palms facing down, pull the shoulders down and away from the ears, lengthen the back of the neck, bend the knees to the chest, and straighten the legs to a vertical position (Figure 7.11A). Stretch through the heels.

This preparatory posture lengthens the lower-back muscles and stretches the muscles at the back of the legs. It can be held anywhere from five to 30 seconds.

From the position shown in Figure 7.11A, exhale, bend the knees, and bring them close to the chest while resting on the back. Then inhale deeply, follow it with an exhale, and slowly bring the knees down toward the left, as shown in Figure 7.11B. Keep the knees off the floor and together, pull the right side of the rib cage back and down toward the right, roll the right shoulder back and down toward the floor, and stretch out through both arms. Hold for five to 15 seconds, breathing deeply, then inhale and bring the knees back to the chest. Repeat the same process to the other side (Figure 7.11C). Go to each side three more times.

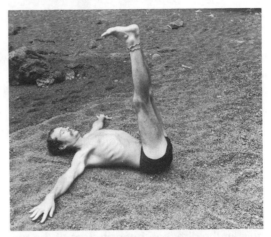

FIGURE 7.11A*

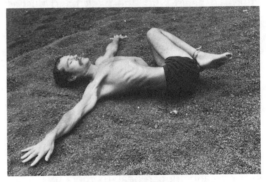

FIGURE 7.11B*

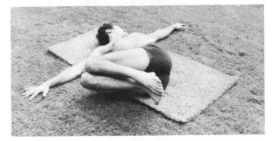

FIGURE 7.11C*

As you are doing this lower-back twisting series, pull the hips away from the shoulders to help maintain length in the lower spine and in both sides of the waist. To add to the spinal twist, the head can also turn in the direction opposite to the one the knees have taken. The turning of the neck and head is an excellent alternative that carries through the rotational movement of the rib-cage area into the neck.

You can also move in and out of each side in a flowing fashion, exhaling to the side and inhaling to the center several times.

Lower-Back Twist with Legs Outstretched

This is an excellent posture to loosen the lower-back muscles, realign the lumbar vertebrae, strengthen the abdominal and thigh muscles, and increase the efficiency of the internal organs of digestion and elimination. To do this posture correctly takes determined effort as well as flexibility, but it is well worth the effort, as it is one of the best postures of all for relieving back tension and strengthening the abdominal muscles.

While lying on the back with the arms stretched out to the side and the palms down, bend the knees and bring them close to the chest; then follow the instructions given for Figure 7.11B, bringing the bent knees to the left. Next straighten out both legs to the left, keeping them a few inches off the floor. Stretch through the heels of both feet and pull the right side of the rib cage back to the right. Keep both arms and shoulders down and the neck lengthened. Turn the head and look to the right hand (Figure 7.12A). Hold for a few seconds.

Inhale, bend the knees, and bring them back to the chest. Exhale and bring the bent knees to the right. Repeat the same process to the other side.

An alternative way to move into the lower-back twist with the legs outstretched is to begin on the back with the legs straightened vertically, as shown in Figure 7.11A, from here exhale, shift onto one hip, and slowly lower the straightened legs to the side of the hip you have shifted onto.

The rib cage pulls back and down in the opposite direction that the legs have gone, and the head turns away from the legs as well

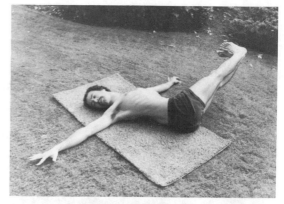

FIGURE 7.12A*

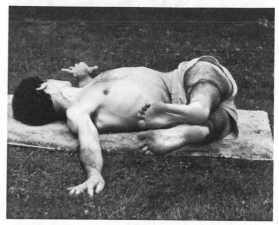

FIGURE 7.12B*

(Figure 7.12B). The main work must be done by the upper abdominal muscles. The spine should remain straight while you are doing this posture. Lengthen both sides of the waistline as the legs are brought to each side. Do the posture in slow motion, exhaling to bring the straightened legs to the side, and inhaling to bring them back to the center. Once the legs have been brought down to the side, hold for five to 10 seconds, extending through the base of the heels and base of the big toes.

Cat Twist

The cat twist is one of the best of all postures for relieving lower-back tension. It helps to

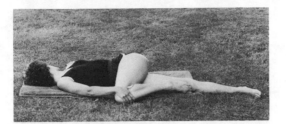

FIGURE 7.13A*

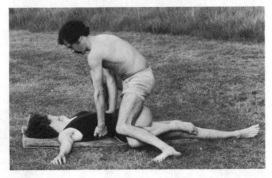

FIGURE 7.13B*

loosen the lower-back muscles and to realign the lumbar vertebrae. I recommend that this posture be practiced morning and evening on a daily basis.

This lower-back twist is very helpful for the organs of digestion, elimination, and reproduction, as well as the adrenal glands. It streches the outer-thigh and outer-buttocks muscles and loosens the hip socket. It is painless for most people to do and effective for all.

Lying on the back, bend the left leg and bring the heel of the foot just above the right knee on the quadriceps muscle. Inhale, bring the right hand to the outside of the left knee, and stretch the left arm straight out to the left (Figure 7.13A). Exhale, bring the left knee down toward the right, stretching straight down through the right side of the torso and leg. Pull back and down to the left with the left side of the rib cage as the knee comes toward the floor. Stretch out through the left arm, lengthen the neck, turn the head, and look to the left.

If you are a beginning yoga student, you have a choice: either bring the crossed-over knee to the floor (as shown in Figure 7.13A) and let the shoulder over which you are looking raise, or keep the shoulder to the floor and do not bring the crossed-over knee all the way to the floor. In order to keep the shoulder down, the shoulder-blade muscles of that side must contract. As the knee is brought toward the floor, the upper abdominal muscles must pull back and away from the bent knee in order to pull the rib cage back and down. When the abdominal muscles pull the lower part of the rib cage back toward the floor, all the internal organs will be stimulated.

Move the knee toward the floor on the exhale, breathe deeply once in the pose, and then come up on the inhale. The pose can be held for five to 20 seconds to either side. Do each side twice, holding the tighter side a bit longer.

The partner adjustment shown in Figure 7.13B is very effective for improving the cat twist. Basically, the partner gives an adjustment that helps to realign the lumbar vertebrae. It is very safe if done slowly and carefully.

Linda begins in the position shown in Figure 7.13A. I place my left shinbone on the outside of her left knee, my left hand underneath her right lower ribs, and my right hand on the topside of her left rib cage. My main work is lifting her right lower rib area from underneath. Meanwhile, I gently push down her left lower ribs with my right hand. Do not push down hard on the topside of the lower ribs, as the floating ribs could be damaged; pulling up from beneath the lower ribs is safe since the floating ribs do not attach to the spine.

My knee gently pushes on the outside of her crossed-over knee, but this is mainly to add stability so that she can turn her rib cage and thus stretch the lower left side of her back.

Work on each side for ten to 30 seconds.

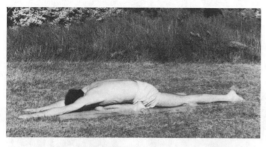

FIGURE 7.14*

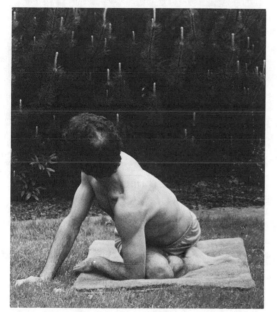

FIGURE 7.15*

Earth Pose

The earth pose stretches the outer-buttocks and outer-thigh muscles, releases tension in the iliopsoas muscles, and lengthens the lower back. It can be very restful.

Place the right heel in front of the opposite hip, stretch the left leg straight back, and stretch the torso out over the bent knee and the hands along the floor. You may have to lift the hip of the outstretched leg to bring the chest over the knee (Figure 7.14).

This forward-stretch posture can be held for 20 seconds to two minutes. It is the preparation for the asymmetrical twist shown in Figure 7.15.

Asymmetrical Twist Starting from earth pose (Figure 7.14), inhale, lengthen the spine, bring the left elbow outside the knee, and place the right hand one to two feet from the right hip. Keeping the torso low to the ground, exhale and turn the rib cage to the right. Pull the right shoulder back and down, expand the chest, and look over the right shoulder as you lengthen the spine and twist more and more. Push against the knee with the left elbow and brace the right hand on the floor to aid the twisting action (Figure 7.15). Work in the pose for ten to 20 seconds; repeat to the other side.

Outstretched-Torso Twist

This pose stretches out the lateral torso muscles nicely. It also stretches the hamstring and inner-thigh muscles and loosens the hip and shoulder sockets.

Bring the right heel into the groin and stretch the left leg out to the side. Inhale, stretch to the inside of the left leg with the torso, reach out with the left hand, and take hold of the inside of the left foot. Exhale, bring the left elbow to the floor inside the knee, lengthen the torso, roll the rib cage under, and bring the right arm over the head to take hold of the outside of the left foot. Turn and look up as you continue to lengthen the torso and rotate the rib cage (Figure 7.16A). Work each side for ten to 20 seconds.

An alternative arm position for the posture shown in Figure 7.16A is to bring the left hand to the right knee. Use the leverage of the

FIGURE 7.16A**

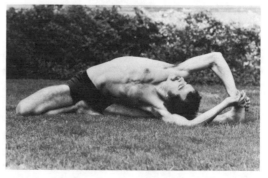

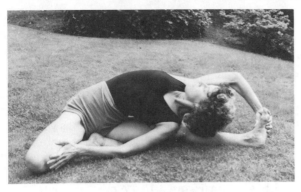

FIGURE 7.16B**

bottom hand to aid in the work of the pose by pushing against the knee, as shown in Figure 7.16B or by gripping the outside of the knee and pulling against it. The goal is to roll the rib cage under.

With Partner One of the main difficulties in doing the outstretched torso twist is to overcome the bunching that occurs between the rib cage and the hip area of the underneath side of the body. Partner work helps to elongate the torso, freeing the body to twist further.

In Figure 7.17, I am pulling Linda's arms up and out over the inside of her outstretched leg and bracing my foot against her foot. Maintaining the same grip, I help her to roll her rib cage under by pulling her top arm back so that her chest begins to turn toward the ceiling. Work each side for ten to 20 seconds.

Twists Out of Lotus

Half-bound Lotus Twist The half-bound lotus twist relieves tension in the upper, middle, and lower back. Beginning in full-lotus position, inhale, lift the chest, exhale, bring one hand behind the back, and clasp the foot with the hand of the same side. (An alternative for the flexible student is to continue to twist further and grasp the outside of the shinbone of the opposite side.) Bring the other hand to the outside of the knee that you have twisted toward. Lift strongly with the chest

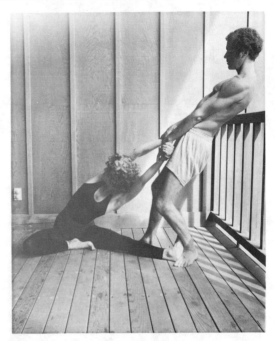

FIGURE 7.17*

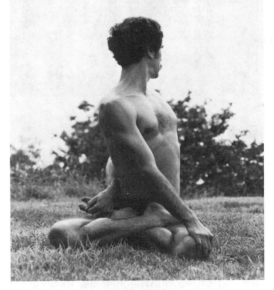

FIGURE 7.18**

and spine; use the leverage of the hands to twist as you look over the back shoulder and repeat to the other side (Figure 7.18). Work in the pose for five to 20 seconds.

Half-Lotus Twist The half-lotus twist brings flexibility to the spine, shoulders, hip socket, knees, and ankles. The position of the arm against the lower back serves as a deep massage, helping to relieve lower-back tension. The half-lotus twist works the shoulder joint to the extreme and opens the chest, allowing full rotational movement of the rib cage and deeper breathing.

The right foot rests in the crease of the left thigh and torso in half lotus. Inhale, lift the chest, exhale, and bring the left hand around behind the back until you can grasp, first the inner thigh of the bent leg, then the shinbone of the same leg. Reach out the right hand to the outside of the left shin, then, if possible, to the outside of the left foot (Figure 7.19A). Straighten the spinal cord; attain length from the base of the spine to the top of the neck. Breathe deeply and continue to lift with each inhale and twist with each exhale. Work for 20 seconds to one minute, release, and repeat to the other side.

The posture illustrated in Figure 7.19B is one of the best of the twists for breaking up tension in the back muscles. As can be seen in the drawing, the left upper-back muscles (latissimus dorsi, trapezius, and rhomboid)

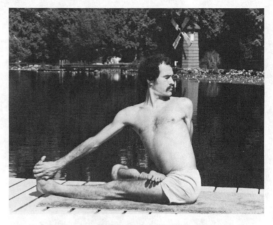

FIGURE 7.19A**

must contract strongly to allow the left hand to grasp the right shin. The right lower-back muscles (most notably the latissimus dorsi) must stretch, along with the buttocks (gluteus maximus) and thigh muscles (quadriceps) of the right leg to get into the pose. Also note the contractive work of the left shoulder (deltoideus) and left upper-arm muscles (biceps). While in any of the postures shown in this book, try to get inside the muscles of the body and feel how you could work them in a less painful and more efficient way.

FIGURE 7.19B

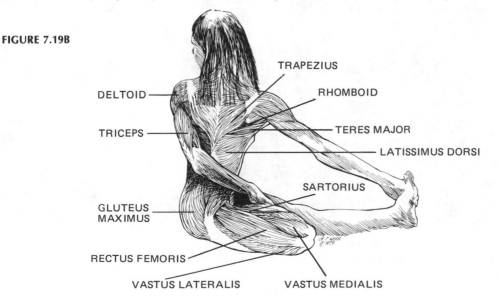

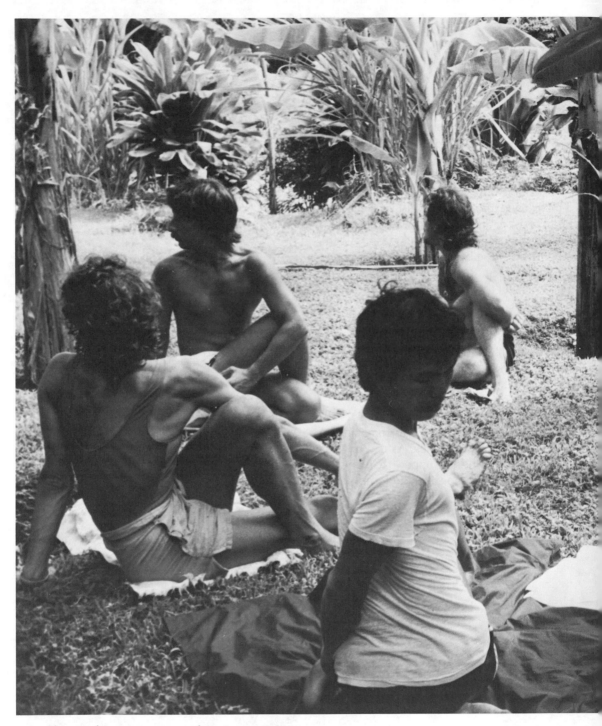

Shown above is a group of yogis practicing a twist in a banana grove located in the Sacred Pool area, Maui, Hawaii. This is a beginner's pose.

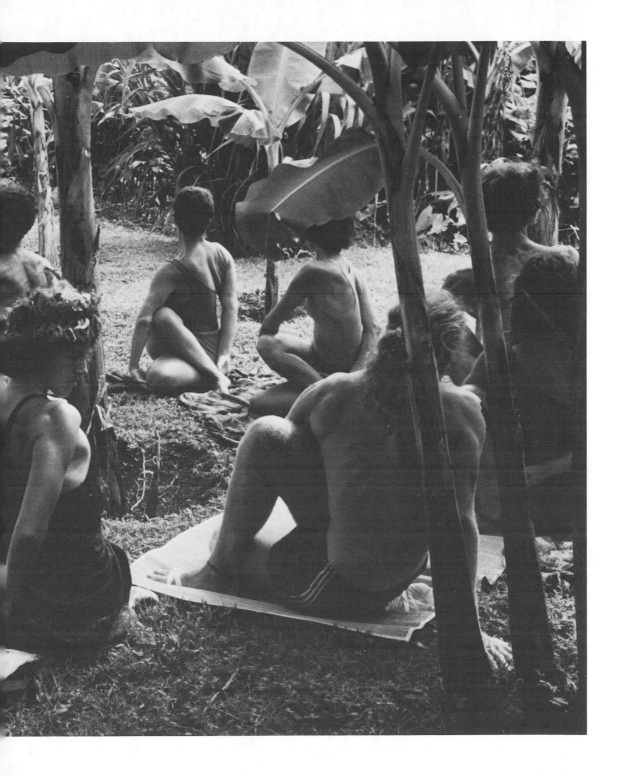

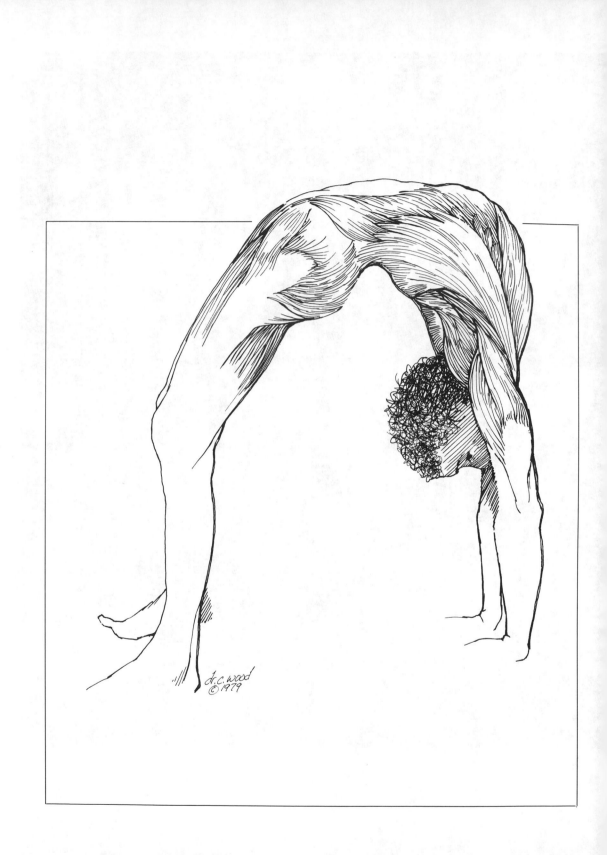

d.c.wood
©1979

EIGHT
backbends

Backbends can elicit a feeling of exceptional well-being as a result of the whole body's becoming supercharged with oxygen. Since each and every cell of the body, including brain cells, must have oxygen to live, performing a set of backbends energizes both the body and the mind. The nervous system is strengthened, the endocrine system is stimulated, the efficiency of the respiratory and circulatory systems is vastly improved, the digestive organs are stimulated, and the eliminative system is improved.

The practice of Hatha Yoga brings with it an answer to the pressing problem of how to keep healthy under the constant pressure of modern living. A supple spine and efficiently working internal organs are two of the main keys to good health. Practice of the backbending postures will increase the suppleness of the spine and the efficiency of the internal organs to a very high degree.

At a muscular level, backbending action stretches the frontside torso and quadriceps muscles to the utmost. The buttocks and upper-back muscles must exert incredibly strong contractive action as the frontside muscles stretch. If the extreme contraction does not take place in the buttocks and upper-back muscles, compression of the discs between the lumbar vertebrae will occur. The pelvis must tuck to the utmost and the chest lift and expand while performing backbends!

A caved-in chest leads to shallow breathing and the retention of tension. To release physical, mental, and emotional tension, a deep, slow, rhythmic breath must be focused upon. For this desired type of breathing to occur, the chest cavity must be able to expand and contract fully. The chest muscles surrounding the rib cage must be free to stretch, and the tightness of the chest-cavity muscles must be released. Backbends free the chest, rib-cage, back, and abdominal muscles, thus allowing improved breathing to occur.

Internal rotation of the shoulder joint is performed by most people throughout the day, as moving forward with the hands and arms is required by most work tasks. After a few years of using the arms and hands almost solely in front of the body, one's shoulders tend to stiffen in a forward position. Backbends help to loosen the shoulder-joint muscles and ligaments and stimulate the production of synovial fluid (lubricating fluid) in these joints. Calcium deposits, bursitis, and general tension through the upper back, neck, shoulders, and arms can be relieved through the rotational movement of the shoulder joints that backbends emphasize.

Backbends also loosen the pelvic-girdle area of the body and free blocked energy in the pelvic basin. Backbends demand that you tuck the pelvis in the most extreme way possible; and in so doing, you loosen the sacroiliac joint. The sacroiliac region of the body must be freed to enable graceful, fluid movement of the lower half of the body.

Beyond the physiological level, the development of greater will power becomes the yogi's main concern. Backbends work directly on the strength of will, because it takes determined effort to do a proper backbend, and fear must be dealt with. Throughout most of our daily life we move in a forward direction and focus on what is in front of us. Backbends take us the other way, toward what is behind our field of vision. Doing backbends helps one to conquer deep-rooted fears and to become a stronger individual.

Of the six main groups of yoga postures (standing, inverted, twists, backbends, forward stretches, and meditational poses), the backbends are the most exhilarating. They feel wonderful when done correctly, and yet —I cannot stress it enough—you must be very careful when doing backbends, because severe backaches can result if they are done without extreme tucking action of the pelvis.

Most backbends should be held for only a few seconds, as it is best to simply move in and out of these poses before you tire and overarch the lumbar area. Until you are very familiar with backbends, it is best to do a few repetitions rather than try to hold one of these demanding poses for more than a few seconds. There are a couple of exceptions that will be pointed out.

Most backbends should be moved into during a deep inhalation. Once in the pose,

you should breathe as slowly and deeply as possible. The backbending position should then be released on the exhale. To move into certain of the most extreme backbends, however, it works best to exhale and then lift into the pose. Try to come out of a backbend gracefully and slowly. It is a good habit to rest on your back with the knees brought to the chest or in some simple forward-stretch pose for a short while after each particular backbending action.

You should not end a yoga workout with backbends. No matter how careful you are, the greatest arching generally will occur in the lumbar vertebrae. This must be "ironed out" through forward stretches and simple relaxation postures on the back to end a yoga session.

Cat–Cow

Cat–cow is a series of wavelike spinal movements that loosen, warm, and energize the spine and the muscles along the spine. Cat–cow can be performed any time during a yoga workout; it is particularly appropriate as a preparation for backbends.

If you desire a supple spine, practice cat–cow daily. These movements can bring relief to some types of nagging backaches and neckaches. The breath and body must work as one during this exercise.

Figure 8.1A shows the abdominal area hanging low like a cow's; thus the name *cow* posture. Figure 8.1B shows the back arching like an angry cat's; thus the name *cat* posture. To get into position, bring the hands under the shoulders and bring the knees together under the hips. Inhale, drop the abdominal muscles, tilt the pelvis upward, drop down between the shoulder blades, and look up, as shown in Figure 8.1A.

From here exhale with force, lift the abdominal muscles, tuck the pelvis under, round the upper back, and bring the chin to the chest, as shown in Figure 8.1B. Cat–cow

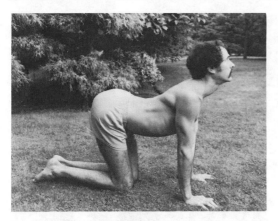

FIGURE 8.1A*

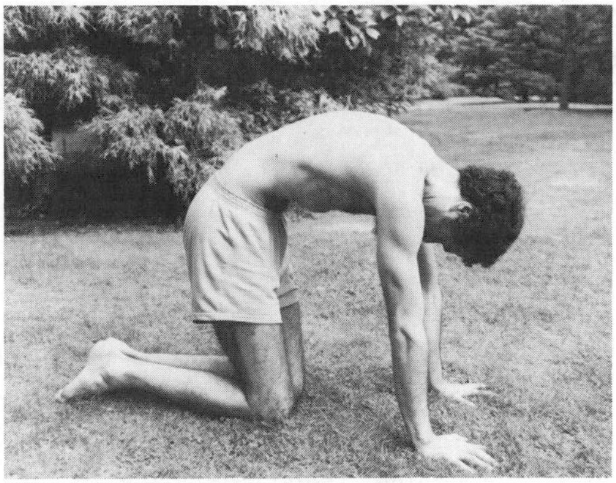

FIGURE 8.1B*

should be performed in a wavelike way by flowing in and out of these two positions. As the abdominal muscles passively drop and round out in cow position, the air will rush in to fill the lungs, the pelvis will tilt upward, and the spine should sway in a wavelike manner from its bottom to its top. The upward lift of the head occurs at the very end of cow.

While performing cat–cow, the main emphasis should be on the exhalation and the movement into cat position. This spinal movement begins as the abdominal muscles lift strongly back toward the backbone and the air is exhaled out. Carrying the movement through brings about a tucking action of the pelvis and a rounding of the back in a wave-like manner from the bottom to the top of the spine. The chin comes down to the chest at the very end of the cat posture.

Cat–cow can be done very slowly or very quickly; in either case, the wavelike rhythm should be maintained. Keep the arms straight throughout the spinal movements and let the breath carry the movement. You can make the movements subtle or do them in a more exaggerated way. Do five to ten rounds of cat–cow, rest in prayer pose, and then do five to ten more rounds. These same basic spinal movements can be done while sitting in the cross-legged position.

Cobra, Bow, and Locust

From among hundreds of yoga postures, the ancient masters agreed upon a set of twelve that stimulate every muscle, nerve, and gland of the body. These "magic" twelve yoga postures are headstand, shoulderstand, plough, fish, peacock, spinal twist (left and right), cobra, bow, locust, sitting forward stretch, corpse, and lotus pose.

At this point I would like to deal with cobra, bow, and locust. These backbends form a set that can be done one after the other, so that they work progressively down the back. The danger of cobra and bow is the tendency to overarch the lumbar vertebrae and underarch the thoracic vertebrae. The danger of locust is, again, compression of the lumbar area of the spine.

The cobra, bow, locust series elicit a wonderful feeling when done properly, but they must be done carefully. The lower back must be protected through strong contraction of the upper-back and buttocks muscles in cobra and bow and through the stretch of the legs in locust.

Cobra   In cobra, the raised head and body resemble the raised hood of a cobra. Cobra loosens the shoulder joints; strengthens the upper back; tones the buttocks muscles; in-

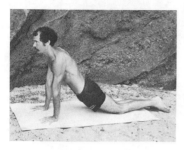

FIGURE 8.2A*

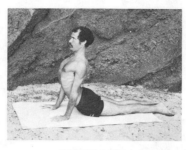

FIGURE 8.2B*

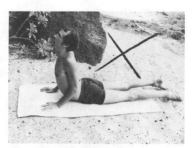

FIGURE 8.2C

creases lung capacity; stretches the thigh, frontside-hip, abdominal, and chest muscles; stimulates the thyroid and adrenal glands; improves kidney functioning; releases blocked energy from the pelvic region; limbers and strengthens the spine; and increases the efficiency of the organs of digestion, elimination, and reproduction. All in all, cobra is a very powerful pose.

From cat position, slide the hands a few inches forward in front of the line of the shoulders, exhale further, squeeze the buttocks firmly, and lower the hips close to the floor in a gliding fashion. Look straight forward and keep the arms straight (Figure 8.2A).

From the position shown in Figure 8.2A, continue to move down with the hips and pull the chest through the arms on a deep inhale. Pull the shoulders back and down. Squeeze the buttocks muscles firmly and try to drive the hips down to the floor while keeping the arms straight. Lengthen the neck by lifting through the back of the head. Hold the cobra pose for a few seconds, taking a couple of deep breaths; then on the exhale unfold the vertebrae down one by one very slowly and rest onto the stomach. Come back to cat position and repeat once again (Figure 8.2B).

Figure 8.2C shows an incorrectly done cobra pose. Painful compression in the lower back and neck areas will occur if the pose is done in this way. Compare with the posture shown in Figure 8.2B to see the differences between an alive pose and a poorly performed cobra.

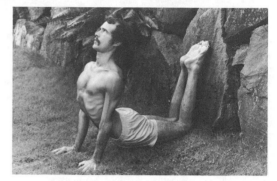

FIGURE 8.3A*

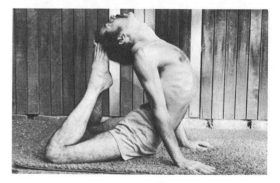

FIGURE 8.3B**

King Cobra   In king cobra the knees are bent and, ideally, the toes and head touch. In the end, the leg, torso, and head form a closed circuit of energy.

To prepare for king cobra, bend the knees and place them against a wall, bring the bottom next to the heels, and the hands on the floor in front of the shoulders. From here, exhale, tuck the tailbone under strongly, and lower the hips toward the floor. Inhale, bring the chest through the arms, expand the chest by pulling the shoulders back and down, keep the knees close to each other, and try to drive the hips and tailbone to the floor (Figure 8.3A). Release the pose after a few seconds.

In the final king cobra posture, the head and toes touch together. Bring the knees 12 to 30 inches apart and the hands underneath the shoulders, and then work in the same manner as described in Figure 8.3B with the knees spread. Arch the neck and point the toes toward the head as you squeeze the buttocks and shoulder-blade muscles. Hold for a few seconds and breathe deeply once in the pose.

Bow In the bow pose the body resembles an arched bow. The benefits of bow are very similar to those mentioned for cobra, but the throat, chest, abdominal, frontside-thigh, and arm muscles are stretched more intensely, owing to the backward-pulling action of the legs upon the arms and back. Also, the shoulder joint is loosened, the thyroid and sexual glands are stimulated, and the upper-back muscles are worked more intensely than in cobra.

There are two ways to do bow. One is to lift the knees high and remain flat on the stomach, as shown in Figure 8.4A. The second way is to lift the chest high and keep the knees close to the floor, as in Figure 8.4B.

To move into bow, lie on the stomach, bend the knees, and take hold of the ankles. The beginner should work on bow with the knees one to two feet apart. The ideal bow (for more advanced students) is to have the knees and ankles in close toward each other.

Referring to Figure 8.4-A, inhale, lift the knees high, flex the ankles, and pull back with the feet. Contract the buttocks and upper-back muscles, relax the shoulders, arch the neck, and look up. Hold for five to 20 seconds, breathing as deeply and slowly as possible.

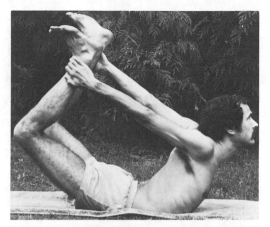

FIGURE 8.4A*

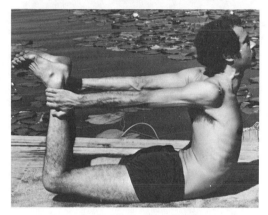

FIGURE 8.4B**

FIGURE 8.4C*

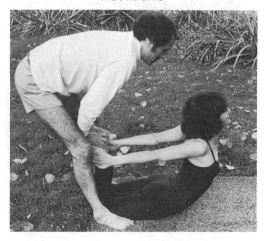

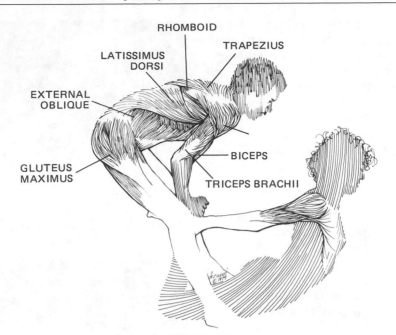

RHOMBOID

TRAPEZIUS

LATISSIMUS
DORSI

EXTERNAL
OBLIQUE

BICEPS

GLUTEUS
MAXIMUS

TRICEPS BRACHII

FIGURE 8.4D

Referring to Figure 8.4B, keep the knees close together and near the floor as you inhale, lift the chest, and pull the flexed ankles back. Tighten the buttocks muscles, push the pubis into the floor, continue pulling back with the feet, expand the chest, stretch the arms, arch the neck, and look up. Hold for five to ten seconds.

Partner work expands the chest cavity and breaks up upper-back tension in bow. In Figure 8.4C, as I pull Gail's flexed ankles back, she must squeeze her buttocks muscles very firmly. The frontside of her body must let go into the stretch. Work for ten to 20 seconds.

The medical illustration of partner work in bow (Figure 8.4D) points out a contrasting element in partner work. One thing you'll note is that the person being adjusted must surrender into the work of the adjustment, as his or her body will be taken to its limit. The fluidity of the lines running through Linda's body points this out. The contrasting element is that the person doing the adjustment must

actively work to move the partner deeply into the pose. Notice the work of the thigh, buttocks, back, chest, and arm muscles of my body here.

Figure 8.4E shows the bow pose done on the side. The advantage here is that it is easier to contract the gluteus muscles than when on the stomach. To do this version, lie

FIGURE 8.4E*

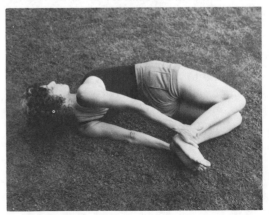

on one side, bend the knees, take hold of the ankles, contract the gluteus muscles, pull the feet back, and look over either the top or the bottom shoulder. Work in the pose for five to 20 seconds and repeat to the other side.

Locust   Locust is a posture that requires a lot of determined effort to perform. Because of the incredible amount of work that must take place in order to lift the legs and because of the end position of the pose, the circulatory system is stimulated and a tremendous amount of blood is brought to the throat and brain. Locust also helps to clear the intestinal tract and can help to relieve constipation. It is a posture that tones and strengthens the leg, buttocks, and lower-back muscles and helps to increase the efficiency of the endocrine system. Locust is not recommended for those with high blood pressure or serious heart ailments.

Half Locust   Half locust involves much less work than full locust, and yet there must be a strong stretch of the legs to avoid lumbar compression. To prepare for half locust, make a fist with the hands and place them so that the palms are under and facing the thighs. With the chin on the floor, contract the buttocks muscles, inhale, lift one leg, contract the thigh muscles, and stretch through the toes of the raised leg. Press the opposite foot to the floor and square the hips (Figure 8.5A). Hold five to 15 seconds and repeat to the other side.

Full Locust   Full locust is an extremely difficult pose for the beginning student to perform. To lift the legs up requires tremendous strength in the hamstring, buttocks, and lower-back muscles, as well as flexibility in the lumbar spine. Even if you can only bring the feet a few inches above the ground, do not be

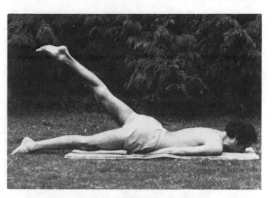

FIGURE 8.5A*

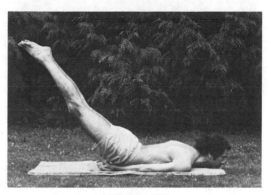

FIGURE 8.5B*

discouraged, because you will get an equally positive benefit with the feet low.

Begin as in half locust, then lift both legs with an inhale. Firm contraction of the buttocks and hamstring muscles is the key. Keep the big toes, ankles, and the knees together as the legs are stretched to the utmost. Point the toes and hold for a few seconds (Figure 8.5B).

Fish

Fish pose gets its name by virtue of the fact that one can float on the surface of a body of water in fish position. Beginner's fish pose can be helpful for the person who has a rigid middle and upper back; it isolates these two areas and forces them to work. Fish also stretches

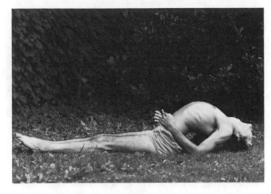

FIGURE 8.6*

the frontside of the neck and the upper-chest muscles quite nicely, and it is good for those with thyroid problems and for those who have a hard time getting air into the upper part of the lungs. It helps to counterbalance the effect that forward stretches, plough, and shoulderstand have upon the neck and back muscles and internal organs.

Be careful not to put too much pressure upon the neck in fish pose. The upper-back muscles should contract firmly, and the top of the head should rest lightly upon the floor. The work of the upper-back muscles can be facilitated by pushing the elbows strongly down into the floor. Fish is one of the few backbends that does not require the buttocks muscles to do any work at all.

Lie on your back, stretch your legs, bring the elbows down by the lower part of the rib cage, make a soft fist with the hands, and bring the forearms to a vertical position. Inhale, push the elbows down, lift the chest, and arch the neck to bring the top of the head to the floor. Contract strongly between the shoulder blades and slide the head back toward the hips (Figure 8.6). Hold for five to 20 seconds, breathing deeply and slowly.

Camel

The camel pose is one of the most highly recommended of the yoga backbends. In this pose the body resembles the hump of a camel, with the sternum (chest bone) being the highest point of the hump. The expansion of the chest cavity and the release of tension in the upper-back muscles are two of the greatest benefits of the camel pose. It also stretches the entire frontside of the body, thus increasing the circulation of blood and oxygen throughout the body, and it helps to bring awareness to the upper-back muscles, such that forward-stooping shoulders can be avoided.

Compression in the lumbar area is difficult to overcome, but certainly not impossible if the buttocks and upper-back muscles are contracted strongly and the chest lifted as high as possible while in camel.

Kneel down and bring the knees together (the beginning student may spread the knees hip-distance apart). Inhale, bring the hands onto the bottom, contract the gluteus muscles tightly, lift the chest, and begin to arch the upper back by drawing the shoulder blades in toward the spine. Keep the chin toward the chest. The elbows pull in toward each other as you lift (Figure 8.7A).

From Figure 8.7A, bring the hands to the heels of the feet. Continuing the contraction of the gluteus muscles and of the muscles between the shoulder blades, let the head hang backward (Figure 8.7B). Breathe as deeply as possible in this position for five to 20 seconds, then come out of the pose slowly, rest the bottom on the heels, and stretch the torso and hands forward in prayer position.

The beginning student can help lessen compression in the lower back by hooking the toes under, bringing the hands to the heels of the feet, and strongly tucking the pelvis (Figure 8.7C). This position can be held for five to 20 seconds, with the buttocks muscles squeezing firmly throughout. Bringing the chin to the chest helps, as the less the curve in the neck, the less compression there tends to be in lower back. Move into this version in the same way as discussed for Figures 8.7A and B.

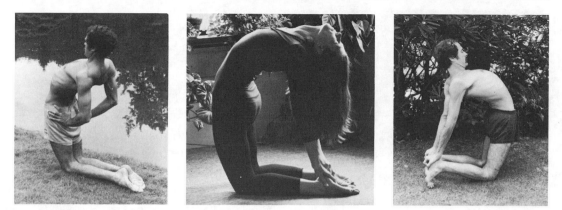

FIGURE 8.7A*   **FIGURE 8.7B****   **FIGURE 8.7C***

Camel with Partners The adjustment shown in Figure 8.8Λ is excellent for those who carry upper-back tension and for those who have a difficult time breathing. The person doing the pulling must be careful not to pull the arms too much and must be correct with the placement and push of the feet. The ball of my top foot has been placed between the space of Linda's shoulder blades, on the contracted muscles. As Linda's chest is expanded through the firm push of my top foot, I help her to avoid overarching in the lower back by the downward pushing action of my lower foot. Notice how she has brought her hips against the wall. Linda breathes deeply and relaxes into the adjustment. Work for ten to 30 seconds.

Those with tight shoulders can get uncomfortable bunching of the muscles at the top of the shoulders when they try to bring their arms up and back in the backbending poses. Partner work can help to relieve this congestion. The partner adjustment shown in Figures 8.8B and C is a very helpful way to awaken the upper-back muscles as the arms are brought back. In Figure 8.8B, I clasp my fingers and place the knuckles of my thumbs between the topside of Linda's shoulder blades to the sides of the spine. While she clasps her hands around my neck, I press in and push the skin between her shoulder blades downward with my knuckles while pulling her arms up.

From Figure 8.8B, I lift up and back with my chest and neck and slowly dig the knuckles of my thumbs down along the muscles of Linda's upper back. *If the standing person lifts up sufficiently, he or she can begin to arch the partner's back without causing compression in the kneeling person's lower back!* Linda tucks her pelvis, breathes deeply, and lets go into the adjustment (Figure 8.8C). Work for ten to 30 seconds.

Both people have to be very flexible to go to the extreme shown in Figure 8.8D. In this version I hold Linda's arms and continue to arch back as she lets go into the stretch. It is very important that I tuck my pelvis strongly and push in and up with my hips while taking Linda back. Breathe deeply and work for ten to 20 seconds.

Figures 8.8E and F point out the muscular work involved in the partner adjustments shown in Figures 8.8C and D. In Figure 8.8E, note the work involved by both Linda's body and mine. The gluteus muscles of both persons must contract; her quadriceps, abdominal, and armpit-area muscles must stretch; and my thigh, upper-back, shoulder, arm and neck muscles must work strongly. As I push the knuckles of my thumbs between Linda's shoulder blades, her lattisimus dorsi, middle

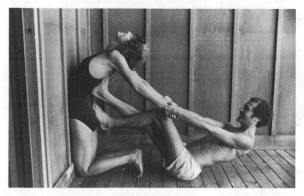

FIGURE 8.8A*

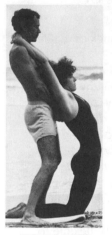

FIGURE 8.8B*

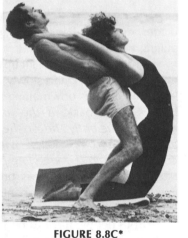

FIGURE 8.8C*

FIGURE 8.8D*

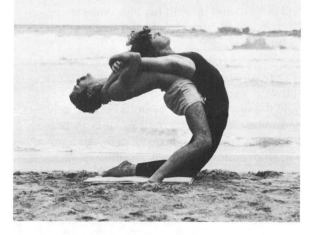

LATISSIMUS DORSI

GLUTEUS MAXIMUS

GLUTEUS MEDIUS

TENSOR FASCIA LATA

ILIOTIBIAL TRACT

VASTUS LATERALIS

BICEPS FEMORIS

FIGURE 8.8E

trapezius, and rhomboideus muscles are drawn in toward the spine and down. This action eases the tension in her deltoideus and upper trapezius muscles as her shoulder joint opens.

It is especially striking to see the muscular work of the adjuster in Figure 8.8F. In this drawing, Chuck Wood, the artist of all these fine biomedical illustrations, contrasts the passive stretching action of Linda's body to the contractive work of my body. Study the drawing to see the exact work of the adjuster in this pose.

In most of the partner work shown in this book, the person adjusting must work much harder than the person being adjusted, who is being taken into an extreme position and must let go into it. The person being adjusted can concentrate on the actual position the muscles and joints have been moved into as his or her body is taken to its limit in the correct way. The adjusted person should then try to reenact the feeling when attempting the posture alone.

The key to the proper performance of the Hatha Yoga postures is to isolate a certain

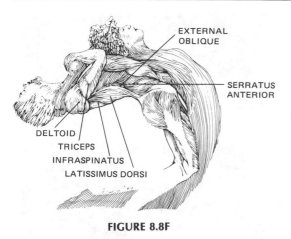

EXTERNAL
OBLIQUE

SERRATUS
ANTERIOR

DELTOID
TRICEPS
INFRASPINATUS
LATISSIMUS DORSI

FIGURE 8.8F

muscle group and contract that set of muscles forcefully while completely relaxing the antagonistic set of muscles, which are being stretched. The stretched muscles are usually the ones that give you the most pain in the yoga asanas. Being taken to the extreme in a partner adjustment is a great way to train certain muscles of the body to let go rather than tense up while performing the asanas. Partner work also breaks up deep-rooted tension in such a way that the posture will be less painful when you do it on your own.

Hanging Over a Partner

Here the underneath person's back gives such support that the top person's chest and abdomen can expand to the fullest. Study the pictures and follow the step-by-step process carefully.

The person underneath must make certain to slide down quite low before lifting the partner. In Figure 8.9A, I place my bottom below Linda's, she bends her arms, and I take hold of her elbows.

In Figure 8.9B, I lean forward and begin to straighten my legs to take Linda off the ground. (An alternative arm position is for both partners to hook the elbows together.) If

the person on top has a tight back or shoulder joint, do not take her any further than shown. The person on top should be passive at this point and let go into the light, airy feeling this position can elicit.

Linda remains passive as I stretch her arms first out and then down (Figure 8.9C). This opens Linda's armpit area and stretches her pectoralis muscles and abdominal muscles more than in the position shown in Figure 8.9B. Work for as long as is comfortable in this position. For the person on top, relaxing into this position for a short while can result in a transcending experience.

In Figure 8.9D, Linda hooks her feet around my thighs and squeezes her buttocks muscles while I stretch the frontside of her body. This enables her to arch more than if her legs were dangling, the net result being a much greater stretch to the thighs, abdomen, chest, and arms. Note the beauty of the united bodies as they bend with each other. Work for as long as is comfortable in this position.

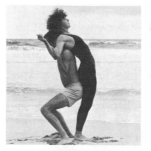

FIGURE 8.9A*

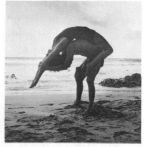

FIGURE 8.9B*

FIGURE 8.9C*

FIGURE 8.9D**

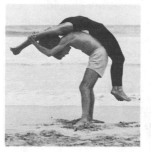

Stretching Side Arch The stretching side arch is a good, safe backbend that will increase the circulation of blood and oxygen throughout the entire body. While lying on one side, stretch the arms up and the legs down as the back arches gently (Figure 8.10). The upper-back and gluteus muscles should contract, as with most backbends.

The stretching side arch is revitalizing for the body when you first wake up in the morning, after corpse pose, or as a preparation for further backbending postures. Hold each side for a few seconds.

Upper Back Arch on Stomach

This is an excellent posture that helps to expand the chest cavity, break up tension in the upper-back muscles, stretch the neck and arm muscles, and stimulate the circulation of blood and oxygen throughout the body. Beginning on your stomach with the legs and feet together and stretched back, interweave the fingers and rotate the wrists so that the heels of the hands pull down and the elbow joint is extended. (An alternative is to pull straight back with the interwoven hands.) Inhale, lift the chest as high as possible, contract the muscles between the shoulder blades, squeeze the buttocks muscles firmly, and pull the hands back and down along the thighs. Look up, arch the neck, breathe deeply and slowly, and remain in the pose for five to 30 seconds (Figure 8.11).

Partner Work In Figure 8.12, I am pulling back Gail's arms as she squeezes her buttocks muscles firmly and relaxes her shoulders. Expansion of the chest cavity and loosening of the shoulder joints occurs through this work. Work for ten to 30 seconds.

Hanging Over a Chair

Hanging over the seat of a chair can be a very effective posture to break up rigidity in the

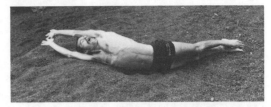

FIGURE 8.10*

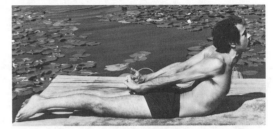

FIGURE 8.11*

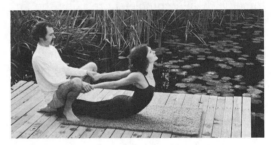

FIGURE 8.12**

back muscles, increase lung capacity, and loosen the shoulder joints. It also stretches the abdominal muscles and benefits the internal organs of digestion, elimination, and reproduction. While hanging over a chair, the chest expands increasingly as the pectoralis, intercostal, serratus anterior, and abdominal muscles are stretched, resulting in deeper, fuller breathing. It can also help to clear up sinus problems.

The chair that is used must have a flat seat and an even edge to hang over. A folding chair is used in the accompanying photo. You can lie sideways across some chairs and achieve the same effects. A bench, bed, or couch could also be used.

Hanging over a chair can be practiced by most yoga students if necessary precautions are taken. The problems that must be overcome are compression of the lower back and neck. It is one of the few backbending positions that can be held for long periods. Experienced yogis can safely hang over a chair for five to ten minutes. The beginning student should not attempt the pose for more than one minute, however, unless he or she is quite flexible already.

As shown in Figure 8.13, bring the feet down with the heels on the floor and the balls of the toes pressing against the wall. It is very important that the edge of the chair touch the bottom edge of the shoulder blades when the legs are stretched, as shown in Figure 8.13.

An excellent arm and hand position to use while arching over a chair is to interweave the fingers and rotate the wrist outward. This works the upper-back muscles, loosens the shoulder joints, and expands the chest cavity more than the arm and hand position shown in Figure 8–13. Pushing the balls of the toes against a wall aids the work of the legs and buttocks muscles and tucking action of the pelvis. Work in the pose for 30 seconds to five minutes, then bring your hands to the side of the backrest and slowly pull yourself up and hang forward over the backrest with your chest and head for one minute or so.

Elongated Bridge

The elongated bridge strengthens the wrists, arms, upper back, buttocks, and legs. It stretches the chest and abdominal muscles, develops the arches of the feet, and is energizing.

From a sitting position with the legs outstretched, place the hands three to six inches behind the buttocks, shoulder-width apart, and point the fingers away from the body. Inhale, push the hands down, and lift the

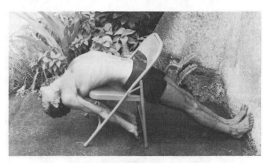

FIGURE 8.13*

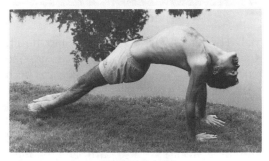

FIGURE 8.14**

chest and bottom as shown in Figure 8.14. Stretch through the legs, point the toes, let the head hang, squeeze the shoulder-blade and buttocks muscles firmly, and breathe deeply. Hold five to 20 seconds, come down, rest, and repeat once more.

Bridge, Holding the Ankles

The benefits of doing bridge pose while holding the ankles are numerous. It stretches the arm, neck, chest, abdominal, and thigh muscles; strengthens and breaks up tension in the upper-back and buttocks muscles; loosens the lower-back area; elongates the neck vertebrae; and aids the circulatory, respiratory, digestive, eliminative, reproductive, endocrine, and nervous systems. It is one backbend that should be done daily.

Lie on the back and bring the heels next to the bottom, hip-distance apart. Take hold of the outside of the ankles, inhale, tuck the

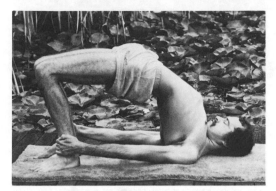

FIGURE 8.15*

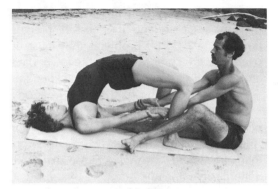

FIGURE 8.16A*

pelvis under, and raise the bottom into the air. Contract the buttocks muscles firmly, grip the ankles solidly, keep the feet parallel, and push the entire soles of the feet against the floor and lift the pelvis as high as possible. Contract the muscles between the shoulder blades and lift the chest (Figure 8.15). Allow the back of the neck, frontside torso, arm, and leg muscles to stretch without resistance.

If stiffness prevents you from holding the ankles, practice the pose by interweaving the fingers, placing the clasped hands between the feet, and pushing against the floor with the straightened arms. You should not raise the heels off the floor in the final pose. A more advanced version of the bridge pose is to bring the feet and knees together while holding the ankles.

Come out of the pose by releasing the ankles, lifting the heels, and uncurling the spine one vertebra at a time until the whole back rests on the floor. Work in the pose for ten to 20 seconds before unfolding down. Repeat the bridge two or three times.

Bridge with Partners Partner work can be very effective in breaking up tension in the upper-back muscles and thoracic vertebrae, in loosening the shoulders, and in stretching the neck, chest, and abdominal muscles in the bridge pose.

Linda brings her feet slightly wider than hip-distance apart and raises up into the

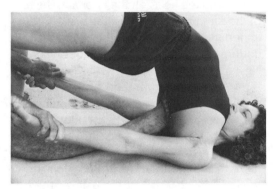

FIGURE 8.16B*

bridge pose on her own. I bring my right leg between her legs, push the ball of my right foot into Linda's upper back, firmly grip her wrists, and stretch her arms, as shown in Figure 8.16A. The adjustment can easily be taken to the extreme, so it is very important to work slowly and carefully. Do not pull the arms so hard that the shoulders raise off the floor. Make sure to push the foot evenly into the muscles of both sides of the upper back (Figure 8.16B). Linda's work is to protect her lower spine by tucking her pelvis and squeezing her buttocks muscles. Work in the pose for 20 to 30 seconds.

Full Backbend (Wheel)

The sanskrit name for this pose, *chakrasana,* translates as *wheel.* The wheel, which I call the full backbend, is one of the most energizing of all the yoga postures. If you can do this pose without overly compressing the lumbar vertebrae, then do it daily. The list of benefits for this pose are essentially the ones given in the introductory backbend discussion. The full backbend epitomizes the backbending postures. It is graceful but takes a lot of work in the thigh, buttocks, upper-back, shoulder, and arm muscles. I have found partner work to be extremely helpful in this pose.

As can be seen in the biomedical illustration (Figure 8.17A), much muscular work is involved in the full backbend. Notice the contractive action in the arm, shoulder, upper-back, buttocks, and thigh muscles. Also note

the incredible stretching action of the chest, abdominal, and frontside thigh muscles. This pose, when done correctly, does not require so much arm strength as it does thigh and buttocks strength.

To move up into full backbend, lie on the back, walk the feet in close to the bottom, and bring them slightly wider than the hips. Place the palms on the floor under the shoulders, point the fingers toward the feet, and take a couple of deep breaths to prepare to lift up (Figure 8.17B). Inhale deeply, tuck the pelvis under forcefully, and lift the hips and the chest as high into the air as possible in a quick motion. Once up, lift the heels to allow

FIGURE 8.17A

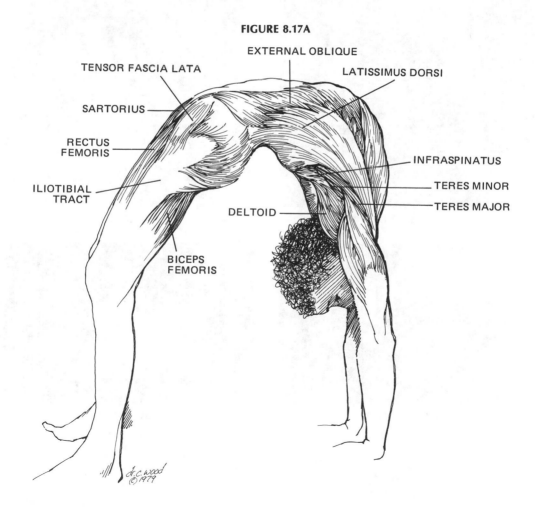

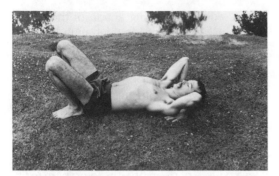

FIGURE 8.17B*

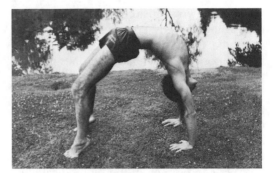

FIGURE 8.17C**

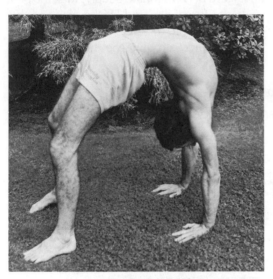

FIGURE 8.17D***

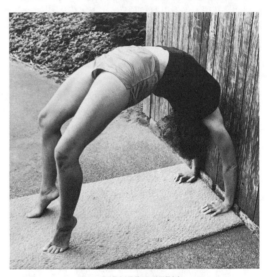

FIGURE 8.17E**

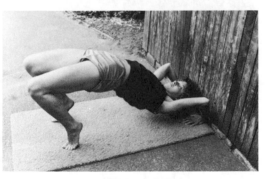

FIGURE 8.17F*

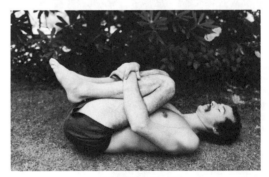

FIGURE 8.17G*

stronger tucking action of the pelvis to occur. Walk the feet in, lift the chest, straighten the arms, and let the head hang loosely (Figure 8.17C). Hold for a few seconds and then come down slowly on the exhale.

The advanced version of the full backbend is shown in Figure 8.17D. Both feet stay parallel and press firmly against the floor in this version. The sacrum and coccyx must tuck to the extreme, and the chest should lift above the straightened arms. Breathe deeply and let the head hang. The key to this posture is to tuck the pelvis under with as much force as possible. Work in this pose for a few seconds and then slowly come down on the exhale. Repeat two to ten times.

The wall can be very helpful in the performance of the full backbend; it braces the hands and keeps them from sliding. All those unfamiliar with the pose should use the wall, as shown in Figure 8.17E by Linda. To come into the pose, bring the top of the head next to the wall as you lie on your back. Place the heels of the hands against the wall with the palms down on the floor. Inhale, lift up into full backbend, and bring the chest toward the wall. Lift the heels, press down with the balls of the toes, squeeze the buttocks firmly, and breathe deeply. Come down slowly, as shown in Figure 8.17F. Repeat one to three times.

To descend from the full backbend, exhale, bring the back of the head onto the floor first, then the shoulders, and slowly lower the spine down one vertebra at a time (Figure 8.17F). The heels must lift and the pelvis must tuck as you come down.

After coming down from the full backbend, bend the knees and squeeze them toward the chest to stretch the lower back muscles and lumbar vertebrae (Figure 8.17G). It is a good idea to rest in this position for one to two minutes. You may want to do a gentle rocking action by pulling the legs in toward the chest and releasing them repeatedly for a short while.

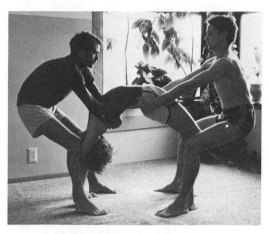

FIGURE 8.18A

The knees-to-chest pose should be done periodically throughout a yoga workout. It is one of the most comforting of all the yoga postures.

Full Backbend with Partners The full backbend is good to do with partners, as compression in the lower back can then be relieved and length in the lumbar spine attained. The person receiving the adjustment does not have to do much muscular work and can surrender into the expansion of the chest cavity and the opening of the shoulder joints. This adjustment results in a rush of oxygen and surge of blood throughout the body for the person being adjusted. It stretches the whole frontside of the body to its limit and frees the breathing muscles to work efficiently.

In Figure 8.18A, Linda begins on her back and lifts up into full backbend with our help. David places his knees to the outside of her knees and brings his hands around her buttocks muscles, fingertips on the sacrum. He pulls Linda's hips up and strongly back. I place the tips of my fingers between her shoulder blades and lift and pull her equally strongly in the opposite direction.

In order to get better work through her thighs, Linda pushes out with her knees against David's inner knees, as he creates re-

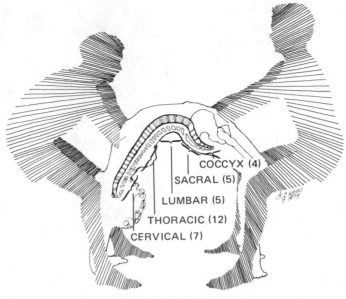

COCCYX (4)
SACRAL (5)
LUMBAR (5)
THORACIC (12)
CERVICAL (7)

FIGURE 8.18B

sistance by pushing in. This helps Linda to tuck her sacrum and coccyx more effectively.

David and I are pulling as hard as we can with reassurance from Linda that her lower back and shoulders feel fine. Work for 20 seconds to one minute.

With the aid of four people and two straps, as shown in Figure 8.18C, the person being pulled can experience a tremendous opening of the chest cavity. It is quite a tug-o'-war, and the winner ends up to be Ed, whom we are pulling. Refer to Figure 8.18A to understand the work of the two inside people performing the adjustment. The straps have gone around my hands and Leslie's and are being pulled in opposite directions. Ed is holding Leslie's ankles as we take him deeply into the pose. Although this may look like torturous treatment, it actually feels marvelous to the backbender. There is an even arch throughout the spine and, if the four adjusters do a good job, no uncomfortable compression should be occurring in the lower back. Work for ten to 30 seconds.

Figure 8.18D shows the most highly recommended way to do a four-person

adjustment in full-backbend position. Chris, the person we are adjusting, has brought her arms between Russ's legs and has taken hold of the outside of Kathy's ankles. The work shown here is basically the same as in Figure 8.18B, except that the backbender is holding the ankles of the outside person. Study Figures 8.18C and D carefully to see how to do this adjustment.

There must be clear communication between the people pulling and the person being pulled. The adjusters should pull lightly at first, and only as the backbender gives approval should the intensity of the opposite pulling action be increased. Work for ten to 30 seconds in the pose.

Figure 8.18E shows a very restful pose that stretches the lower-back muscles. I am sitting on Linda's ankles and gently pushing her knees down. This relieves tension in the lower back after vigorous backbends. Hold for 30 seconds to one minute.

Full Backbend—Feet Raised Performing the full backbend with the feet raised on a bench or chair helps to expand the chest,

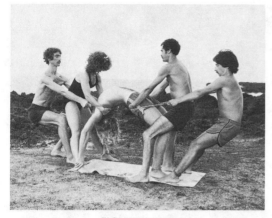

FIGURE 8.18C*

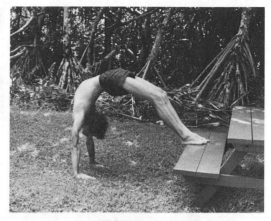

FIGURE 8.19***

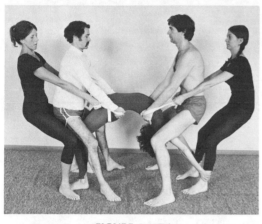

FIGURE 8.18D*

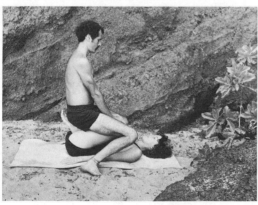

FIGURE 8.18E

opens the shoulder joints, and works the up-per-back muscles more than when the feet

are on the floor. To get into the pose shown in Figure 8.19, Terry begins on his back with his bottom underneath the bench seat and the feet on the edge of the seat. He then lifts up into the full backbend on the inhale and brings the chest further and further forward above the straightened arms. Work in the pose for ten to 20 seconds and come slowly down.

Forearm Backbend

Forearm backbend gives the same benefits as full backbend, and it works more deeply on the upper back and shoulder joint. Forearm backbend will give more openness to the arm-pit and chest areas, and you will need more flexibility to do it correctly than you will for the full backbend.

The forearm backbend can be done with or without the aid of a wall. I'll describe the pose with the use of a wall (Figure 8.20A); however, the instructions apply also to Figure 8.20B, except when the wall is mentioned.

Lie on your back with the knees bent, bring the feet close in to the buttocks and slightly wider than the hips, with the head four to six inches from the wall. Bend the elbow and place the palms of the hands on the floor under the shoulders with the fingers pointing toward the feet (as the full-backbend prepara-tion). Inhale, roll back onto the forearms, lift the hips, and bring the elbows to the floor and

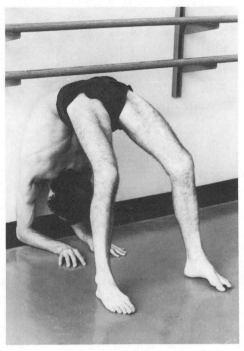

FIGURE 8.20A*

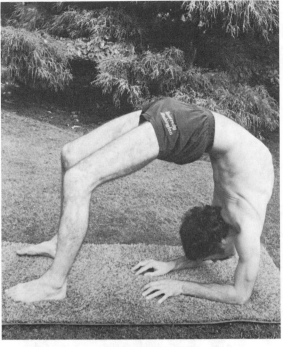

FIGURE 8.20B*

against the wall in a quick motion. The arm position is like headstand arm position, except that the hands are slightly separated. Take all the weight off the head and neck by pushing down strongly with the forearms, tuck the pelvis, and lift the chest as you walk the feet in. Try to bring the chest to the wall and look toward the hands. Hold for a few seconds before coming down slowly. Rest, then repeat one or two more times.

Massage-in-Prayer Pose After doing a set of vigorous backbends, or in between backbends, the partner adjustment shown in Figure 8.21A feels wonderful. While I rest in prayer pose, Linda pushes the heel of her left hand firmly down into my lower-back and sacrum areas. At the same time, she brings the heel of her right hand onto my upper-back muscles and pushes down and away from her left hand. The result of this action is that my

spinal cord and back muscles stretch out nicely. The main work of the adjuster is to push against the top of the sacrum very firmly so that the lower back receives the greatest stretch. Work for ten to 30 seconds.

Prayer pose serves as an excellent position for massage. The back muscles stretch and stand out in such a way that they can be worked on at a very deep level. In Figure 8.21B Linda strokes her thumbs·along the muscles of my back. She begins low in the back and slowly and deeply slides her thumbs up the muscles along the sides of the spine. She kneads to the inside of my shoulder blades in the upper-back area. The tops of the shoulders and neck can also be worked on in this position. Work for one to five minutes.

In Figure 8.22, my three-year-old niece, Trisha, does the cobra with me. Many of the yoga postures come naturally to young children.

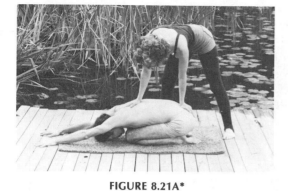

FIGURE 8.21A*

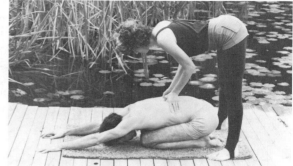

FIGURE 8.21B*

FIGURE 8.22*

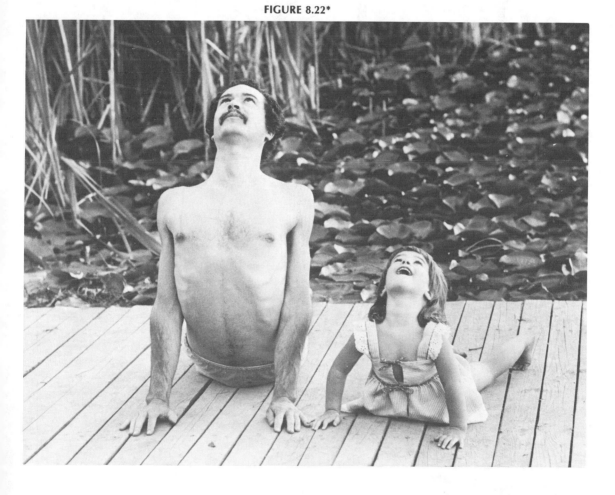

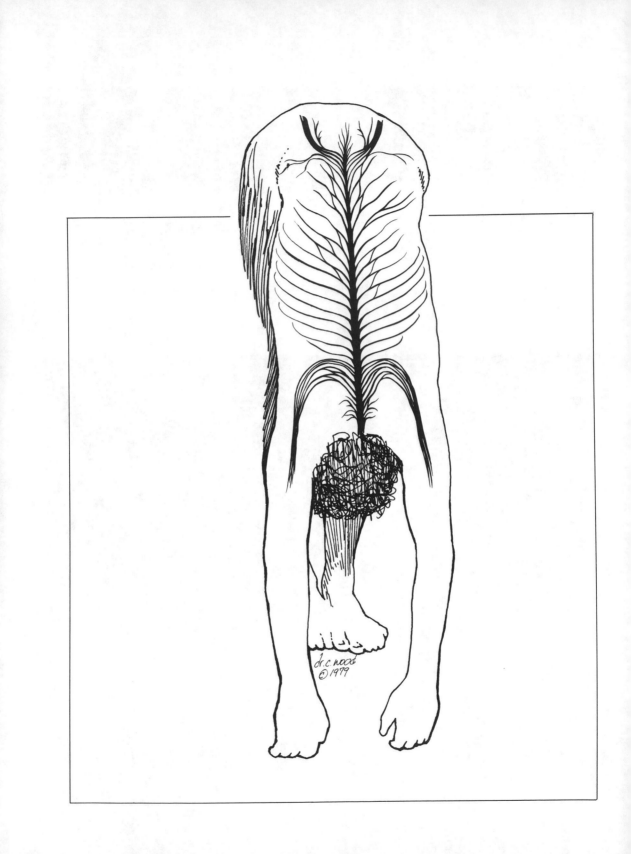

NINE
forward stretches

The main sitting-forward stretch, *paschimot-tanasana* (which I call the doudle-legged forward stretch), is one of the top-ranking yoga postures for developing physical, mental, and spiritual well-being. The double-legged forward stretch elongates the whole backside of the body to the utmost, thus increasing the circulation of blood throughout the body. Paschimottanasana and other forward-stretching postures can directly lengthen the spinal column more effectively than any of the other main groups of yoga asanas.

The forward-stretching postures awaken a strong flow of energy through the legs and buttocks area. Those of us who spend the majority of the day sitting or standing need to periodically stretch our leg muscles so that the blood will begin to move through the arteries, capillaries, and veins more efficiently. Those who engage in vigorous exercise such as jogging, bicycling, tennis, racketball, and basketball will get the blood moving through the legs, but the net result of such leg work is that the hamstring and calf muscles tighten up. Those who jog or engage in other forms of vigorous athletic exercise need the counterbalancing effect that the forward stretches have upon the legs.

It has been my experience that the majority of people begin yoga practice in search of a way to relieve backaches. The forward bends (I use the terms *forward bend* and *forward stretch* interchangeably) help to stretch the back muscles and lengthen the space between the vertebrae. These postures, when performed correctly, can be quite beneficial to those with lower-back problems, since the direct result of holding such poses is a release of tension in this area of the back.

The forward stretches tremendously aid the internal organs of digestion, elimination, and reproduction. During a forward stretch the abdominal muscles are turned inward and inverted. This services as a deep massage to the internal organs. The stomach, liver, kidneys, pancreas, gallbladder, and intestines are all stimulated as one stretches the torso, arms, and legs forward. Foodstuff is digested much more efficiently through daily practice of the forward-stretching postures. The nerves of the sexual organs, prostate, uterus, bladder, and large intestines are stimulated during a straight forward stretch as well. A possible increase in sexual vitality is accompanied by greater control over the sexual energy. An increase in the efficiency of the organs of elimination results in the release of toxic wastes. Constipation can be greatly relieved through daily practice of the forward stretches.

It should be pointed out that all the major systems of the body are improved through the practice of forward stretches, including the endocrine system. The amount of hormones secreted by the endocrine glands depends largely upon the condition of the circulatory system. Forward stretches improve the circulation of blood throughout the body and help to balance the production of hormones by the endocrine glands.

One of the greatest benefits of the forward stretches is that they strengthen and calm the nervous system. Many of the forward bends can be held for minutes at a time. The double-legged forward stretch can be held five to ten minutes by the advanced practitioner. The longer one of these postures is held, the more you move toward a peaceful frame of mind. It is possible to lose yourself and leave the world of daily problems during a long forward bend.

During forward bends you should adopt an attitude of submissiveness. Resisting the stretch at the back of the legs will only make the pain worse. The approach you need in performing the more vigorous standing postures and most of the backbends is exactly opposite that needed to move deeply into the forward stretches. The tranquility of the forward-stretching postures occurs as you surrender into the pose with your body and mind.

It is inevitable that the beginning yoga student will experience a great amount of pain at the backside of the knees when first attempting the forward-stretching asanas. There are aids that beginners can use to help them move into the straight-legged forward bends with less pain. Partner work, straps, moving in and out of many forward stretches in dance-like fashion, correct use of mental imagery,

and proper breathing are aids that I will discuss. It is important to realize that we must submit into the stretch of the forward bends by relaxing the whole backside of the body. It is especially important to allow the stretch to move evenly throughout the entirety of the backside of the legs, from the ankle right up through the buttocks muscles.

When dealing with a lot of stretch at the back of the legs, it is helpful to try to visualize the anatomical position of the muscles and ligaments that are causing you pain, and talk to them, telling them to relax and let go into the stretch. In yoga we become aware of how the body functions from the inside out. Rather than focusing on the hundred or more reasons that you could think of to justify breaking the pose, picture the muscular stretching action that is occurring and consider how beneficial this is to the nervous and circulatory systems. Only one main active muscular contraction should occur in the later stages of the forward bends, that being deep within the frontside of the hip socket. The torso should fold foward over the legs like a pocketknife. The deeper the fold between the legs and the trunk of the body, the more the spine and torso can stretch forward.

You must focus your attention upon the breath during moments of intense stretch. Breathing slowly and deeply calms the mind and allows certain nerves to release some of their excess activity; this, in turn, allows certain muscles to release some of their unnecessary patterns of holding. Most advanced students of yoga report that the forward-stretching postures actually feel marvelous. As the accumulated tension in the back of the legs is broken up, the main focus of attention can go to the wonderful feeling of elongation that occurs along the spine and lower back muscles.

You should move into a forward stretch on an exhale. This allows the abdominal area to flatten and the back to stretch out more.

Once in the pose, breathe slowly, deeply, and steadily. At the beginning of the asana try to reach out a little further with each exhale. Finally, when your limit has been reached, hold the stretch and allow a deep, slow, rhythmic breath to take over. Near the end of the pose, try to stretch a little further with each complete exhale before coming out of the posture on an inhale.

Forward stretches are good postures to do periodically throughout a yoga workout. The standing forward stretches work well in between the more vigorous standing poses. The sitting forward stretches and those done on your back can give the elongation of the spine that the back needs in between the backbends. Forward stretches feel good after inverted poses and help to evenly distribute the energy after a set of twisting postures. Do forward stretches often throughout your yoga workout! They also calm the mind and prepare you for corpse pose or the sitting breathing practices that should be done to complete a yoga session.

The first half of this chapter will be concerned with sitting forward stretches and forward-stretching postures done on the back. The second half will be concerned with hip-opening postures. The hip-openers, like the forward stretches, are performed through a combination of leg- and spine-stretching movements. The hip-opening postures are different in that they emphasize external rotation of the hip socket(s) and stretching of the inner-thigh muscles. The benefits of the hip-opening postures will be discussed individually, posture by posture, in the second section of this chapter. For the most part, the benefits of the forward-stretching postures will not be discussed individually, since the main benefits of the asanas have already been discussed in general terms. The benefits of the various forward stretches do not vary too much from posture to posture. Doing many different forward stretches adds variety and interest and

allows you to work longer on them.

Sitting Forward Stretches

Double-Legged Forward Stretch The double-legged forward stretch epitomizes the forward-stretching postures. The step-by-step process of how to correctly move into the pose is shown here in Figures 9.1A and B. Begin by sitting upright with both legs stretched forward. Bring the heel of the hands behind the bottom, push against the floor with the straightened arms, lift and expand the chest, and lengthen through the spine as shown in Figure 9.1A. Contract the quadriceps muscles, stretch through the back of the legs, and begin to lean forward.

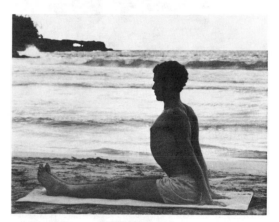

FIGURE 9.1A*

FIGURE 9.1B*

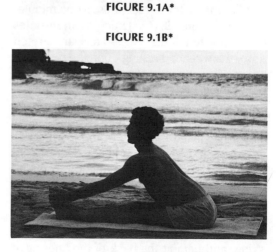

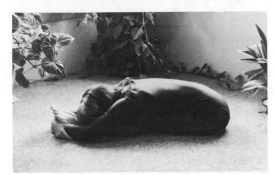

FIGURE 9.1C

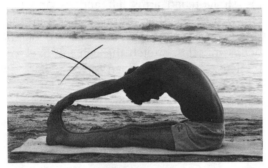

FIGURE 9.1D

Figure 9.1B shows the continuation of the forward-folding movement of the torso. The chest cavity should continue to expand as the hands reach out and take hold of the feet. The shoulders should be drawn back and down, and the back of the knees should be kept against the floor as the spine stretches. Hold this pose for ten seconds to one minute.

In Figure 9.1C, Janice demonstrates the completed double-legged forward-stretch pose, the forehead resting upon the two shinbones. The principle of moving into the pose is that the head should not touch the legs until the abdominal muscles first touch the thighs and the chest is brought close to the knees. Janice has taken the pose to the extreme by wrapping her arms around the feet as she holds her forearms. The progression would be to bring the hands to the heels, then reach out further and wrap the wrists around the ankles. It helps to point the toes while in the completed pose, as the stretch through the hamstring, and pain at the back of the knees can

be lessened. Work in the double-legged forward stretch for ten seconds to ten minutes. The lengthy list of benefits resulting from the performance of this pose is given in the introductory forward-stretch discussion.

Figure 9.1D illustrates the double-legged forward stretch done incorrectly. The main problems are the concavity of the chest and roundedness of the back, which restrict the breathing capacity of the lungs and compress the discs on the anterior side of the spine. The sitting forward stretch done in this manner does not relieve back tension; rather, it aggravates the tense muscles.

The sitting forward stretch will lengthen the spine if done properly. Do not sink back onto the gluteus muscles; rather, lift the chest in such a way as to sit on the front part of the sitting bones. The upper-back muscles must initially draw in toward the spine to aid the lift and expansion of the chest.

Straight Forward Stretch with Strap

The most direct way for the beginning yoga student to correct the problems illustrated in Figure 9.1D is shown in Figure 9.2. If you cannot reach your feet while maintaining a straight spine, use a strap. The first motion of the spinal column should be to lift upward rather than to stretch forward. Once the spinal column has acquired straightness, the chest should reach out toward the feet. Notice the deep fold that occurs in the hip socket, the contraction of the quadriceps muscles, and the stretch through the backside of the legs. The back of the knees should touch the floor. Work in this pose for 20 seconds to one minute.

One-Legged Forward Stretch
Begin by bending one knee and placing the foot in the groin, as shown in Figure 9.3. Bring both hands behind the bottom, push the hands down, inhale, and lift the chest. Continuing to expand the chest cavity, exhale, reach out with the spine and the arms, and take hold of

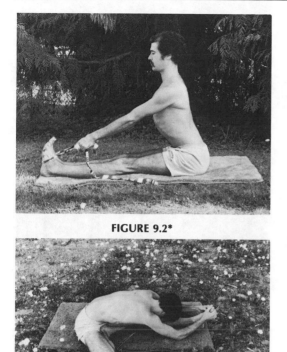

FIGURE 9.2*

FIGURE 9.3*

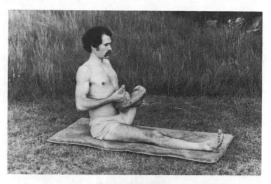

FIGURE 9.4A**

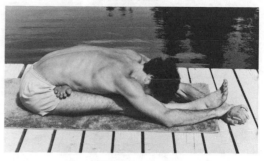

FIGURE 9.4B**

the outstretched foot with the hands. The hips should remain square, both sitting bones should rest evenly on the ground, and the muscles along both sides of the spine should stretch evenly. The one-legged forward stretch with the foot to the groin can be held anywhere from ten seconds to one minute. Repeat the posture to the other side for the same length of time.

Half-Lotus Forward Stretch
Demonstrated in Figure 9.4A is the preparatory action for the half lotus forward stretch. Inhale, lift the left foot up close to the navel, and then place the heel into the fold between the right leg and the torso.

Complete the pose by reaching both hands to the foot of the outstretched leg and continuing to expand the chest as you exhale

and stretch forward (Figure 9.4B). Keep the toes of the straightened leg pointing upward.

The heel of the bent leg pushes in deeply against the eliminative organs, thus helping to activate them more than would the straight forward stretch. Stretching out over one leg at a time can be more restful than the double-legged forward stretch. Both should be incorporated into a yoga workout. Hold the pose shown for ten seconds to three minutes and repeat to the other side.

United Forward Stretch
A partner can help you to achieve a better forward stretch than you could achieve on your own. Set this adjustment up by bringing your feet against your partner's and clasping wrists. Inhale, pull your partner slightly up as you pull him or her forward, and at the same time, try to keep your back straight (Figure 9.5A). Bend your knees if it is difficult to hold onto your partner's wrists while pulling forward. With straightened legs and a straight back, exhale

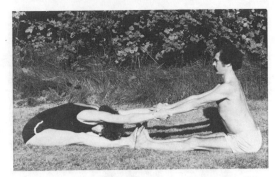

FIGURE 9.5A*

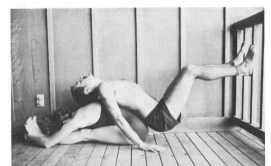

FIGURE 9.6A*

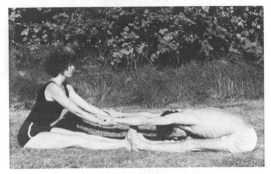

FIGURE 9.5B*

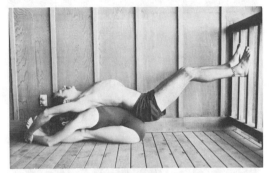

FIGURE 9.6B**

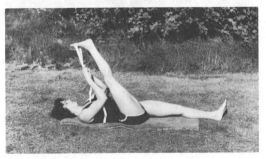

FIGURE 9.7A*
FIGURE 9.7B*

and let your partner pull you forward (Figure 9.5B). The two of you should go back and forth three or four times, holding each end of the stretch for five to 20 seconds. United forward stretch is exceptional for stretching out the arms, legs, and spine. Work with the breath in this adjustment; inhale to pull your partner and exhale as you are pulled.

Double-Legged Forward Stretch (Lying on Another)
The position demonstrated in Figure 9.6A allows the person underneath to stretch out the backside of his or her body completely. It is especially beneficial for the underneath person's lower back.

As shown in Figure 9.6A, I have placed my sacrum (the sacrum is the flattened bone centered at the topside of the buttocks area) on top of Linda's sacrum and my feet against a railing (the feet could go against a wall just as easily), knees bent. I push my hands onto the floor, gently rest my back upon hers, and

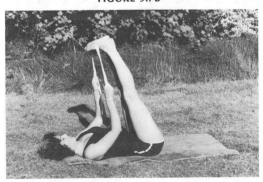

slowly begin to push my feet against the railing. It is important for Linda to give me accurate feedback as to what she needs to further her stretch in the way that is least painful to her. At first I carry most of my body weight on my hands. Graudally I put more and more weight onto Linda's back and push my sacrum into hers. Work in this pose for 20 seconds to one minute.

In Figure 9.6B, I am pushing my feet against the railing rather firmly and have brought my sacrum just above the backside of Linda's hip bone. Slowly I can work my way up Linda's lumbar vertebrae, pressing my sacrum into the space between the vertebrae where she needs the greatest release. I have reached my hands over her head and taken hold of her feet. This position can be held for 30 seconds to one minute.

Forward Stretches On Back

Leg Stretches on the Back with a Strap
Place the strap around the right foot, lift the right leg, stretch the left leg down along the floor, stretch through both heels, and contract the quadriceps muscles of both legs (Figure 9.7A). Work toward attaining a deep fold in the hip socket of the right leg as the left leg reaches down. Pull the shoulders down and lengthen the back of the neck. Breathe deeply and slowly. Work for ten seconds to one minute and repeat to the other side.

A strap should be used as shown in Figure 9.7B, if you cannot keep the lower back down as you are holding the ankles of the straightened legs. Place the strap around both feet, stretch through the heels, pull down against the floor with the top of the sacrum, drop the shoulders onto the floor away from the ears, and lengthen the entire spine. Work 20 seconds to two minutes and slowly try to bring the legs toward the chest.

Leg Stretch on the Back with Partner
In Figure 9.8, I press my hands into the hip

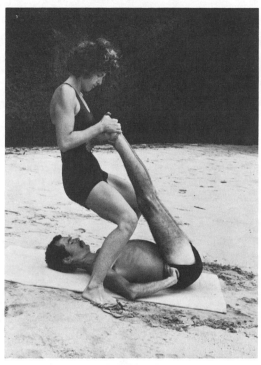

FIGURE 9.8*

socket while Linda pulls up through my heels and brings my legs toward my head. This partner adjustment is helpful in achieving a better stretch through the back of the legs and lower-back area. Work for 30 seconds to one minute.

Leg Stretches on the Back for Flexible Students
In the pose shown in Figure 9.9A, a more advanced version of the pose shown in Figure 9.7-A, the key is to push the hips down and extend through both legs while maintaining length along the spine. Hold for ten seconds to two minutes. Repeat to the other side.

The posture shown in Figure 9.9B is the final version of the pose discussed in Figure 9.7B. Janice holds the heels of her feet, presses her lower back to the floor, and pulls her straightened legs down to her chest. This pose increases the circulation of blood, oxygen, and nerve energy throughout the body.

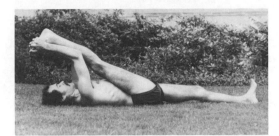

FIGURE 9.9A**

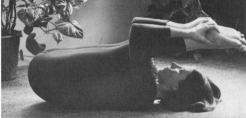

FIGURE 9.9B**

The key is to fold like a pocketknife and extend all along the spine and through the back of the legs from the buttocks to the ankles. Press the lower back down on the floor for a maximum elongation. Hold for ten seconds to three minutes.

Dog Stretch with a Strap

Dog stretch with a strap can be held for five minutes or longer. The longer it is held, the more the spine, back muscles, and leg muscles stretch out. It is a very restful way to improve your forward stretches. It also relieves upper- and lower-back tension, helps to open the shoulder joints, brings blood into the brain and pituitary gland, stimulates the adrenal glands, and helps the digestive and eliminative organs. It can be practiced by all yoga students and can be done at any time during a yoga workout.

In Figure 9.10A, a sash is tied to the railing and the body rests over the strap in dog-stretch position. Notice the placement of the strap—at the fold between the trunk and

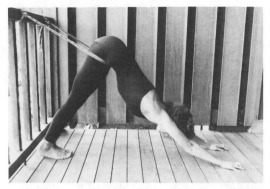

FIGURE 9.10A*

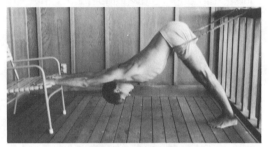

FIGURE 9.10B*

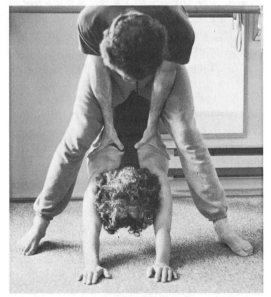

FIGURE 9.10C*

the thighs. Once in the strap, the work of the lower half of the body is to tilt the pelvis upward and to stretch the heels toward the floor. Stretch out through the arms, relax the shoulders, and let the rib cage drop down. Hold for 30 seconds to five minutes, allowing gravity to stretch you out more and more.

To loosen the shoulder joints and flatten the upper back more than in the position shown in Figure 9.10A, it is helpful to place the hands on the seat of a chair as shown in Figure 9.10B. With this aid the shoulder-blade muscles can be activated and tension in the upper back and shoulder joints relieved.

Dog stretch done in a strap provides an ideal position in which to deeply massage another person's back. In Figure 9.10C, I push my thumbs down into Linda's back to help break up muscular tension. Deep massage can help to loosen muscles that have been tight for years.

Familiarize yourself with the back muscles by looking over medical illustrations in Figures 3.4A and 3.5B. As shown in Figure 9.10C, I am stroking deeply and steadily with my thumbs, first of all following the muscle fibers that run laterally on either side of the spine from the bottom of the spine to the shoulders. Once in the shoulder-blade and shoulder-joint areas, I follow the contour of these upper-back muscles by digging down quite deeply with my thumbs and fingertips. This type of message helps to free the back muscles for further yoga work.

Cobbler Pose

This pose resembles the way cobblers sit in India. It is a good pose for those with tight hip joints to practice, as it loosens the hip sockets, stretches the inner-thigh muscles, and yet it does not place stress upon the knee joints. It is especially beneficial for women and can help to regulate the menstrual cycle. Cobbler pose is helpful for anyone with problems in the pelvic region.

To move into cobbler pose, sit upright, bring the soles of the feet together, pull the heels as close to the groin as possible, interweave the fingers, and clasp the hands around the toes. Using the feet for leverage, lift and pull the chest forward, straighten the

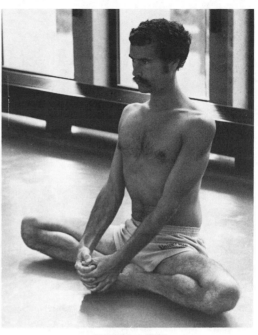

FIGURE 9.11*

spine, and draw the knees toward the floor (Figure 9.11). Work in the pose for 20 seconds to two minutes, breathing deeply.

Forward-Stretching Cobbler Pose

In the outstretched cobbler pose, the lower back gets a good stretch, the internal organs are stimulated, the groin muscles are lengthened, and the hip socket is opened wider and wider by the force of gravity. It is good for kidney and urinary-bladder problems as well.

From the position shown in Figure 9.11, pull the shoulders down and back through a contraction of the muscles between the shoulder blades, lift out with the chest, and slowly fold forward. Work toward bringing the abdomen to the feet and extending the spine as far as possible (Figure 9.12). The spinal cord should remain straight and the soles of the feet together as you fold forward in this posture. Ideally, the knees would go all the way down to the floor. The outstretched cobbler can be held for ten seconds to one minute.

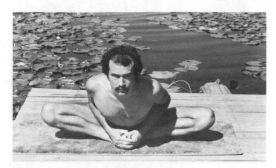

FIGURE 9.12**

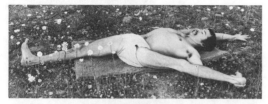

FIGURE 9.13A**

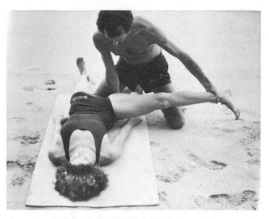

FIGURE 9.13C*

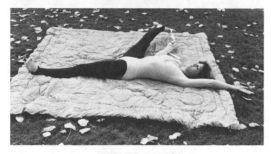

FIGURE 9.13B*

tain equal length to the right and the spine elongated as the left foot is brought higher and higher (Figure 9.13A). Contraction of the quadriceps muscles of both legs will facilitate the stretch through the back of both legs. Work for 30 seconds to two minutes. Repeat to the other side.

One-Legged Outstretched Hip-Opener with Aids

If you cannot straighten the leg that is opening to the side while holding it with the hand, then the use of a strap is very helpful. In Figure 9.13B, Linda bends her right leg, places the strap around the foot, rolls her right bottom under, and straightens her right leg out to the side. After the leg has opened to the side, cinch down on the strap and work toward the foot with the hand. Stretch through the left leg, the spine, and the arm. Work in the pose for 30 seconds to one minute and repeat to the other side.

Figure 9.13C, I am trying to roll Linda's right buttock under as she stretches her right leg out to the side. To open the hip socket properly, the external rotator muscles in the buttocks area should work, and a partner can facilitate this action. Linda's left buttock pulls down against the floor and her left leg stretches straight down. Work for 20 seconds to one minute per side.

One-Legged Outstretched Hip-Opener

This marvelous posture dramatically increases the blood circulation in the legs and arms, loosens the hip sockets, tones the buttocks and thigh muscles, and stretches the spine.

Bend the left knee, take hold of the outside of the foot with the left hand, roll under with the left buttock, straighten the left leg, stretch out through the left heel, and bring the leg to the side. Contract the buttocks muscles of the right leg and stretch through the heel of the right foot. The right side of the body should form a straight line and be extended to its limit. The waist of the left side should main-

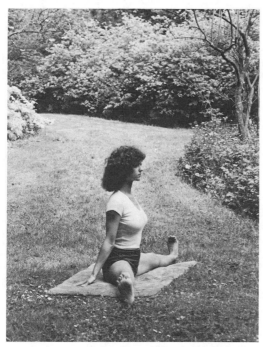

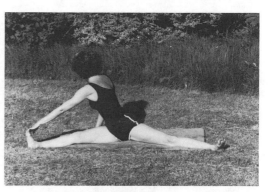

FIGURE 9.15*

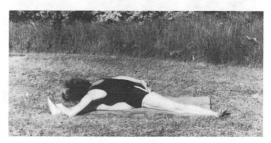

FIGURE 9.14**

FIGURE 9.15B**

Side Splits

The side splits helps to bring blood and oxygen into the pelvis and inner-thigh areas, loosens and opens the hip joints, stretches the hamstring and inner-thigh muscles, and releases bound-up energy in the pelvic region of the body. Those who wish to trim their legs down should do this pose daily. A fairly advanced degree of flexibility is a prerequisite.

In Figure 9.14, Diann demonstrates the vertical side splits. With the hands behind the bottom, she lifts the hips and moves the trunk forward, thus spreading her legs wider apart. Notice how she stretches through the heels and the base of the big toes to get maximum work out of her leg muscles. Work in the pose for five to 20 seconds before going on to the twisting side splits.

Twisting Side Splits The twisting side splits are good for the lower and upper back, the internal organs, and the legs. From the position shown in Figure 9.14, inhale and turn the torso until it faces over the right leg. Bring the right hand to the outside of the right thigh, and use it as a brace to enable the chest to lift. Bring the left hand to the outside of the right foot, and use that arm for leverage to twist the rib cage further and further to the right (Figure 9.15A).

From the position shown in Figure 9.15A, exhale, pull the rib cage to the right just above the right thigh, and stretch the chest out over the right knee (Figure 9.15B). Notice the extension occurring through both legs, the stretch of the spinal column, and the way the left hand pulls against the outside of the right foot. Work in the pose for five to 20 seconds and repeat to the other side.

Forward-Stretching Side Splits The benefits of the forward-stretching side splits above and beyond those already mentioned for vertical side splits are increased loosening

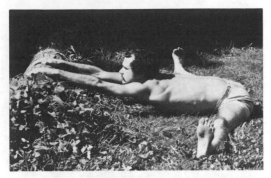

FIGURE 9.16A**

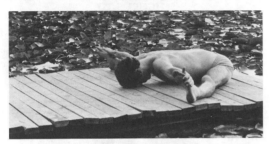

FIGURE 9.16B***

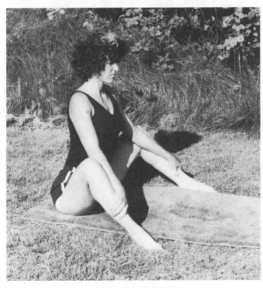

FIGURE 9.16C*

of the hip sockets, increased stretch to the inner thighs and hamstring muscles, and greater stretch to the buttocks and lower-back muscles.

The key to the forward-stretching side splits is to tilt the pelvis upward as you extend through the legs and fold forward. To help the expansion of the chest, the extension of the spine, and the tilt of the pelvis, it helps to hold onto something that is higher than ground level, as shown in Figure 9.16A. Work in the pose for 20 seconds to one minute.

The final version of the forward-stretching side splits is shown in Figure 9.16B. You complete the energy circuits by gripping the outer edges of the feet with the hands. Notice the straightness of the spine. This pose can be held for one minute or longer.

Figure 9.16C illustrates the preparatory pose for the forward-stretching side splits. Sit upright, bend the knees, and spread the feet apart. Hold onto the inner shinbone, lift the chest, and slowly slide the heels out. Tilt the pelvis back, lift through the chest, and work slowly toward the final pose.

Forward-Stretching Side Splits with Partners

Forward-stretching splits are a difficult pose that can be greatly aided through partner work. In Figure 9.17A, I

FIGURE 9.17A**

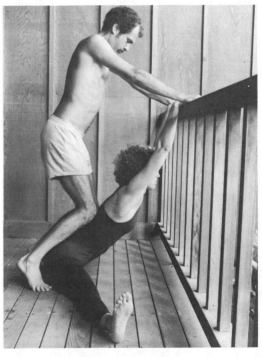

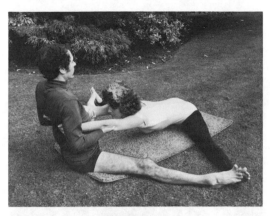

FIGURE 9.17B**

gently and carefully push my knees up into Linda's middle back to try to flatten out the back. She supports her hands upon a railing to bring herself forward on the sitting bones and to aid the lift of her chest. Work for ten to 30 seconds.

Another helpful way in which partners can work together in the forward-stretching side splits is shown in Figure 9.17B. Stretch and spread the legs, place the bottom of the feet together, join arms, and then slowly and carefully pull each other back and forth. The person being pulled forward should exhale; the person pulling should inhale. Go back and forth three or four times.

Side Splits on Back

Stretch the legs out to the sides with a strap around the bottom of each foot. While in the position shown in Figure 9.18A, relax the back muscles, push the hips against the floor, contract the quadriceps muscles, stretch through the heels of both feet, and slowly bring the feet toward the floor. Breathe deeply and work in pose for 20 seconds to one minute.

Grasp the heels, stretch out through the back of the legs, and try to bring the toes to the floor. The feet should be brought toward the line of the shoulders, the hips pulled down, and the lower-back area flattened against the floor (Figure 9.18B). You may need to hold the calf muscles to do this pose.

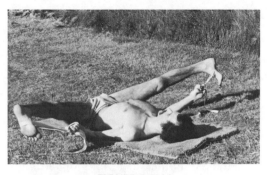

FIGURE 9.18A*

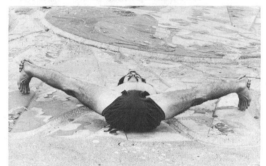

FIGURE 9.18B***

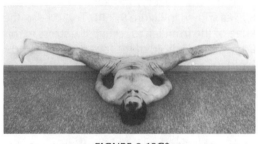

FIGURE 9.18C*

Work for ten to 30 seconds, rest, and repeat.

The most relaxing way to practice the side splits is to lie on your back, bring the bottom next to the wall, and rest the outstretched legs against the wall (Figure 9.18C). This position can be held for long periods, since little muscular work is involved. You should relax the inner-thigh muscles and back muscles and allow the breath to become the main focus of attention. Stretch through the heels of the feet and allow gravity to take the legs down. Hold for one to three minutes and come out of the pose very slowly.

Front Splits

The front splits release locked energy in the pelvic region, loosen the hip sockets, stretch and tone the leg muscles, and loosen the iliopsoas muscles. Both the front splits and side splits are very challenging poses that must be approached cautiously.

Stand with the heels placed about three feet apart, turn the hips and feet to the right, slide the feet further apart, fold forward, and bring the hands down next to the right foot. Bend the left knee to the floor and slide the right foot in front of the hands. Try to square the hips by bringing the front hip back and the left hip forward as you spread into the splits. Lift the chest as you push down firmly with the hands (Figure 9.19A).

If the hip of the back leg can be brought close to the floor and both legs stretched totally from the position shown in Figure 9.19A, you may be ready to stretch the torso out over the front leg. Fold deeply into the hip of the front leg and extend the spine out over the leg, as shown in Figure 9.19B. Try to relax the knee of the front leg to relieve the stress in this area, and take hold of the foot with the hands. Hold for a few seconds before trying the other side.

If the hip of the back leg is on or very close to the floor from the position shown in Figure 9.19A, you can stretch the arms and spine straight up and extend through the fingers. The key action is to lift upward with the torso and squeeze down with the buttock of the back leg. In Figure 9.19C, notice the line of the spine and arms and the squareness of the hips. Work for a few seconds and repeat to the other side.

Thunderbolt Posture

There are numerous names for this posture, such as *adamant, adamantine, diamond, kneeling pose, hero's pose, thunderbolt,* and *sitting-between-the-heels pose.* It can be used as a meditation posture, since the body

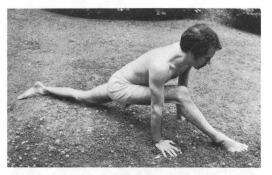
FIGURE 9.19A*

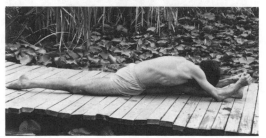
FIGURE 9.19B***

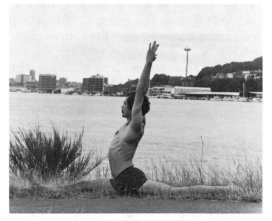
FIGURE 9.19C***

is brought into a straight and stable position. From a physical point of view, this pose stretches the quadriceps muscles, loosens the knee joints, develops arches in the feet, and creates flexibility in the ankle joints. Few other postures stretch the quadriceps muscles as much as this pose does. Once you become comfortable in this pose, the steadiness and solidity of the body helps to calm the mind and the nervous system.

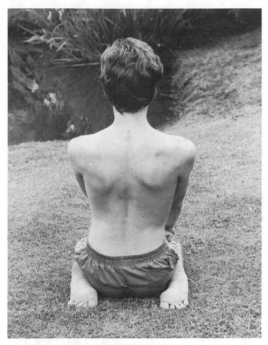

FIGURE 9.20A**

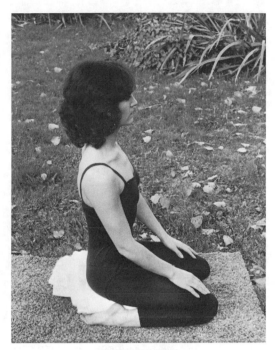

FIGURE 9.20B*

Shown in Figure 9.20A is the upright thunderbolt posture. From a kneeling position, spread the feet apart, sit between the feet, and slowly let the bottom rest onto the floor. Keep the heels against the hips and in line with the toes. In all the thunderbolt positions, the tops of all ten toes should rest on the floor. Pay special attention to the fourth and fifth toes of each foot. Let the knees spread hip-distance apart. (The flexible student may bring the knees together.) Lift up through the torso and straighten the spine. Breathe deeply in the pose for 30 seconds to five minutes.

A thickly folded blanket can be placed between the feet and underneath the bottom to help relieve the stress of the stretch along the quadriceps muscles in the upright thunderbolt. Notice the straightness of Gail's spine in Figure 9.20B. The shoulders should drop down away from the ears, and the back of the head should lift. The hands can rest on the thighs. Remain in the pose for 20 seconds to three minutes, breathing deeply.

Supine Thunderbolt Position The supine thunderbolt is a wonderful pose for relaxing the nervous, digestive, eliminative, and reproductive systems, increasing blood circulation throughout the entire body, stretching the quadriceps muscles, loosening and realigning the knee joint, and improving the arches of the feet. It can help menstrual problems as well.

From the upright thunderbolt posture, with the knees spread hip-distance apart, use the elbows for a brace and recline into a supine position. Once in the supine position, there are two main arm positions: one is stretching the arms straight back, as shown in Figure 9.21A, and the other is clasping the elbows with the hands above the head.

It is very difficult to tuck the pelvis under in this pose, but this is exactly what should be done. Contract the buttocks muscles, flatten the abdominal muscles, and stretch the lower-back muscles to aid in the tucking of the pelvic girdle. Then relax into the position at-

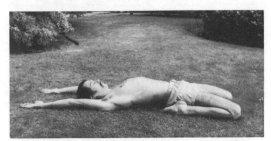

FIGURE 9.21A**

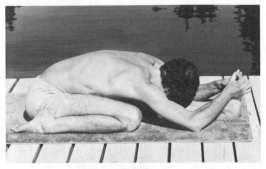

FIGURE 9.22A*

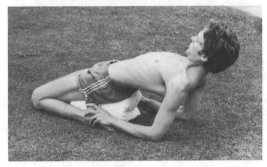

FIGURE 9.21B*

tained. The advanced student can bring the knees together while in the supine thunderbolt. Breathe deeply in the pose for 20 seconds to two minutes.

The stretch of the quadriceps muscles across the knee joints can be quite uncomfortable in the position shown in Figure 9.21A. The beginning student can work toward the supine thunderbolt position gradually, as shown in Figure 9.21B. Place a thickly folded blanket between the heels, lean back onto the elbows, keep the chin up, and hold for ten to 30 seconds.

Half Thunderbolt Forward Stretch

When done to both sides, the half thunderbolt forward-stretching postures can bring about a nice balance to the leg muscles by stretching the backside of the outstretched leg and the frontside of the bent-knee leg in alternate fashion. These postures stretch the spine and back muscles and loosen the ankle, knee, and hip joints.

Sit upright, bend the right knee, bring the right heel against the right hip (half thun-

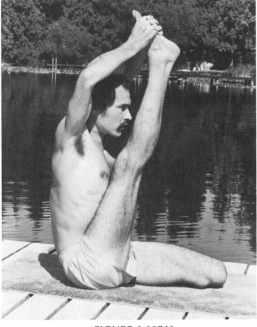

FIGURE 9.22B**

derbolt), and stretch the left leg forward. Inhale, lift the chest, exhale, stretch the torso out forward between the thighs, and take hold of the left foot (Figure 9.22A). Stretch through the backside of the left leg, extend forward with the spine, try to keep both sitting bones down on the floor, and try to relax the quadriceps muscles of the right leg. Work in the pose for ten seconds to one minute, breathing deeply. Repeat to the other side after going on to the position shown in Figure 9.22B.

It is easier to keep both sitting bones down in the upright half thunderbolt forward stretch than in the posture shown in Figure 9.22A. Sit upright with the left foot next to the left hip in half thunderbolt, bend the right leg, take hold of the right foot with both hands, lift the chest, drop the shoulders, ano straighten the right leg (Figure 9.22B). Try to bring the chest to the knee and the spine to a vertical position. Work in the pose for ten to 30 seconds and repeat to the other side.

Yoga Nidra

Yoga nidra is the yogic sleep posture. (The feet behind the head serve as the yogi's pillow.) This pose stimulates the entire nervous system because of the tremendous stretch it gives to the spine. Yoga nidra stretches the neck, hamstring, and lower-back muscles, as well as the lumbar, thoracic, and cervical spinal vertebrae. It is a good asana to do after vigorous backbends. It opens the hip joints and serves as a deep massage to the internal organs of digestion and elimination. All in all, it is a very powerful pose.

The preparatory position for the yoga nidra pose is shown in Figure 9.23A. Lie on the back, bend both knees to the chest, let the knees drop open, and take hold of the right foot with both hands. Lift the head and upper back off the floor and bring the right shoulder in front of the right knee. Slip the foot behind the head and let it rest behind the neck.

Continuing from the pose just described, take hold of the left ankle and slip it behind the right ankle. Flex the ankles of both feet and hook the ankles and feet together, as shown in Figure 9.23B. Bring the arms forward, push the upper arms down against the hamstring muscles, and pull the lower back toward the floor. Bring the hands onto the floor behind the bottom, lift the chest, push the head and neck back, and pull the elbows to the floor (Figure 9.23C). Breathing is difficult in this pose, but holding the pose gives you good practice for breathing in a "tight" situation. In the beginning, simply move in

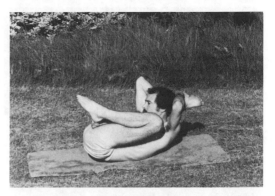

FIGURE 9.23A**

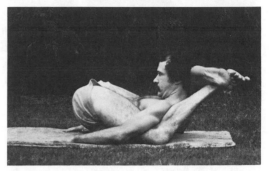

FIGURE 9.23B**

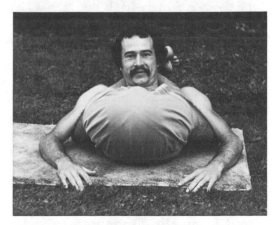

FIGURE 9.23C**

and out of the yoga nidra pose briefly; then repeat with the position of the feet reversed. After several months of practice, it may be possible to rest the head back upon the ankles as if you were resting comfortably on a big pillow for a minute or longer.

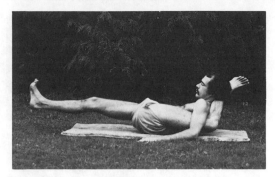

FIGURE 9.24**

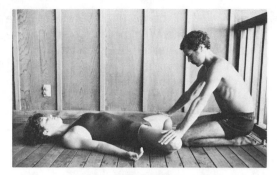

FIGURE 9.25A*

Half Yoga Nidra

Like the full yoga nidra, half yoga nidra takes a great deal of perseverance to master, but once you can do it with grace, it should become a part of your daily routine. This pose can help to correct swayback and also can give great relief to lower-back problems for the flexible student.

The preparatory actions for moving into the half yoga nidra are described with reference to Figure 9.23A. Bring the flexed left ankle behind the neck, push the upper left arm down against the left hamstring muscles, continue to hold the left foot with the right hand, and stretch straight down with the right leg. The leg should not be straightened until the left foot is firmly secured at the nape of the neck. If you can straighten the leg, extend through the back of the leg and reach out with the foot as shown in Figure 9.24. Pushing the foot of the straightened leg against a wall makes this posture easier. Work in the pose for 20 seconds to one minute. Repeat to the other side.

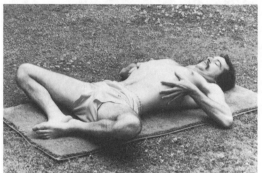

FIGURE 9.25B*

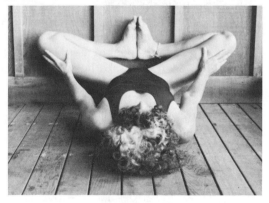

FIGURE 9.25C*

Bent-Knee Hip-Openers

The bent-knee hip-openers bring energy into the pelvic region, aid the urinary system, can help balance the menstrual cycle, stretch the inner-thigh muscles, and release tension in the hip sockets. Those who have trouble bringing the knees to the floor in the sitting cross-legged position should work on the following poses to help open the hip sockets.

In Figure 9.25A, I am gently and gradually pushing down on the inside of Linda's knees while she breathes deeply and relaxes into the pose. With each exhale I can put a tiny bit more pressure on Linda's legs. Linda's work is to totally let go in the pose. I can continue to push down as long as her legs are continuing to drop a little lower as I push. The person being adjusted must guide the adjuster. Work for 20 seconds to two minutes.

With the soles of the feet together and the heels close to the groin, allow the knees to drop open and stretch the arms along the floor past the head, or place the hands on the side of the rib cage, as shown in Figure 9.25B. This is a good posture for deep breathing and meditational work. A yoga session can be ended with this pose, since it is relaxing and allows you to concentrate for extended periods. Hold for one to ten minutes, maintaining attention on the breath.

Another good way to end a yoga session is to rest on the back with the bottom against a wall and the knees opened. Bring the feet together and push the knees toward the wall (Figure 9.25C). If it is hard to keep the soles of the feet together while opening the knees, then allow the heels to move apart, and keep only the little toes together. This is a very restful pose for the back muscles and can be held one to five minutes.

Prayer Pose Prayer pose is one of the most relaxing of all the yoga postures. It should be done periodically throughout an asana workout. It stretches the back and quadriceps muscles, elongates the spine, develops better arches in the feet, increases blood circulation in the arms and hands, has a soothing effect upon the organs of digestion, elimination, and reproduction, and has a very calming effect on the mind.

To move into prayer position, sit onto the heels in an upright position, stretch the abdomen and chest out over the thighs, rest the front of the body on the thighs, bring the forehead onto the floor, and stretch the arms forward. The bottom should remain on the heels as you stretch forward (Figure 9.26).

This is an excellent pose in which to practice deep, slow, rhythmic breathing. With the chest and rib cage resting on the thighs, it is easy to bring awareness to the expansion

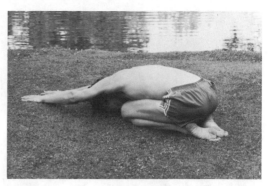

FIGURE 9.26*

and contraction of the lungs. Prayer pose can be held for 20 seconds to three minutes.

MEDITATIONAL POSTURE

For more than three thousand years, the master yogis have espoused sitting on the floor in a cross-legged position. The yogis say that a straight spine must be maintained in order for the body to be truly comfortable. Many of the ancient sages and rishis sat in the lotus position meditating for hours daily and continued this routine for years on end. Do you not think they would have found the optimum position in which to sit through all their years of experimentation?

To maintain a straight spine for long periods of time in the cross-legged sitting position, strong back muscles and flexibility in the joints are required. To be specific, sitting straight in a cross-legged position demands flexible hip, knee, and ankle joints, as well as upper-back strength and an uplifted spine. The Hatha Yoga postures are aimed at making the body pliable and strong so that good alignment of the spine can be maintained for meditational purposes. The most basic principle of yogic meditation is this: to be able to concentrate on one object at a time, you must first of all be able to still the body. Only after the body is stilled can the mind be stilled.

People all around us, rich and poor

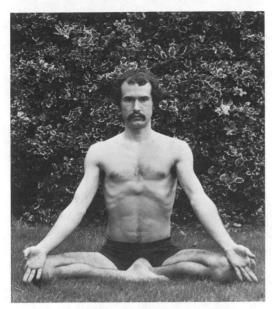

FIGURE 9.27A*

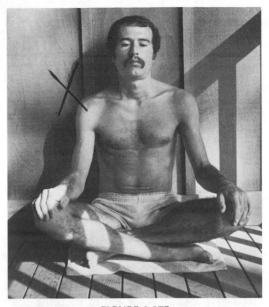

FIGURE 9.27B

alike, are seeking a way to relieve the despair and stress of their lives. The spiral of this despair, which manifests as mental tension, emotional anxiety, physical disorders, or all three, can be broken quite abruptly through yoga practice. I wish to relay to you the ray of hope that each and every person is capable of reaching a state of consciousness in which peace is found. Peace of mind is available to one and all, but to find it we must work toward it. The work of calming the mind begins with the very concrete process of learning how to straighten and still the body.

Cross-Legged Sitting Posture

With practice, the cross-legged sitting pose, as shown in Figure 9.27A, can become the most comfortable of all sitting postures.

It is best to spread the knees as far apart as possible, with one heel in front of the pubis and the other heel in front of the first heel, while doing the cross-legged sitting pose. Ideally, both knees would rest on the floor, as this provides a very stable base.

Note the differences in the positioning

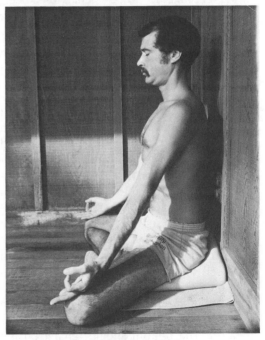

FIGURE 9.27C*

of the feet, knees, head, neck, shoulders, and spine as compared with the pose demonstrated in Figure 9.27B.

In Figure 9.27B, the cross-legged sitting

posture is shown with the neck, head, and shoulders slouched and the chest caved in. Sitting in this position for prolonged periods will result in backaches, shallow breathing, and unclear thinking.

If you have trouble opening the hip sockets enough to bring the knees to the floor in the cross-legged sitting posture, sit on a thickly folded blanket, as shown in Figure 9.27C. This will bring you forward onto the sitting bones and will allow the knees to drop toward the floor, the chest to lift, and the spine to straighten. Notice the straight line of the spinal column, the carriage of the head, neck, and shoulders, and the overall grace of the pose.

CORPSE POSE

The body resembles a corpse in this pose, hence the name. To get into it, lie flat on your back with legs and arms outstretched and the whole body relaxed (Figure 9.28). Corpse pose should be held for three to ten minutes at the conclusion of a Hatha Yoga workout. (Refer to the corpse pose discussion in Chapter 4 for body-positioning instructions.)

The corpse position renews both the body and the mind. You will also find it helpful to do brief periods of corpse pose between certain of the more vigorous yoga postures, as it allows energy to be distributed evenly throughout the body. This brings to balance the work of the individual yoga poses and integrates the full set of postures.

Corpse is a pose of total receptivity, but do not be deceived by the simplicity of the asana. Although no muscular effort is involved, it is said to be the most difficult posture in all of yoga to master. Therefore, some helpful instruction must now be given.

We all have certain areas of the body that are very tense. Our tension patterns have been built up over the course of many years and cannot be released simply by strength of

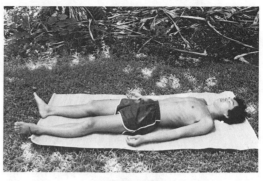

FIGURE 9.28*

will. Deep relaxation of the body will not occur until the mind becomes peaceful. The most difficult work of corpse pose is to appease the thoughts moving through the mind.

The master yogis say that the mind controls the body and that the breath controls the mind. To slow down the relentless onslaught of thoughts, the breath must be made slow, deep, steady, and rhythmic. The rhythm of the breath should become the main focus of attention during the first few minutes of corpse pose. (Refer to Chapter 3 for a full discussion of yogic breathing.) You can time the breath while in corpse, breathing in for a set number of counts, then out for a like number. This timed breath can be done for the first two minutes or so of corpse pose.

The inhale and the exhale should both proceed from the bottom to the top of the lungs. Thus, if you were breathing in and out for six counts, you would breathe two counts into the abdomen, two counts into the lower rib-cage area, and two counts into the upper chest in continuous wavelike fashion. The exhale would consist of two counts from the abdomen, two counts out of the lower rib-cage area, and two counts out of the upper chest in wavelike fashion.

As you breathe deeply and slowly in corpse pose, you can view the various parts of the body from a detached vantage point. You should eventually feel that you can pull far enough away from the physical body to get an overview of it. From above the body you will be able to relax the tense areas of the body more readily.

The mind has incredible potential, but if its potential is to be realized, the thoughts must be focused. We cannot force the mind to settle down, but we can give it something interesting to focus on. We need to center our thoughts upon internal harmony. The breath is the key that will move us toward a recognition of the harmonious vibrations within.

After working on a deep, rhythmic breath for a while, you might begin to hear the lub-dub of the heart. To help you to feel this pulsation you can retain the in-breath for a few counts after each inhalation. Once the rhythm of the heartbeat is clearly heard, attention can then shift to the circulation of blood through the body.

The breath will quite naturally become lighter, softer, and finer as the rhythm of the heartbeat becomes the main object of concentration. It is just during the first few minutes of corpse pose that a deep, slow, carefully controlled breath should occur. As the mind moves toward a meditative state, the breath will naturally find a rhythm suitable to the type of concentration you become involved with.

Concentrating upon the pulsation of

FIGURE 9.29

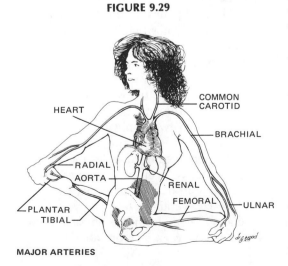

MAJOR ARTERIES

blood throughout the body allows us to become aware of the life force being carried to the individual cells of the body. We eventually might be able to feel, from the inside out, that each cell has its own existence and that all cells are also interconnected in one body. The system that most directly ties all the cells together is the circulatory system, as it is through the bloodstream that oxygen, nutrients, and carbon dioxide are exchanged at the cellular level.

A good corpse-pose exercise is to experience the way the entire circulatory system works. To do this you must consider how the respiratory system is linked with the circulation of the blood. Air comes into the lungs with the inhale, and from the lungs the blood vessels pick up oxygen molecules and carry them to the heart. Then the heart pumps oxygen-filled blood throughout the body by means of an intricate system of arteries, arterioles, and capillaries. The blood picks up food nutrients along the way from the digestive system.

At the cellular level, the oxygen and nutrients are exchanged through the blood for carbon dioxide. This takes place within the capillary system. Thus the cells get the nourishment they need and release the toxic buildup of carbon dioxide. The carbon-dioxide-laden blood is then returned to the heart through the venous system. From the heart the toxins are sent to the lungs, and from the lungs they are expelled with the exhalation of the breath.

The circulatory system (Figure 9.29) is a closed system, which is in contact with each and every cell in the body. There are two loops: a small one, which goes from the heart to the lungs, then back to the heart, and a large one, which goes from the heart throughout the entire body, then back to the heart. The human body is a magnificent machine, and quite obviously the heart is a most vital force in the operation of this machine. The circulatory system is a very fascinating subject for meditation.

Focusing on the electromagnetic energy moving through the body is a bit more subtle, but the longer you stay in corpse pose, the deeper you should look within your body and within your mind. There exists a detailed nerve network, which you should be able to feel within. Consider the brain, the spinal cord, the nerve centers, the electromagnetic energy being generated from these control points, and the way in which this energy moves through the body by means of an intricate web of nerves. This exercise of concentration settles the mind, enabling it to move beyond its normal, everyday thoughts.

I find it helpful to connect the breath with the flow of nerve energy. A way to do this is to draw the electrical energy in toward the spine on the inhale and send it throughout the body in the exhale. If you retain the in-breath, a good exercise is to visualize the spine as a cord of light that becomes increasingly luminous as you retain the inhalation. Try spreading the light and the electromagnetic energy on the exhale, so that the whole body becomes illuminated and energized.

In the initial stages of corpse-pose practice you should focus the mind on the workings of the body in a very concrete way. Breath, heartbeat, and nerve energy provide such a focus. However, these subjects should be approached from a subjective point of view, rather than trying to recall anatomy and physiology books or lectures. The books and lectures are useful, but one must transcend the rational mind to gain a true sense of freedom and relaxation. Hopefully the creative aspect of your consciousness will awaken while in corpse pose.

Approach the inner workings of the body as an explorer discovering new territory. For example, I have compared the electromagnetic energy moving through my body to glacial water flowing down a stream—down a vast system of streams, into imposing rivers, and on to the majestic ocean. These images have led me to a consideration of the workings of the mind, causing me to liken the individual drops of water to individual thoughts: both come and go in a brief moment. I have likened the stream of water to the stream of consciousness, to the continuity of consciousness, to the continuity underlying the appearance of change. I have come to understand that there is a divine plan that allows continual change and unchanging eternity to exist simultaneously.

Through relaxation and meditation we allow the creative aspect of our consciousness to awaken. We must allow these inspirational thoughts to flow freely. As molecules of water make their way from melting glaciers, down small streams and larger rivers to the vast ocean, so do our creative thoughts lead us to seek other minds, to blend with other minds, to melt into a planetary awareness that, in turn, empties into the all-pervading cosmic consciousness of humankind.

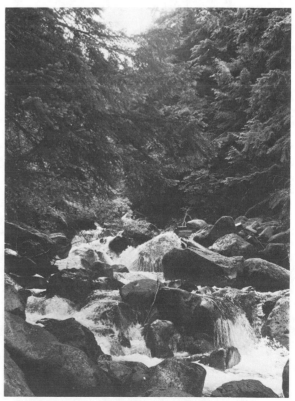

V

MEDITATION

In the final chapter of the book, Chapter 10, themes for meditation will be discussed. The first part of the chapter goes into a discussion of the seven main energy centers of the body and associates a type of consciousness with each. The goal of this section is to present a map of the mind to help you act in a very conscious way while involved in the everyday world. The final section ends with a personal meditation that should serve as inspiration for you in your own internal work.

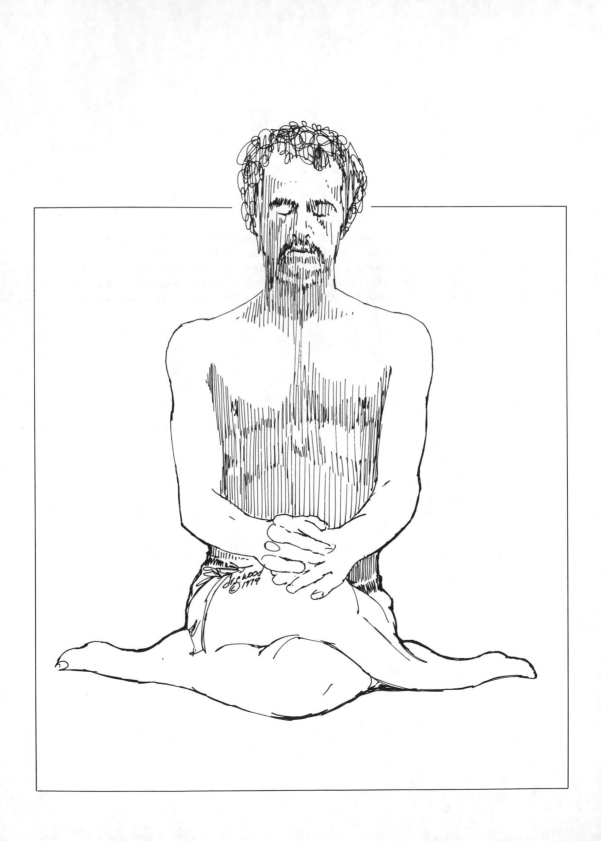

TEN
ego, mind, and meditation

CHAKRAS

There are seven main energy centers along the spinal cord; these are called *chakras*. Each chakra, when activated, releases a unique type of energy. Furthermore, a particular type of consciousness is associated with each chakra. Thus, in working with the chakras we are dealing with energy and with consciousness. The higher we go up the chakra system, the more refined the energy input we encounter and the higher the level of consciousness to which we attune.

The yogis say that the controlling mechanism behind the nervous and endocrine systems of the physical body is the chakra system. The main vortices of the chakras lie deep within an energy channel called *sushumna,* which is the subtle body's equivalent to the spinal cord. As along the spinal column there are nerve centers called plexuses out of which the nerves of the body emanate, so along the sushumna there are energy centers called chakras out of which the subtle nerves of the body emanate.

Sushumna is the central channel through which a very potent type of energy moves. This energy is composed of measurable energy such as electromagnetism and light photons, and also of a type of unmeasurable energy called prana. According to the yoga masters, prana is the vital, essential energy of the universe. It has been found by the yogis that the spinal chakras are the main centers in which the vital energy accumulates within the human body. The seven main chakras are muladhara, swadishthana, manipura, anahata, vishuddha, ajna, and sahasrara.

The positions of the chakras correspond to points along the spinal column. *Muladhara,* the first chakra, is located at the very base of the spine. *Swadishthana,* the second chakra, is located a little higher up in the region of the sacrum. *Manipura,* the third chakra, resides at the navel center. *Anahata,* the fourth chakra, can be found at the level of the heart. *Vishuddha,* the fifth chakra, is located at the top of the throat. *Ajna,* the sixth center, is just slightly above the space between the two eyebrows. *Sahasrara,* the seventh chakra, is situated at the crown of the head.

A close comparison can be made between the endocrine glands and the chakras.

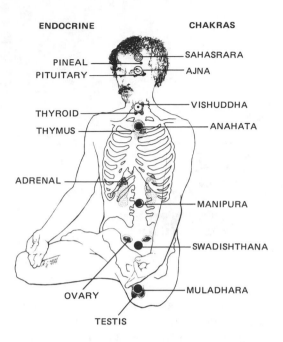

ENDOCRINE   CHAKRAS

PINEAL   SAHASRARA
PITUITARY   AJNA

                    VISHUDDHA

THYROID
THYMUS   ANAHATA

ADRENAL

                  MANIPURA

                  SWADISHTHANA

OVARY   MULADHARA

TESTIS

FIGURE 10.1A

FIGURE 10.1B

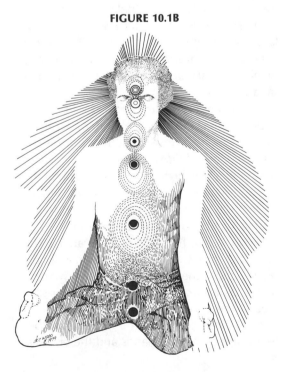

In this comparative scheme (Figure 10.1A), the sex glands are related to the bottom two chakras, the adrenal glands correspond to the third chakra, the thymus gland corresponds to the fourth chakra, the thyroid and the parathyroid glands correspond to the fifth chakra, the pineal gland corresponds to the sixth chakra, and the pituitary gland, which is the master gland of the endocrine system, corresponds to the seventh chakra, which is the crown chakra of the chakra system.

It must be pointed out that the chakras are located along the ethereal counterpart of the spinal cord and cannot be seen through normal vision. Stilling the body and refocusing one's attention to the internal body processes of breath, heartbeat, and the flow of electromagnetic energy will help to bring the mind to a state of rest, so that the prana may begin to move up sushumna, awakening the higher chakras.

Let us now proceed to a consideration of the chakra centers as they relate to levels of consciousness. To quote Ram Dass:

> If you start from the viewpoint that the whole universe is pure energy and then look into the human body, down through the chakras, you can see that energy focused in different parts of the psychic body defines different realities, that each chakra has its own reality and that reality becomes quite solid. As energy goes out from that chakra, it reinforces the reality of that plane.[1]

As discussed in the first chapter of this book, new-age meditation in its higher stages allows one to view the physical universe from a new vantage point. Our duty is then to return to the body–mind–personality complex and act upon the vision received in the meditative state. In the higher stages of meditation, life can be seen as unified and perfect, but the problem is that for most people on the earth-plane, life appears to be quite disorga-

[1]Alan Mesher, "Straight Talking with Ram Dass: An Interview," *Yoga Journal, No. 26,* May–June, 1979, p. 16.

nized and imperfect. Trying to act in a very conscious way while out and about in everyday world can be a very disheartening experience. It is helpful to earmark the possible levels of consciousness in which we and others may find ourselves during the course of a day. Each of us passes in and out of innumerable levels of consciousness throughout our waking hours; however, each person has a particular chakra center in which he or she most often resides. Most people spend the greatest majority of their lives involved in the type of consciousness associated with the first, second, or third chakras.

Muladhara, the First Chakra

At the base chakra one's thoughts are concerned with physical survival. Here one thinks about food, shelter, and the need for self-preservation. Individual separateness from the rest of the world is emphasized at this level. The advantage to being here is that everything is definite, solid, and concrete.

Viewing things from the first chakra level, each person is an individual who must look out for himself. Here the notion of survival of the fittest applies. The way to work through this level of reality is to actually achieve success on the material plane. It is not possible to devote one's life to spiritual matters until food, clothing, shelter, and transportation matters have been taken care of. The advice of Pir Vilayat Inayat Khan is to achieve some degree of material satisfaction first, as only then will you really be free to work on your evolvement as a spiritual being. What is more, achievement on the physical plane will give you greater power to work on the higher planes.

Swadishthana, the Second Chakra

Sensory gratification is dealt with at the second chakra. The principle that if a little is good, then a lot more is better, is the trap of this chakra. Indulgence in food, drink, drugs, sex, parties, gambling, and other stimulating activities earmark the person who resides at the second chakra. The problem here is that one desire leads to another, and there seemingly is no end. This is the level of consciousness that catches many people the greater part of their lives. Only if one's higher nature overcomes the lower-nature desire system can the spiral of indulgence be broken.

If we can mindfully work through temptations, we can gain a tremendous feeling of accomplishment. We are constantly put to the test, and if we pass the test, we become initiated into a higher order, into a deeper level of life. More understanding is attained by going through the test than if we were not tested. There is a net gain as we work through each test, because we become the master of those planes we overcome. We can then help those who are stuck on the lower planes.

During moments of clarity we begin to realize that much of our suffering is the result of our lower-nature indulgences. We must pass through second chakra level of consciousness if we hope to attain peace of mind. To begin with, we can look logically at the impossiblility of fulfilling the countless desires of the senses. Hierarchically, the rational mind is one step above the senses and can overrule certain of the impulses. The only way to truly rise above the sensory-gratification level is to finally say no to many of the pulls of the senses. The practice of Hatha Yoga and meditation helps to give us this power to say no. It is easy to let go of earthly wine when we begin to taste divine wine. We are enabled to overrule the craving for constant material-plane enjoyment when the ecstasy of the higher planes begins to be felt. The cosmic dimension of our being becomes the true overseer as we find freedom from the tyranny of the senses.

Manipura, the Third Chakra

The person whose energy is centered in the third chakra is a person involved in power and control struggles. Attempting to gain control over other people seems to be the only effective way to gain power in the physical world, yet the attempt, if unsuccessful, leaves one vulnerable to feelings of inferiority and inadequacy. On the other hand, the problem with actually gaining influence and power is that the more one has, the more one wants. The person snared by the third chakra level can never acquire quite enough power. Here we see the business executive who forsakes friendship for advancement. Here political backbiting takes place. Here are the major tyrants and the petty tyrants.

There is a great loneliness behind the power-centered ego. Until this level of awareness is transcended, one is destined to suffer. The ego-minded person will invariably try to build an empire of some sort; but there is no peace to be gained here, because as soon as the power structure shows signs of success, its builder begins to fear that it will somehow tumble. Eventually, of course, not only the empire but the person must succumb to death.

According to yoga theory, the root of our problems is false identification with the ego. The ego depends upon other egos for recognition and yet, by nature, must fight these other egos in its struggle for power. This dependence on the one hand and antagonism on the other causes grief and suffering. The higher levels of reality, where unity and peace pervade, simply cannot be perceived by the individual ego. One must become detached from the ego-self to reach the cosmic perspective.

It is also true that we must maintain an ego in order to function in the everyday world, as the development of ego is the protective force that allows us to deal with large numbers of people and to accomplish great tasks. The ideal situation would be to let the degree of the ego needed be determined on a moment-to-moment basis by a power that is higher than our own.

There are two main ways to deal with someone who is forcing an ego confrontation. One is to fight this person with the strongest ego that can possibly be mustered. The other is to detach oneself from involvement with that person. A highly evolved being will generally refuse to fight another being on the battleground of ego versus ego. The whole thrust of a spiritual person's life is toward union rather than separation.

That we should move into the unity of life is a glorious concept, but when we really get down to the heart of the matter it is the thoughts of the mind that hold us back. All day long the mind runs off thoughts that have little to do with unity, and we simply cannot disregard these thoughts. We must shed some light on what the responsibility of the mind actually is.

Certainly, in order to function efficiently in the everyday world, we need to rely on the rational thought process. The rational mind may actually be our greatest physical-plane asset. With it we can meet the needs of the first chakra level, overcome the mindless desires besetting us on the second chakra level, and achieve some degree of success in the world such that we gain respect from those around us. We must go beyond the rational thought process, however, if peace of mind is to be found.

There is an intuitive aspect of our being that senses the truth without having to analyze all the pros and cons. There exists a collective consciousness of mankind, a universal flow of ideas, which is a wellspring for discovery and creativity. Meditation enables us to tap into this vast reservoir. We will not find true peace until we lose our sense of separateness and go beyond the third chakra level of awareness.

We have found that ego gratification and rational mind processes are dealt with at the level of third chakra consciousness. Emotions also fall within the sphere of the third chakra consciousness.

The yoga method of dealing with emotions is very specific and extremely effective both in daily living and in meditation. The key is slow, deep, rhythmic breathing. Whenever we find ourselves out of balance emotionally, it is time to focus all attention on the breath. I cannot emphasize it enough—the internal work of slow, deep, rhythmic breathing is the way to achieve a state of serenity.

Try this the next time you are emotionally upset: (1) inhale for a set number of counts—say, three, (2) hold for brief moment, and (3) exhale to a count of three. A few of these breaths will quickly calm you down. Both the inhale and the exhale should be smooth and steady from beginning to end.

While in the meditative state, if you want to view life from atop the mountain rather than getting stuck down in the valley, treat emotions as just a passing show. They are merely temporary clouds passing through the clear sky of the serenity of our being. As the wind clears the clouds from the mountain, so deep, rhythmic breathing will clear the emotions from one's being.

During meditation it is advisable not to wrestle with one's emotional nature, as any particular emotion could gain power during the struggle. Envy, self-pity, guilt, anger, frustration, and fear are the main emotions that we must watch over carefully. Rather than trying to destroy them, merely be mindful of their appearance and disappearance. They will lose their power in time if we just watch them.

Handling emotions that come up while we are involved in our individuated personality structure requires a slightly different approach from when handling emotions that occur while we are in a meditative state. Purposefully detaching from our emotions in meditation leads to sublimation, but while we are out and about in the everyday world there is a danger of repression if we deny our emotions their logical due outlet.

When we are in the world of action, we should enjoy our positive emotions but not get carried away by them. Riding the waves of emotion can result in a high experience, but what goes up must eventually come down. As for the negative emotions, they must be liberated in a healthy way. Physically active forms of liberation include Hatha Yoga, dance, athletics, Tai Chai, and creative dramatics. Emotions can also be freed vicariously by viewing drama, reading literature, and listening to music; or they can be freed directly through one's own artistic endeavors.

When we are attuned to the third chakra we identify with our ego, rational mind, personal emotions, and personality structure. The problems associated here form an endless stream. The yogis teach that we cannot pull ourselves out of the fog through our limited ego–mind–personality structure. To find our freedom we must lose ourself into the collective whole. Then we can come back into the manifested world as an expression of the totality. To go beyond the prison of our ego-personality structure we must move into the higher chakra centers.

Anahata, the Fourth Chakra

As consciousness moves to the fourth chakra, the spiritual ascent has truly begun. As the prana and electromagnetic energy move out of the lower three chakras and into the heart center, our concern turns toward that of brotherhood. Compassion is the word that characterizes the consciousness of the person who dwells in the heart center.

It is much easier to feel the peaceful unity associated with the heart chakra while immersed in meditation than while out and about in the world. At the soul level, it is often easier to attune to another being in the quietude of meditation than in the person's physical presence. Personality and ego often get in the way of communion between souls. It is a mistake to think that physical distance is a barrier between two people, as neither consciousness nor love has boundaries.

While deeply engrossed in a meditative state we can accumulate vast amounts of cosmic energy, and this energy can be shared with others. From within a state of tranquility we can send vibrations of pure love to acquaintances and friends. From the heart center we can send out light and love throughout the entire universe.

These are very beautiful thoughts, but how do we deal with the problems of the everyday world? How do we deal with those around us who are trying to maneuver and manipulate us?

It is extremely difficult to maintain a universal outlook when dealing with the survival, sexual, and power-struggling efforts of those caught in the bottom three chakras. The compassionate being's duty is to help another recognize the divine qualities that this other person has latent within him or her. It is a mistake, however, to think we can do anything more than point another toward the source that feeds us all. We must keep our own attunement high if we are to help those around us. We can serve as a lamp for another. Whether the light of the lamp is used or not depends on the other person.

While working from the fourth chakra we must be careful, as there is quite a tendency to act in an undiscriminating way at this level of awareness. Having our heart center open in a quiet place with friends is safe and desirable. On the other hand, in the company of cantankerous people it is advisable to veil our gentleness, so that we will not be taken undue advantage of. We must have faith that the transmission of truth occurs at a deeper level than the ego-personality level. We can open our whole being up to another who has no intention to use the energy gained for manipulative purposes. However, if the person we have come into contact with is deeply engrossed in the first, second, or third chakra, then we may have to present ourselves in a way that is unyielding to the demands of his ego while still being yielding to the vibrations of his innermost self. The person whose heart center is open should stand as a wellspring of light and love and truth for the *higher nature* of others to feed from.

Vishuddha, the Fifth Chakra

The fifth chakra is the level at which the creative mind dwells. As the vishuddha center opens, an overwhelming impulse to create moves through one's consciousness. This chakra is the center that poets, musicians, artists, and philosophers ideally should be in during their work. However, the spark of genius cannot be forced through an act of individual will power. The most the artist can do is create a receptive atmosphere and hope that the creative impulse of the collective consciousness will channel through him.

If the purpose of life is to evolve, we must give expression to the creativity of the innermost self. How can we discover new ideas except by quieting the mind and allowing a previously unheard aspect of our being to express itself? A truly creative thought is not a deduced thought; rather, it is an impulse of sudden insight. After the flash of new realization occurs, the rational mind will try to make sense of it.

While you are in the consciousness of the fifth chakra, you will find yourself committed to a reality that does not depend on the praise of others for its sustenance. The artist, poet, musician, or philosopher who truly resides at this level does not care if his or her works are recognized by the outer world or not. He or she is driven by a force that comes from deep inside.

The person who is blocked at the fifth chakra will have trouble expressing his or her innermost feelings. Communicating meaningful concepts to others will be difficult if this center is undeveloped.

The formation and sustenance of a close relationship can be a most creative endeavor. The beauty of relationship is that two or more people who actually do unite form a new whole that adds to the creation. If we do not keep our attunement high, a relationship can be the cause of our greatest grief. Our salvation in relating to another is to rise above the limitations of the self and to merge into the place inside where we all vibrate together as one; then relationship can be creative.

We are not so vulnerable to the power-play of another's ego at the fifth chakra as at the fourth. While residing at the vishuddha chakra we have an easier time walking away from the person who tries to force an ego battle and loving that person from afar. Here we act spontaneously, creatively, and with vision.

Ajna, the Sixth Chakra

The sixth chakra is the center of pure intelligence. With the opening of the ajna center, one grasps the fundamental laws of the universe. The goal of meditation is to gain panoramic vision of all the various levels of reality. What the sixth center has, above and beyond the fifth chakra, is a *conscious* understanding of all the lower levels of reality at once. A great joy and sense of gratitude result from this new understanding of the total picture.

From the sixth chakra, knowledge of the past, present, and future is brought into harmony. What is most amazing about the new vision of the universe is the simplicity of the overall picture. Here one realizes that the clouds of the lower levels of reality were phantoms of one's imagination. The purpose of life is made clear.

Associated with the ajna chakra is the organ of perception called the *third eye*. Intuitive understanding characterizes the person whose third eye has been opened. Emanating from the third eye is a beam of light that cannot be seen or measured except by another with third-eye vision. This beam of light penetrates the illusions of the physical universe, giving one the power to see the essential qualities that lie behind appearances. Thus, part of the intuitive understanding of the sixth chakra occurs because of the penetrative qualities of the higher mind.

The other aspect of intuition is the ability to become a totally receptive channel to other people's messages. At the sixth chakra there no longer exists an individual consciousness that must interpret, categorize, separate, and try to make sense of things as the whole picture makes sense of the parts. There is pure receptivity here, and it is the cosmic intelligence that rules.

The separations and boundaries that have been constructed by man are seen as illusionary. There is nothing but a continuous flow of consciousness, and there is perfect order to this flow. This is the collective consciousness of humankind. This is the cosmic stream of intelligence and understanding. Here we begin to realize that we are all moving within a vast ocean. What is this ocean? To discover the answer, we must traverse one more level of reality.

Sahasrara, the Seventh Chakra

With the opening of the sahasrara chakra, the person reaches the end of his quest and unites with pure spirit. As the ajna chakra is the center of pure intelligence, so the sahasrara chakra is the center of pure spirit.

The most important question each person must ultimately ask is: "Who am I?" From the crown chakra the answer comes through: "I am a wave of infinite power, infinite wisdom, and infinite bliss." No further explanation is forthcoming—or desired.

What has been added by the seventh center above and beyond the sixth is a feeling of eternal peace. The sahasrara chakra is often referred to as the thousand-petaled lotus of light. The halos pictured around certain saints are the representations of the aura of light that

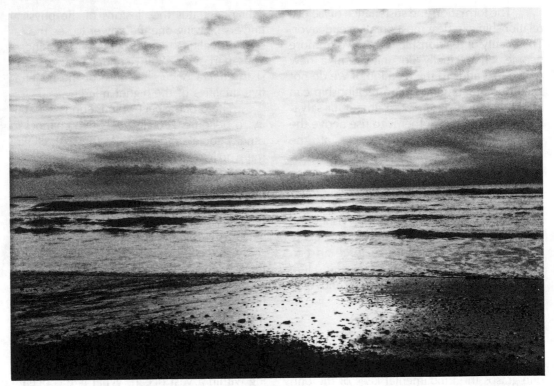

FIGURE 10.2

emanates from the crown chakra. The peace that surrounds these beings is available to one and all.

The end of the soul's quest is the opening of the sahasrara chakra, but it is also the beginning of a new mission—endless service to all other manifested souls who are seeking the light of truth. To serve others we must come back into one of the chakra centers below the seventh. Ideally, we would relate to others from the sixth, fifth, and fourth chakra centers. Please recognize, however, that our duty in serving others is to communicate with them at their highest level of understanding, not ours. We must speak the language that is understood.

MEDITATION ON MAUI

I would like to relay the stages of a meditation that occurred on the morning of September 2, 1978, on the island of Maui, Hawaii. This personal meditation will help to shed light on the ideas discussed earlier in the chapter.

I sit here and my thoughts race around and around, yet they are leading nowhere. I need to calm my mind. I hear the ocean waves washing to and fro, and compare the rhythm with my breath. The wave washing up the shore is like the exhale. The inhale is like the water being pulled back to the sea. I retain the breath after inhaling, and visualize the retention as a new wave building up. As I look out, it can be seen that each wave begins far out at sea and slowly moves in toward the shore. The wave builds slowly until it becomes very large and begins to crest. It then curls and crashes and sweeps its way up the beach. I continue to contemplate the movement of the waves and watch my breathing process for a long while. My thoughts attach onto other things, but still a part of me watches the inhale, the retention, and the exhale and likens them to the stages of an ocean wave. I hear the melodious sound of the in-and-out motion of the waves. There is perfect rhythm to the ceaseless action of the water before me.

I listen, watch, and wait—listen, watch, and wait. There is nothing else to do. My mind continues to spin off thoughts, and I watch the process as my mind clings to various thought patterns. There is a wish that some creative thoughts will begin to come through my mind, thoughts that will be stimulating and intriguing. Yet, I feel that it does not really matter exactly what thoughts actually do come through my mind, because I do know that everything is happening just as it must. If boredom is my lesson for the moment, then all I can do is simply be with the boredom. If anxiousness is the lesson, then I must be with the anxious feelings until they pass. I ask to be cradled by the divine force and ask for guidance. I pray that the energy flowing through me will wash away my petty ego concerns.

I feel the wind blowing about me and liken the clouds in the sky to the thoughts that are moving through my mind. I hear the words and harmony of a beautiful song sung by an old friend. "Let the wind blow through you, it will renew you, let the waves wash over, over, and over." The words are heard again and again. I try to attune to the message of the words and to the vibrational beauty of the melody.

I begin to tap a deeper level of my mind. Memories of experiences of the recent past begin to surface, and these lead to memories of a more distant past. I listen, watch, and wait—and notice that the process is beginning to feel quite comfortable. Nonetheless, there is felt the necessity to focus my mind on a clear meditative theme, so I begin to consider the seven chakras along the spine—muladhara, swadishthana, manipura, anahata, vishuddha, ajna, and sahasrara.

I consider the different elements associated with the different chakras. At the base of the spine is muladhara, the earth connection. A current of energy can be felt entering my body through the base of the spine. From the core of the earth, I draw the electromagnetic earth energy up my spine and continue to draw it up the spine on the inhale. I draw the earth energy slowly up through the chakras until it has reached the top of the head. On the exhale I imagine the electromagnetic energy dropping slowly back down to the bottom of the spinal column. A dull throbbing can be felt at muladhara chakra after dropping back down. Again, I move the electromagnetic current, the earth energy, slowly up and down the spinal chakras (up with the inhale, down with the exhale) before electing to concentrate at the next center, swadishthana.

The second chakra is located a little higher in the pelvic girdle and is associated with the element water. This is an easy element to relate to today with the ocean before me. The second chakra is more of an outlet for energy than the base chakra, which is more of an inlet for energy. I open my eyes and gaze at the ocean and consider the vastness of the ocean, whose magnificence is beyond comprehension. I draw the viscous, flowing feeling of water from the second chakra slowly up the spine on the inhale and feel the energy moving up to the crown of the head and beyond. The vast feeling of the ocean overwhelms my mind. I hold the breath until the exhale must occur and then allow the energy to drop slowly back down to the swadishthana chakra. Again, there is a pulsing, throbbing sensation at this chakra center, and there occurs a very strong desire to move into the higher chakras.

My concentration moves to the navel center, manipura chakra. The element fire is associated with this center, and I begin to feel a lot of sensation here. This is a receptive center for the pranic inflow and is the power center of the physical body. There is a pulsation taking place at this center that beats at the same rhythm as the heartbeat. It is much more comfortable to remain fixed within manipura than to dwell within either of the first two chakras. I hope that the flames will burn away my ego's concern for personal power. I let the warmth of the fire energy spread throughout the abdominal area and hope that any locked-up emotions, such as anger, envy, greed, and self-pity, will be released. I begin to move the prana up the spine on the inhale and bring it back down to manipura on the exhale.

Next, my concentration proceeds to the heart center, anahata chakra. Here the element air works the strongest. Anahata is an outlet for energy and is a strong center from which to project. I understand that the individual personality–ego structure is supposed to dissolve while residing in the region of the heart. I draw the pranic energy into the heart on the inhale and send a radiant form of the energy out on the exhale. I sincerely feel there is no place that this energy sent out from my heart cannot reach. The prana emanates from the anahata center, as do the sun's rays, in all directions at once.

Next comes the throat center, vishuddha chakra, which is associated with the element ether. The throat center is an inlet for prana and is especially strong for attuning to the fourth-dimensional sound current. I feel the prana moving up my spine as if it were a stream of water; then, after the energy begins to flow smoothly, I try to withdraw into the throat center and listen to the sound current passing through. I begin to hear the fourth-dimensional vibration, which the yogis call the *Om.*

I have been taught that a second stage of meditation upon vishuddha chakra would be to draw the vibrational current in through the top of the head and then sit back and listen to the *Om,* so I try this as well. I hear the subtle sound quite well today, but am not

sure if it is more like the sound of a stream of water or the sound of the ocean waves. I do not try to pinpoint exactly what it sounds like, because it could be likened to many things, such as a waterfall, or soft rain, or leaves blowing in the wind, or honeybees buzzing. All I am certain of is that it is soothing to hear this subtle music.

Beyond the vibrational current of the fifth chakra is the cosmic intelligence of ajna chakra, the sixth chakra. It is said that when one resides at the sixth center, consciousness functions in a universal way. I ask the fundamental metaphysical question: Is there order beyond chaos? From the cosmic mind the answer comes that there is perfect order to every aspect of the universe, and that each person is unfolding exactly as he or she must. The cosmic intelligence sends out the message that the glory of the heavens is real, and that we must pass through chaos to understand and appreciate the true perfection of life. I see that there is suffering all around me on the physical plane, and I also see that I am not actually of this world.

Visions of beings of light come before me. Great masters come to me and transfer their radiance and magnetism to my form. All is wonderful. A profound silence surrounds me and a deep reverence for the beauty of life engulfs me.

I wait in stillness, realizing that there is one last breakthrough to be made. The crowning glory of our being is to consciously know God. I pray with all my heart and soul for divine grace. "Oh, God, rest me in thy arms. Oh, God, dissolve the I in me which separates us."

After a while of waiting, it seems as if I am pulled through a black hole and into a whole new dimension. I cannot describe my feelings of wonder and awe except to say that it is like the beginning of creation. I am surrounded by many-colored sparks of light, all glimmering like diamonds in the celestial light display. Now, it has occurred that the person who I thought I was has been shattered. An incredible power that comes from the divine source is felt. New understanding occurs. The wisdom cannot be denied, as the thoughts are more than thoughts—they are truth.

Within the consciousness of the One, there are no problems. It is quiet, still, and peaceful here. There is no longer a striving ego to deal with. All form has fallen away. Energy, light, love, and intelligence remain. Everything is moving toward a great fulfillment.

While immersed in the light of truth, a bond is made. There is work to be done on the physical plane, and the force now being felt will provide direction for that work. "Have faith in the divine guidance, as it will always be with you, wherever you are."

The pull of the moment shifts; now there is a desire to be with people. Energy descends into the physical form. I realize that I have been called to a mission—the same mission described so beautifully by the poet Kahlil Gibran:

You may have heard of the Blessed Mountain.
It is the highest mountain in our world.
Should you reach the summit you would have only one desire, and that to descend and be with those who dwell in the deepest valley.
That is why it is called the Blessed Mountain.[2]

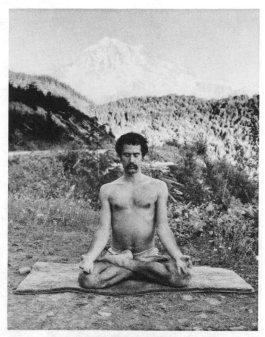

FIGURE 10.3A

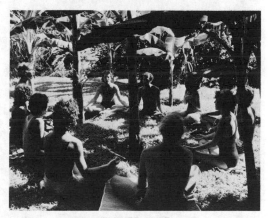

FIGURE 10.3B

[2]Reprinted from *Sand and Foam,* by Kahlil Gibran, by permission of Alfred A. Knopf, Inc. Copyright 1926 by Kahlil Gibran and renewed 1954 by Administrators C.T.A. of Kahlil Gibran Estate, and Mary G. Gibran.

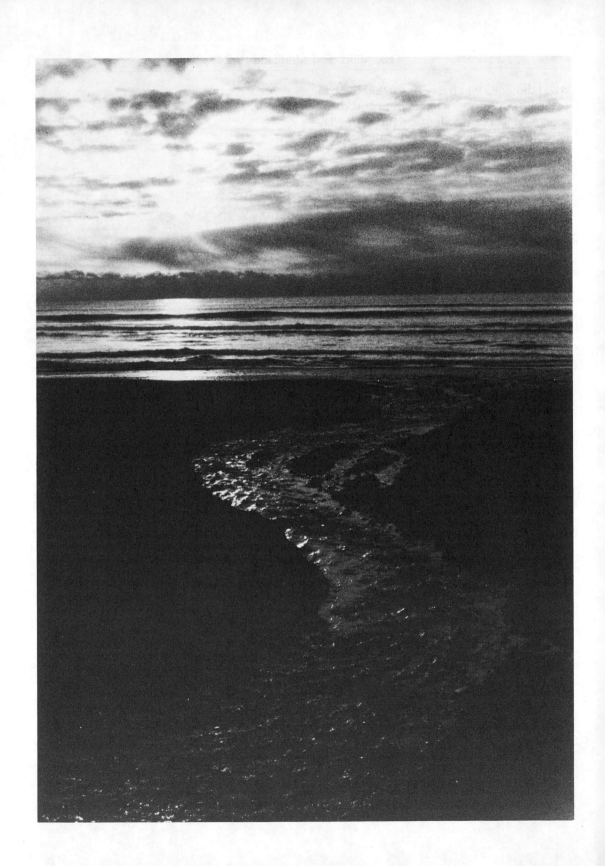

appendix

As thorough as this book is, it just begins to scratch the surface of yoga instruction. Each person has a unique body, and each of you will run into unique problems while attempting the asanas shown. It is very difficult to learn the yoga postures without personal instruction. I recommend that each of you find a teacher to help you correctly move into the postures presented in *Yoga for a New Age*. If a qualified yoga teacher is not available, I strongly urge you to read carefully *all* the information that I have given regarding each particular posture, study the pictures thoroughly, and stay on the cautious side in your practice. Improvement in yoga comes about through daily practice and time.

YOGA ROUTINES

Sixteen yoga routines are presented in this section. These routines are geared mainly for the beginning student who has had some yoga experience and for the intermediate student. All postures used in the 16 appendix routines have been pictured and described in Chapters 5 through 9, except for a few postures taken from Chapter 3. The 16 routines given in this appendix are well-rounded sets that add depth to the simpler routines given in Chapter 4, "Yoga for Beginners."

If you are a beginning student with little or no experience, start with the six sample routines given in Chapter 4. They are basic sets designed to exercise every part of the body. All postures used in the Chapter 4 routines have been pictured and described in Chapter 4.

The 16 appendix routines progress from moderately difficult to longer and more difficult routines. The standing postures are strongly emphasized in the first six routines. Routines 1 through 6 can be attempted by the beginning yoga student, provided that the routines given in Chapter 4 have already been carefully worked through. Both the intermediate and beginning student should work through these first six routines one by one.

Routines 7 through 10 are also geared for the beginning student who has had some experience and for the intermediate student. Routine 7 emphasizes work with a bar, wall, and partner. Parts of this routine may be impossible to practice because of a lack of wall space, a bar, or a partner. Routines 8 and 9 turn away from the standing-posture emphasis, whereas routine 10 comes back to a full-fledged set of standing postures.

Routines 11 through 16 are geared for the intermediate student of yoga. These routines incorporate many of the intermediate postures pictured in Chapters 5 through 9, though not all. These last six routines do not need to be followed in any particular order.

All 22 routines presented in this book should serve as a springboard for your own creative yoga work. Your goal should be to come up with unique routines that work well for you. This book is meant to serve as an inspiration to a *continuing* study of yoga. Your practice will be greatly enriched by attempting new postures regularly.

How to Use the Routine Figure Numbers

A figure number is listed after every posture in each of the 16 routines. Let us look at a specific example to explain how to work with the photographs and figure numbers. In routine 1 the sixth posture is listed as follows:

6. Standing rotations (Figs. 5.11 through 5.16).

You would attempt to perform all the standing rotational postures listed, provided that your body is able to do them. It is helpful to practice the postures in front of a full-length mirror as you attempt to simulate the pictured asanas one by one.

In Figure 5.16, a partner adjustment is called for. Of course, if you are practicing by yourself, this partner work cannot be done. However, since it is very beneficial to practice with a partner and to try the adjustments shown throughout Chapters 5 through 9, I highly recommend that you find a partner to work with occasionally.

Let us look at another example to see how to work with the figure numbers. In rou-

tine 8 the sixth posture is listed as follows:

6. Sitting twists (Figs. 7.2 through 7.4C).

When attempting this series of twists, you should pick from it the twists that your body is able to do at this time. If you feel too much stress while attempting one of the twists, come out of the pose, study the picture and explanation carefully to see where you might have gone wrong, and then attempt it once more. You may need a teacher to instruct you on some of the fine points of the pose, so if the posture feels harmful to you, skip it and go on to the next posture in the routine.

Be forewarned that even a routine from among the first ten may take you more than an hour to perform the first few times through. One suggestion is to focus on just a few of the postures of a particular routine day by day; do this concentrated work until all the postures of the routine have been worked on in a thorough way. Read the introductory discussions in Chapters 5 through 9 and the main descriptions of the postures over and over again, as this will help in the performance of the individual asanas.

routine 1.

Overall body-loosening routine for beginning students.

1. Cat–cow *(Figs. 8.1A and B).*
2. Dog stretch *(Figs. 6.2A–C).*
3. Classical sun salutation *(Figs. 5.3A–M).*
4. Standing-posture warmup *(Figs. 5.2A–C).*
5. Tree *(Fig. 5.17A).*
6. Standing rotations *(Figs. 5.11 through 5.16).*
7. Resting forward stretch (*Figs. 5.32A and B).*
8. Chair twists *(Figs. 3.10A–C).*
9. Office yoga postures *(Figs. 3.11A through 3.14).*

10. Bridge *(Fig. 8.16).*
11. Corpse pose *(Fig. 9.28).*

routine 2.
Twist emphasis for beginning and intermediate students.

1. Cat–cow *(Figs. 8.1A and B).*
2. Standing-posture warmup *(Figs. 5.2A–C).*
3. Standing rotations *(Figs. 5.11 through 5.16).*
4. Triangle *(Figs. 5.19A and B).*
5. Warrior I *(Figs. 5.20A and B).*
6. Extended lateral angle *(Figs. 5.21A and B).*
7. Revolving lateral angle *(Fig. 5.26B).*
8. Sitting twist *(Fig. 7.3B).*
9. Bent-knees lower-back twist *(Figs. 7.11A–C).*
10. Lower-back twist with legs outstretched *(Figs. 7.12A and B).*
11. Knees to chest *(Fig. 8.17G).*
12. Cat twist *(Fig. 7.13A).*
13. Leg stretches on back *(Figs. 9.7A and B).*
14. Bent-knee hip-opener on back *(Figs. 9.25B and C).*

routine 3.
Warmup routine for runners or basic morning routine for beginning yoga students.

1. Standing-posture warmup *(Figs. 5.2A–C).*
2. Modern-day sun salutation *(Figs. 5.4A–I).*
3. Classical sun salutation *(Figs. 5.3A–M).*
4. Standing rotations *(Figs. 5.11 through 5.16).*
5. Standing forward stretches with feet apart *(Figs. 5.36A–C).*
6. Triangle *(Figs. 5.19A and B).*

7. Warrior I *(Figs. 5.20A and B).*
8. Extended lateral angle *(Figs. 5.21A and B).*
9. Resting forward stretch *(Figs. 5.32A–C).*
10. Revolving lateral angle *(Fig. 5.26B).*
11. Lower-back twist with bent knees *(Figs. 7.11A–C).*
12. Cat twist *(Figs. 7.13A and B).*
13. Knees to chest *(Fig. 8.17G).*
14. Bent-knee hip-opener on back *(Fig. 9.25B).*

routine 4.
Stretches for hamstring and lower-back muscles after running; geared for beginning and intermediate yoga students.

1. Modern-day sun salutation *(Figs. 5.4A–I).*
2. Standing-posture dance *(Figs. 5.41A through 5.43B).*
3. Elephant swing *(Fig. 5.44).*
4. Standing forward stretches with feet apart *(Figs. 5.36A–C).*
5. Resting forward stretch *(Fig. 5.32C).*
6. Warrior I *(Figs. 5.20A and B).*
7. Extended lateral angle *(Figs. 5.21A and B).*
8. Standing rotations *(Figs. 5.11 through 5.16).*
9. Double-legged forward stretch *(Figs. 9.1A and B).*
10. Sitting twists *(Figs. 7.3B through 7.4B).*
11. Shoulderstand with wall *(Figs. 6.15A–D).*
12. Plough *(Fig. 6.25A).*
13. Knees to chest *(Fig. 8.17G).*
14. Lower-back twist with bent knees *(Figs. 7.11A–C).*
15. Cat twist *(Figs. 7.13A and B).*
16. Knees to chest *(Fig. 8.17G).*
17. Bent knees on back *(Fig. 9.25B).*

routine 5.
General loosening routine for beginning and intermediate yoga students.

1. Sitting twists *(Figs. 7.3B-7.4B)*.
2. Lower-back twist with bent knees *(Figs. 7.11A-C)*.
3. Bridge pose *(Fig. 8.15)*.
4. Knees to chest *(Fig. 8.17G)*.
5. One-legged stretch on back *(Fig. 9.7A)*.
6. One-legged outstretched hip-opener *(Fig. 9.13B)*.
7. Side splits on back *(Fig. 9.18C)*.
8. Triangle *(Figs. 5.19A and B)*.
9. Rotating triangle *(Figs. 5.25C–E)*.
10. Warrior I *(Figs. 5.20A–E)*.
11. Extended lateral angle *(Figs. 5.21A and B)*.
12. Warrior II *(Figs. 5.22A–C)*.
13. Revolving lateral angle *(Figs. 5.26A–D)*.
14. Resting forward stretch *(Figs. 5.32A and B)*.
15. Squat posture *(Figs. 5.31A–C)*.
16. Shoulderstand with wall *(Figs. 6.15A–D)*.
17. Bent-knee hip-opener with partner *(Fig. 9.25A)*.
18. Massage in prayer pose *(Fig. 8.21B)*, or prayer pose *(Fig. 9.26)*.
19. Corpse pose *(Fig. 9.28)*.

routine 6.
Day-in and day-out routine for beginning and intermediate students.

1. Standing posture warmup *(Figs. 5.2A–C)*.
2. Classical sun salutation *(Figs. 5.3A–M)*.
3. Triangle *(Figs. 5.19A–F)*.
4. Warrior I *(Figs. 5.20A–E)*.
5. Extended lateral angle *(Figs. 5.21A–D)*.
6. Warrior II and III *(Figs. 5.22A through 5.23D)*.
7. Resting forward stretch *(Figs. 5.32A and B)*.
8. Standing-posture dance *(Figs. 5.41A through 5.43B)*.
9. Standing rotations *(Figs. 5.11 through 5.16)*.
10. Cat–cow *(Figs. 8.1A and B)*.
11. Camel *(Figs. 8.7A and C)*. or Bridge *(Fig. 8.15)*.
12. Prayer pose *(Fig. 9.26)*.
13. Outstretched leg twists *(Figs. 7.2 through 7.3B)*.
14. Sitting and outstretched-leg twists *(Figs. 7.3B through 7.4B*
15. Double-legged forward stretch *(Figs. 9.1A through 9.2)*.
16. Leg stretches on back with strap *(Figs. 9.7A and B)*.
17. One-legged outstretched hip opener *(Figs. 9.13A and B)*.
18. Bent-knee hip-openers *(Figs. 9.25A and B)*.
19. Knees to chest *(Fig. 8.17G)*.

routine 7.
Routine with bar, wall, and partner emphasis for beginning and intermediate students.

1. Full-body warmup *(Figs. 5.5A–D)*.
2. Triangle preparation *(Fig. 5.6)*.
3. Leg stretch on bar *(Fig. 5.7A)*.
4. Twisting leg stretch with bar *(Figs. 5.8A and B)*.
5. Classical sun salutation *(Figs. 5.3A–M)*.
6. Standing forward stretches *(Figs. 5.36A-C)*.
7. Prayer pose *(Fig. 9.26)*.
8. Ninety-degree handstand with wall *(Figs. 6.34A–C)*.
9. Resting forward stretch *(Figs. 5.32A and B)*.

10. Shoulderstand with wall *(Figs. 6.15A–D)*.
11. Lower-back twist with bent knees *(Figs. 7.11A–C)*.
12. Lower-back twist with legs outstretched *(Figs.7.12A and B)*.
13. Cat twist with partner *(Figs. 7.13A and B)*.
14. Forward stretch on back *(Figs. 9.7A through 9.9B)*.
15. Twisting side splits *(Figs. 9.15A and B)*.
16. Sitting twists with partners *(Figs. 7.8A–C)*.
17. Bent-knee hip-opener *(Fig. 9.25C)*.
18. Side splits on back *(Fig. 9.18C)*.
19. Corpse pose *(Fig. 9.28)*.

routine 8.
General loosening routine for beginning and intermediate students.

1. Classical sun salutation *(Figs. 5.3A–M)*.
2. Modern-day sun salutation *(Figs. 5.4A–O)*.
3. Resting forward stretch *(Figs. 5.32A–C)*.
4. Standing-posture dance *(Figs. 5.41A through 5.43B)*.
5. Swayback exercise *(Figs. 5.30A–C)*.
6. Sitting twists *(Figs. 7.2 through 7.4C)*.
7. Squatting twists *(Figs. 7.7A and B)*.
8. Asymmetrical twist *(Fig. 7.15)*.
9. Knees to chest *(Fig. 8.17G)*.
10. Bridge, holding ankles *(Fig. 8.15)*.
11. Prayer pose *(Fig. 9.26)*.
12. Camel *(Figs. 8.7A–C)*.
13. Hare pose *(Figs. 6.16A and B)*.
14. Bow pose *(Figs. 8.4A and B)*.
15. Knees to chest *(Fig. 8.17G)*.
16. Forward stretches on back *(Figs. 9.7A through 9.9B)*.

17. Hip-opener with bent knee *(Fig. 9.25B)*.
18. Corpse pose *(Fig. 9.28)*.

routine 9.
Inverted-posture emphasis for beginning and intermediate students.

1. Cat–cow *(Figs. 8.1A and B)*.
2. Forearm dog to forearm lift *(Figs. 6.1A and B)*.
3. Dog stretch *(Figs. 6.2A–C)*.
4. Ninety-degree forearmstand with wall *(Figs. 6.30A and B)*.
5. Ninety-degree handstand with wall *(Figs. 6.34A and B)*.
6. Headstand *(Figs. 6.3A through 6.7)*.
7. Prayer pose *(Fig. 9.26)*.
8. Shoulderstand *(Figs. 6.15A–D)*.
9. Shoulderstand twisting routine *(Figs. 6.22A–F)*.
10. Plough *(Fig. 6.25B or 6.26C)*.
11. Knee-to-ear pose *(Figs. 6.27A and B)*.
12. Bridge from shoulderstand *(Figs. 6.28D and E)*.
13. Lower-back twists *(Figs. 7.11A through 7.13A)*.
14. Earth pose *(Fig. 7.14)*.
15. One-legged forward stretch *(Fig. 9.3)*.
16. Double-legged forward stretch *(Figs. 9.1A through 9.2)*.
17. One-legged outstretched hip-opener *(Figs. 9.13A and B)*.
18. Side splits on back *(Fig. 9.18C)*.
19. Bent-knee hip opener *(Fig. 9.25C)*.
20. Corpse pose *(Fig. 9.28)*.

routine 10.
Standing-posture emphasis for beginning and intermediate students.

1. Cat–cow *(Figs. 8.1A and B)*.
2. Classical sun salutation *(Figs. 5.3A–M)*.

3. Standing rotations *(Figs. 5.11 through 5.16).*
4. Triangle *(Figs. 5.19A and B).*
5. Warrior I *(Figs. 5.20A and B).*
6. Extended lateral angle *(Figs. 5.21A–D).*
7. Half moon *(Figs. 5.24A–E).*
8. Resting forward stretch *(Figs. 5.32A and B).*
9. Rotating triangle *(Figs. 5.25A and B).*
10. Revolving lateral angle *(Figs. 5.26B–D).*
11. Resting, forward stretch *(Figs. 5.32A–C).*
12. King dancers' pose *(Figs. 5.28A–C).*
13. Chair pose *(Fig. 5.29).*
14. Swayback exercise *(Figs. 5.30A–C).*
15. Cat-cow *(Figs. 8.1A and B).*
16. Earth pose *(Fig. 7.14).*
17. Prayer pose *(Fig. 9.26).*
18. Plough *(Fig. 6.25B or 6.26B).*
19. Knee-to-ear pose *(Figs. 6.27A and B).*
20. Corpse pose *(Fig. 9.28).*
21. Three-part yoga breath *(Figs. 3.20A through 3.21C).*

routine 11.
Inverted posture emphasis for intermediate students.

1. Dog stretch *(Figs. 6.2A–C).*
2. Handstand walking up the wall *(Figs. 6.35A–D).*
3. Handstand with wall *(Figs. 6.36A through 6.37C).*
4. Prayer pose *(Fig. 9.26).*
5. Headstand *(Figs. 6.3A through 6.7).*
6. Headstand variations *(Figs. 6.10 through 6.12).*
7. Hare pose *(Figs. 6.16A and B).*
8. Neck rolls *(Fig. 6.17).*
9. Tranquility pose *(Fig. 6.18).*
10. Shoulderstand *(Fig. 6.21).*

11. Shoulderstand twisting routine *(Figs. 6.22A–F).*
12. Plough *(Fig. 6.26B or C).*
13. Knee-to-ear pose *(Figs. 6.27A and B).*
14. Bridge from shoulderstand *(Figs. 6.28A–E).*
15. Knees-to-chest pose *(Fig. 8.17G).*
16. Double-legged forward stretch *(Figs. 9.1A–C).*
17. Half lotus forward stretch *(Figs. 9.4A and B),* or one-legged forward stretch *(Fig. 9.3).*
18. Earth pose *(Fig. 7.14).*
19. Asymmetrical twist *(Fig. 7.15).*
20. Outstretched torso twist *(Figs. 7.16A and B).*
21. Bent-knee hip-opener with wall *(Fig. 9.25C).*
22. Corpse pose *(Fig. 9.28).*

routine 12.
Shoulder- and hip-loosening routine for intermediate students.

1. Cat–cow *(Figs. 8.1A and B).*
2. Full-body warmup *(Figs. 5.5A–D).*
3. Triangle preparation *(Fig. 5.6).*
4. Leg stretch on bar *(Figs. 5.7A and B).*
5. Twisting leg stretch with bar *(Figs. 5.8A and B).*
6. Side stretch with bar *(Fig. 5.10).*
7. Standing-posture dance *(Figs. 5.41A through 5.43B).*
8. Standing forward stretches with feet apart *(Figs. 5.36A–C).*
9. Standing front splits *(Fig. 5.39).*
10. Twisting side splits *(Figs. 9.15A and B).*
11. Prayer pose *(Fig. 9.26).*
12. Hanging over a chair *(Fig. 8.13).*
13. Prayer pose *(Fig. 9.26).*
14. Full backbend *(Figs. 8.17A–G).*
15. Earth pose *(Fig. 7.14).*

16. Asymmetrical twist *(Fig. 7.15).*
17. Steer pose *(Figs. 7.10A–C).*
18. Half yoga nidra *(Fig. 9.24)* or leg stretches on back *(Figs. 9.7A through 9.9B).*
19. Full yoga nidra *(Figs. 9.23A–C).*
20. Shoulderstand *(Fig. 6.21).*
21. Shoulderstand twisting routine *(Figs. 6.22A–F).*
22. Plough *(Fig. 6.26C).*
23. Bent-knee rest pose on back *(Fig. 9.25B).*
24. Corpse pose *(Fig. 9.28).*

routine 13.

Back-loosening routine for intermediate students.

1. Cat–cow *(Figs. 8.1A and B).*
2. Dog stretch *(Figs. 6.2A–C).*
3. Ninety-degree forearmstand with wall *(Figs. 6.30A and B).*
4. Forearmstand *(Fig. 6.29).*
5. Prayer pose *(Fig. 9.26).*
6. Assymetrical twist *(Fig. 7.15).*
7. Sitting twists *(Figs. 7.4A through 7.5B).*
8. Twisting side splits *(Figs. 9.15A and B).*
9. Side splits *(Fig. 9.14).*
10. Outstretched torso twist *(Figs. 7.16A and B).*
11. Cat–cow *(Figs. 8.1A and B).*
12. Ninety-degree handstand with wall *(Figs. 6.34A–C).*
13. Handstand *(Figs. 6.35A through 6.37C).*
14. Shoulderstand *(Fig. 6.21).*
15. Knees-to-chest *(Fig. 8.17G).*
16. Bridge *(Fig. 8.15).*
17. Full backbend *(Figs. 8.17A–G).*
18. United forward stretch *(Figs. 9.5A and B).*

19. Plough pose *(Fig. 6.26C).*
20. One-legged outstretched hip-opener *(Figs. 9.13A and B).*
21. Side splits on back *(Figs. 9.18A and B).*
22. Twisting side splits *(Figs. 9.15A and B).*
23. Forward-stretching cobbler pose *(Fig. 9.12).*
24. Knees-to-chest *(Fig. 8.17G).*
25. Corpse pose *(Fig. 9.28).*

routine 14.

Backbend emphasis for intermediate students.

1. Classical sun salutation *(Figs. 5.3A–M).*
2. Standing-posture dance *(Figs. 5.41A through 5.43B).*
3. Ninety-degree handstand with wall *(Figs. 6.34A and B).*
4. Ninety-degree forearmstand *(Figs. 6.30A through 6.31).*
5. Back arch on stomach *(Fig. 8.11).*
6. Bow *(Figs. 8.4A–E).*
7. Prayer pose *(Fig. 9.26).*
8. Locust *(Figs. 8.5A and B).*
9. Prayer pose *(Fig. 9.26).*
10. Massage in prayer pose *(Figs. 8.21A and B).*
11. Lower-back twist with bent knees *(Figs. 7.11A–C).*
12. Lower-back twist with legs outstretched *(Figs. 7.12A and B).*
13. Cat twist *(Figs. 7.13A–C).*
14. Knees to chest *(Fig. 8.17G).*
15. Bridge, holding ankles *(Fig. 8.15).*
16. Forward stretch on back *(Figs. 9.9A and B).*
17. Full backbend *(Figs. 8.17A–G).*
18. Forearm backbend *(Figs. 8.20A and B).*

19. Knees to chest *(Fig. 8.17G).*
20. Plough pose *(Fig. 6.26C).*
21. One-legged outstretched hip-opener *(Figs. 9.13A and B).*
22. Half yoga nidra *(Fig. 9.24)* or leg stretches on back *(Figs. 9.7A through 9.9B).*
23. Full yoga nidra *(Figs. 9.23A–C)* or knee-to-ear pose *(Figs. 6.27A and B).*
24. Side splits on back *(Fig. 9.18C).*
25. Corpse pose *(Fig. 9.28).*

routine 15.
Forward stretch and twist emphasis for flexible students.

1. Cat–cow *(Figs. 8.1A and B).*
2. Dog stretch *(Figs. 6.2A–C).*
3. Double-legged forward stretch *(Figs. 9.1A–C).*
4. Half-lotus twist *(Figs. 7.19A and B).*
5. Half-lotus forward stretch *(Figs. 9.4A and B).*
6. Half-bound lotus twist *(Fig. 7.18).*
7. Double-legged forward stretch *(Figs. 9.1A–C).*
8. Heroic twist *(Fig. 7.9B).*
9. Steer pose *(Fig. 7.10A–C).*
10. Double-legged forward stretch *(Figs. 9.1A–C).*
11. Twisting side splits *(Figs. 9.15A and B).*
12. Forward stretching side splits *(Figs. 9.16A and B).*
13. Front splits *(Figs. 9.19A and B).*
14. Earth pose *(Fig. 7.14).*
15. Asymmetrical twist *(Fig. 7.15).*
16. Hare pose *(Fig. 6.16B).*
17. Bridge pose *(Fig. 8.15).*
18. Shoulderstand *(Fig. 6.21).*
19. Shoulderstand twisting routine *(Figs. 6.22A–F).*
20. Plough *(Fig. 6.26C).*

21. Knee-to-ear pose *(Figs. 6.27A and B).*
22. One-legged outstretched hip-opener *(Figs. 9.13A and B).*
23. Half yoga nidra *(Fig. 9.24)* or leg stretches on back *(Figs. 9.7A through 9.9B).*
24. Full yoga nidra *(Figs. 9.23A–C)* or knee-to-ear pose *(Figs. 6.27A and B).*
25. Bent-knee hip-opener on back *(Fig. 9.25B).*
26. Corpse pose *(Fig. 9.28).*

routine 16.
Day-in and day-out routine for flexible students.

1. Headstand *(Fig. 6.9).*
2. Headstand twisting routine *(Figs. 6.13A–E).*
3. Prayer pose *(Fig. 9.26).*
4. Shoulderstand *(Fig. 6.21).*
5. Shoulderstand twisting routine *(Figs. 6.22A–F).*
6. Plough *(Fig. 6.26C).*
7. One-legged forward stretch on back *(Fig. 9.9A).*
8. One-legged outstretched hip-opener *(Fig. 9.13A).*
9. Half yoga nidra *(Fig. 9.24).*
10. Double-legged forward stretch on back *(Fig. 9.9B).*
11. Forward stretching cobbler pose *(Fig. 9.12).*
12. Twisting side splits *(Figs. 9.15A and B).*
13. Forward stretching side splits *(Figs. 9.16A and B).*
14. Half-lotus twist *(Fig. 7.19A).*
15. Grasping-ankle twist *(Figs. 7.5A and B).*
16. Grasping-wrist twist *(Fig. 7.6).*
17. Camel pose *(Figs. 8.7A and B).*
18. Prayer pose *(Fig. 9.26).*
19. Full backbend *(Figs. 8.17A–G).*

20. Forearm backbend *(Figs. 8.20A and B).*
21. Knees to chest *(Fig. 8.17G).*
22. Double-legged forward stretch on back *(Fig. 9.9B).*
23. Supine thunderbolt *(Fig. 9.21A).*
24. Half thunderbolt forward stretch *(Figs. 9.22A and B).*
25. Double-legged forward stretch *(Figs. 9.1A–C).*
26. Corpse pose *(Fig. 9.28).*
27. Meditation *(Fig. 9.27A).*

index